Second Edition

Hypospadiology

Repairing Hypospadias Better

Warren Snodgrass, MD
and Nicol Bush, MD, MCS

OH Press
Dallas, Texas

ISBNs: 979-8-9894235-8-3 (pbk); 979-8-9894235-7-6 (hc);
979-8-9894235-9-0 (ebk)

Cover art courtesy of Dr. Pierre Mouriquand
Author photos by Steve Riley Editions
Cover and book design by Mayfly book design

Library of Congress Catalog Number: 2024920653
First Printing: 2025

The goal of repair is to make the abnormal anatomy of hypospadias into the normal anatomy of a penis.

Contents

Related Conditions

Complications and Reoperations

Managing Penile Skin

Follow-Up

Getting Better

Foreword

Although hypospadias is a common birth defect, it is a rare condition that affects only one-half percent of newborn males. Severe hypospadias affects only one-tenth of those. The first candidates for specialty certification as pediatric urologists self-reported to the Board of Urology performing a median of one distal repair a month and two proximal repairs a year (Kogan and Feustel, 2011).

Hypospadias repair is challenging, and results in more complications than any other surgery that pediatric urologists routinely perform. In part, this is predicted by the low surgical volume, as many studies find that surgeons and centers that perform complex operations frequently often have better outcomes. One practical step to address this situation is for groups to designate a surgical team to manage proximal hypospadias and reoperations, which account for most complications.

These complications usually result from mistakes a surgeon makes. All hypospadias repairs consist of a series of steps, and the ways that urologists perform those steps can vary widely. However, not all the ways in which these steps are performed give the same result. So another way to improve outcomes is for surgeons to analyze their own work and determine if they have the less than 10% and 25% complication rates for distal and proximal repairs, respectively, that the literature suggests we should achieve. Those who have more should next review their methods step by step in comparison to others with better results to see how they can improve. We refer to this process as the 3Ps: Prospective data collection (to easily and accurately learn results), Periodic outcomes review (to know about complications sooner), and Practice changes (to do better). We frequently apply this personal quality improvement to our own work, and continue to learn ways to do hypospadias repairs better.

This second edition of *Hypospadiology* describes and illustrates each step of the operations that achieve the best results. We have learned so much since the first edition was published in 2014 that the entire book has been rewritten. If you are using different operations than we describe, we encourage you to tally your results and confirm they are as good as we report – or otherwise change. If you are performing TIP and STAC but have higher complications than reported here, we encourage you to use this book to help identify steps you could do better. We have done that, which is why the second edition is so different than the first!

Today some urologists have decided that distal hypospadias is a mostly "cosmetic" problem. And many urologists have given up trying to repair proximal hypospadias into a normal penis, suggesting parents accept a coronal, or lower, meatus, "mild" persisting curvature, and/or an overall abnormal appearance. Data prove that both are wrong.

Boys born with hypospadias want to grow into men with a normal penis. Therefore, the goal of every surgeon who undertakes this work must be to consistently turn the abnormal anatomy of this birth defect into a normal penis – defined as having straight erections, a meatus at the tip of the glans, and symmetric penile skin covering the shaft.

We believe that *Hypospadiology II* will help us all do better meeting this challenge.

Warren Snodgrass, MD
Nicol Bush, MD, MCS

References

Kogan BA and Feustel PJ: What can we learn from pediatric urology certification logs? *Urology* 78: 147, 2011

Algorithm for Primary Hypospadias Repair

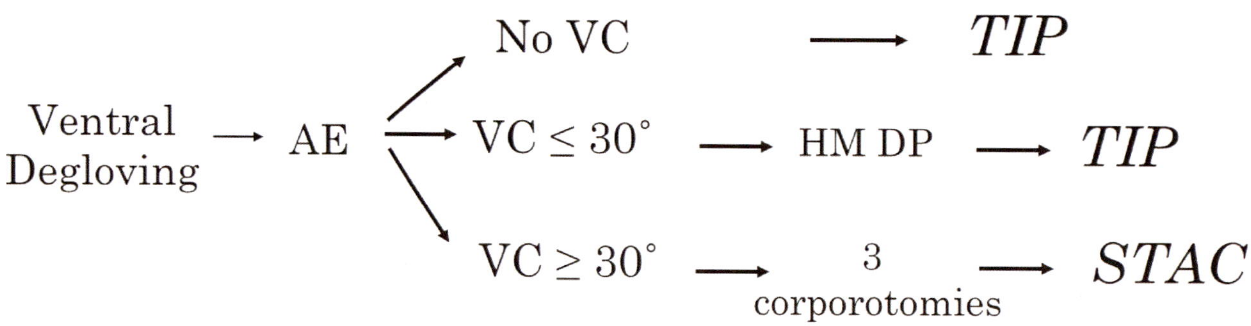

All hypospadias can be repaired by tubularizing the incised urethral plate or a graft neoplate. The decision between TIP and STAC is determined by the degree of ventral curvature.

AE = artificial erection **HM DP** = Heineke-Mikulicz dorsal plication

VC = ventral curvature **STAC** = STraighten And Close

Key Lessons In Hypospadiology II

Goal of Hypospadias Repair

The goal of every repair is to change the abnormal anatomy of hypospadias into a normal penis.

That means penile curvature must be straightened, shaft skin needs to be symmetrically distributed circumferentially, and the meatus should be at the tip of the glans with normal glans fusion enclosing it. These need to be accomplished through incisions confined to the median raphe and circumcision lines, and without leaving visible scars on the glans.

We pediatric urologists must always keep in mind that our work will impact the patient with hypospadias throughout his entire life. Every man wants to have a normal penis. Every surgeon repairing hypospadias should always strive to achieve that goal.

Ventral Penile Curvature

A hypospadias repair is not successful if the penis remains bent, even if the urethroplasty manages to heal without complications. Ventral curvature (VC) of only 20° is sufficient to cause sexual dysfunction and the worry that accompanies it (Menon et al, 2016). But many (perhaps most) patients with persistent or recurrent VC also develop urethroplasty complications, and VC is the most common underlying problem that creates them. Consequently, every patient with a complication undergoing reoperation should have artificial erection done to confirm the penis is straight before proceeding with the correction (Snodgrass & Bush, 2019).

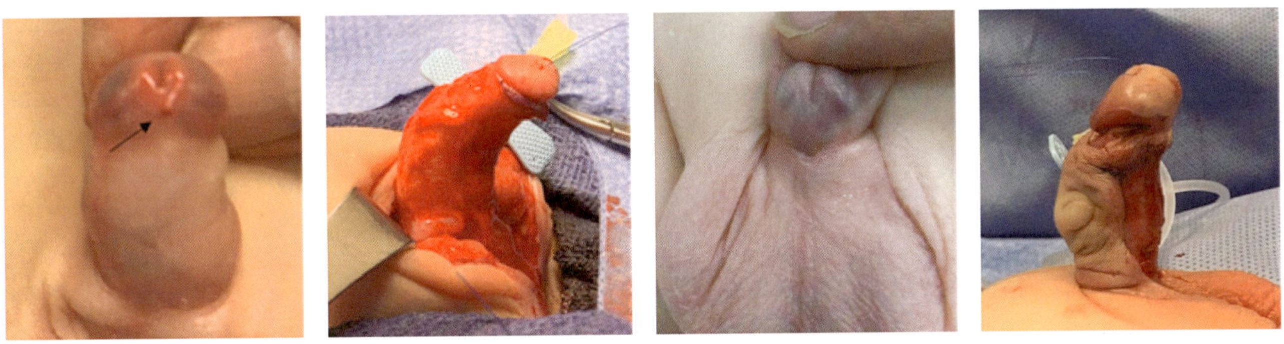

Figure 1. The extent of VC, *not meatal location*, determines the appropriate urethroplasty.
A,B, this patient had a coronal meatus with normal-appearing ventral shaft skin which gave no visual clue that there was VC greater than 30°. As discussed in Chapter 2, this curvature should *not* be corrected by dorsal plication, but rather by 3 ventral corporotomies. This hypospadias should be considered a proximal variant and repaired by STAC as described in Chapter 8 or a STAC-TIP discussed in Chapter 10. C,D, another patient had a meatus at the penoscrotal junction, yet when the penis was degloved ventrally and the scrotal transposition up onto the penile shaft was taken down, the penis was straight. TIP repair is the best urethroplasty option and is described in Chapter 6.

The central role of VC in hypospadias repair is summarized by the following statement and illustrated in Figure 1:

The degree of VC after the penis is degloved, and *not* the meatal location, classifies the severity of hypospadias and determines which repair to use.

Up to 30% of patients with a distal meatus also have penile curvature (Stojanovic et al, 2011; Bush & Snodgrass, 2022). In at least half of these the curvature measures less than 30°, which can reliably be corrected by a Heineke-Mikulicz dorsal plication and TIP repair. The others with VC measuring 30° or more should be considered proximal variants best straightened by 3 ventral corporotomies and either STAC repair as described in Chapter 8, or the variation of STAC-TIP explained in Chapter 10. We recommend that surgeons *not* use dorsal plications to straighten VC more than 30° even when the meatus is located on the glans.

Because VC can be caused by either short ventral skin or short tunica albuginea sheath enclosing the erectile tissue (so-called corporal disproportion), no surgeon can accurately determine preoperatively if the penis will straighten when the skin is released, or remain bent and need corporotomies to make it straight. Accordingly, we inform all parents of boys with a distal meatus that it is possible VC will be found once the operation is underway, and that changes the repair from 1 to more than one operation.

When VC is suspected preoperatively, degloving should first be done *ventrally*, rather than circumferentially.

Whether the meatus is distal or proximal, it is better to begin the operation with a ventral midline skin incision (Figure 2) when VC is suspected. Then, if the penis is bent < 30°, and the family desires circumcision, circumferential degloving is completed. However, when VC is 30° or more, STAC is done without complete degloving so that the foreskin can be maintained until the 2nd stage to use for the urethroplasty graft.

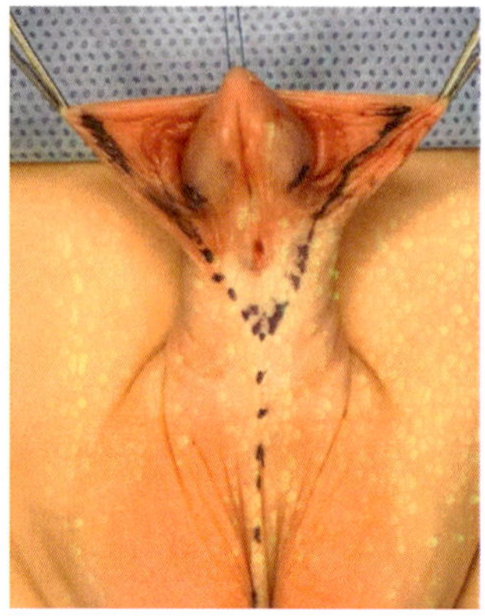

Figure 2. Ventral degloving incision when VC is suspected.
When VC is suspected, this ventral degloving incision should be made. It provides excellent exposure and can be converted to full degloving if the penis is straight or has less than 30° VC to complete distal TIP repair with circumcision. If ≥ 30° VC is confirmed, ventral degloving facilitates STAC repair with preservation of the foreskin for urethroplasty grafting at the next operation. The incision is marked distally along the edge of the prepuce staying approximately 3mm from the corona to preserve the mucosal collar, then alongside the urethral plate, and finally down the midline raphe to the penoscrotal junction or lower.

Because the extent of curvature determines management, VC should be measured objectively.

We explain in Chapter 2 why VC of 30° or more should be straightened using 3 ventral corporotomies, whereas curvature less than 30° can be durably corrected by Heineke-Mikulicz dorsal plication. However, as shown in Figure 3, 30° of curvature is not visually impressive and many surgeons encountering such a penis after degloving would perform dorsal plication to straighten it. We began using a goniometer, which is an orthopedic instrument for measuring angles, to objectively determine the extent of bending, and soon realized that we were *underestimating* VC that ranged from 25° to 40°.

VC < 30° is corrected by a Heineke-Mikulicz (Yachia) dorsal plication.

Plication done through a dorsal midline stab incision into the tunica albuginea of the corpora is reported to more durably straighten VC than Baskin plication, which is done without a tunica incision (Yachia, 1990;

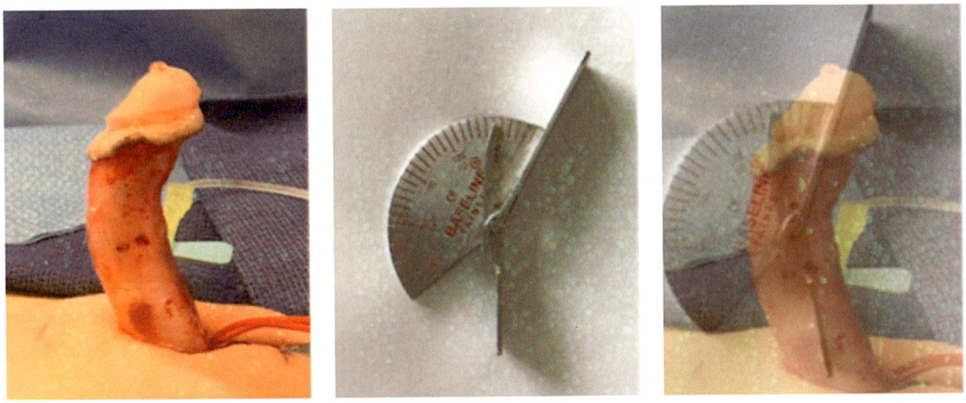

Figure 3. 30°ventral curvature measured with a goniometer.
A, this penis has 30° VC. Before we started using the goniometer we would certainly have done a dorsal plication and TIP repair. That would have put this boy at risk for recurrent VC and related urethroplasty complications. B, finger goniometer after the base has been shortened by 1cm to facilitate measuring the prepubertal penis, which is described in Chapter 3. C, superimposed image showing the correct alignment of the goniometer. The fulcrum is centered at the point of maximum curvature and the distal arm placed at the correct site for the meatus.

Poulsen and Kirkeby, 1995). This method is further discussed in Chapter 2, and shown in Figure 4.

VC ≥ 30° is straightened using 3 ventral corporotomies

30 or more degrees of VC generates too much tension in the ventral aspect of the corpora during spontaneous erections for a dorsal plication stitch to withstand. Surgeons who are not convinced by this statement might imagine the impossibility to significantly bend an erect penis, and then consider the force a suture would have to overcome to hold a bent penis straight during an erection postoperatively. It is not surprising, then, that most of these patients develop recurrent VC after dorsal plication done by any method (Snodgrass & Bush, 2017), which is usually apparent within several weeks after surgery.

Durable straightening is achieved by ventral lengthening, which relieves tension along the shorter side of the tunica albuginea sheath enclosing the erectile tissues. One method makes a single corporotomy and grafts the resulting tunica defect. However, a single incision may not suffice for VC in proximal hypospadias, which averages 70° and can range to 135°. Furthermore, any graft has the potential to contract. We reported that 33% of patients we evaluated after

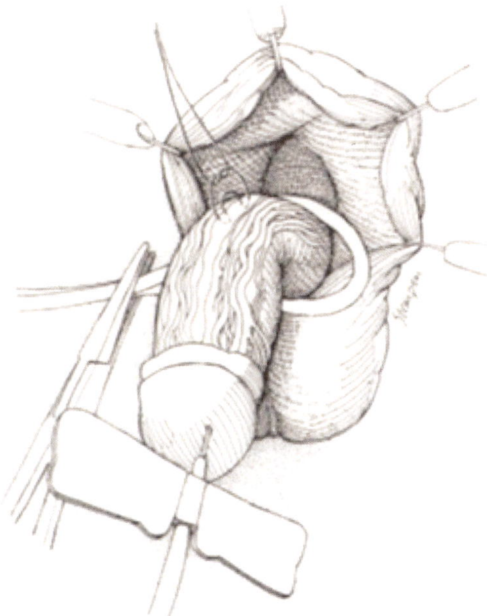

Figure 4. Heineke-Mikulicz (Yachia) midline plication.

An 11-blade makes a 2mm long puncture through the tunica albuginea of the corpora in the midline opposite the point of maximum curvature. This incision is then closed using 4-0 Prolene, including 2mm of the tunic above and below it. The knot is buried into the incision, which is then covered by a small dartos flap to prevent overlying skin from scarring to it. Straightening is confirmed with another artificial erection.

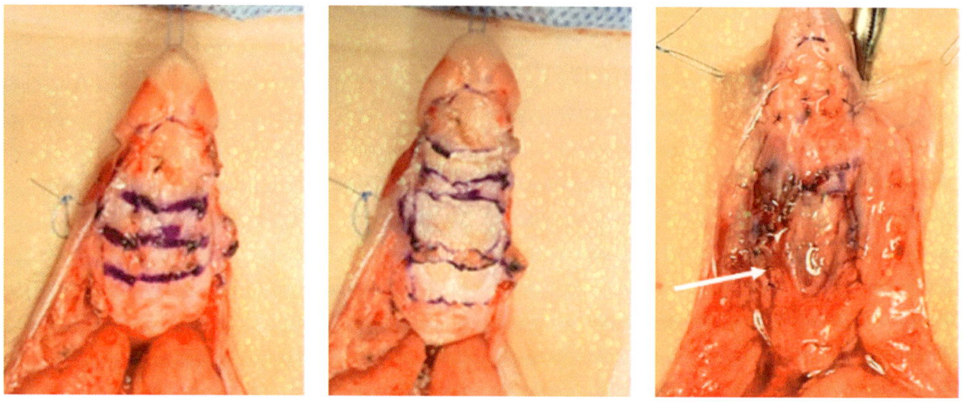

Figure 5. 3 ventral corporotomies to straighten VC ≥ 30°.
A, the point of maximum bending is determined by artificial erection and then marked (middle line). Similar marks are made approximately 4mm proximally and distally. B, incisions are made through the tunica albuginea, exposing, but not damaging, the erectile tissues. These extend from approximately 3 to 9 o'clock. C, the incisions are then covered by dartos tacked to the corpora around their perimeter and to the intervening isthmuses between them to contain any bleeding. The arrow indicates the proximal urethrostomy, which in this case reached past the most proximal corporotomy incision.

single incision corporotomy with grafting had recurrent VC that averaged 54° (Snodgrass & Bush, 2019).

We have done ventral lengthening via 3 transverse corporotomy incisions across the region of greatest curvature for 25 years. These patients undergo staged repairs, and straightening is confirmed at each operation, as well as during any reoperation for a complication. Recurrent VC occurs in less than 2% (Snodgrass & Bush, 2017; 2024). We use the same method for older teens and adults, with none reporting subsequent erectile dysfunction. These corporotomies are shown in Figure 5, and described in greater detail in Chapter 2.

Failure to durably straighten VC is the *most common cause* of urethroplasty complications.

We reported that an astonishing 85% of patients with complications after proximal hypospadias repair had persistent or recurrent VC that averaged 50°, ranging from 30° to 90° (Snodgrass & Bush, 2019). This occurred in 83% who initially had chordee excision, 70% after dorsal plication, and 33% following single corporotomy with corporal grafting. These patients presented with typical urethroplasty complications, including fistulas, strictures, and/or glans and wound dehiscences, some of which were recurrent.

From this experience we learned that many complications following distal repairs are also due to persistent or recurrent VC. Therefore, artificial erection should be done in every hypospadias reoperation.

Figure 6 highlights 2 typical patients with recurrent complications, one with fistulas and the other, glans dehiscences. Neither of their primary surgeons identified their associated penile curvature, nor tested for it with artificial erection. Judging from the operative reports we review, performing a repair of a urethroplasty complication without checking an erection is a common practice, and WS similarly was not taught to suspect recurrent VC or to routinely perform artificial erections when repairing complications.

Recurrent VC develops *early* after repair, and can usually be recognized by the characteristic appearance of the penis.

We have encountered recurrent VC as early as 6 weeks after surgery, and the patients we reported with VC after proximal repairs presented at a median of 12 months postoperatively (Snodgrass & Bush, 2019). This bending can be identified by a typical "hunched over" appearance of the penis as shown in Figure 7. The bent penis resists being lifted cephalad and snaps back into this position as soon as it is released. These findings have consistently indicated that the penis is bent again, and so should prompt reoperation to correct it.

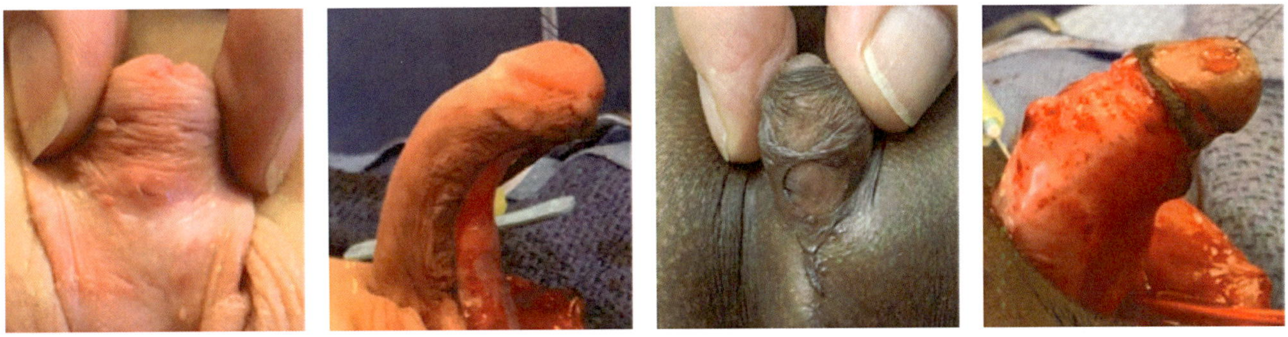

Figure 6. Urethroplasty complications due to recurrent ventral curvature.
A, patient with recurrent fistulas after 2 prior fistula closures found in B to have VC measuring 60°. C, patient with recurrent wound dehiscence from 55° VC seen in D. In both of these cases the initial surgeon did not suspect recurrent VC and did not repeat an artificial erection during attempted repair of the fistula or dehiscence. Tension generated by postoperative erections caused the fistulas and wound dehiscence to recur.

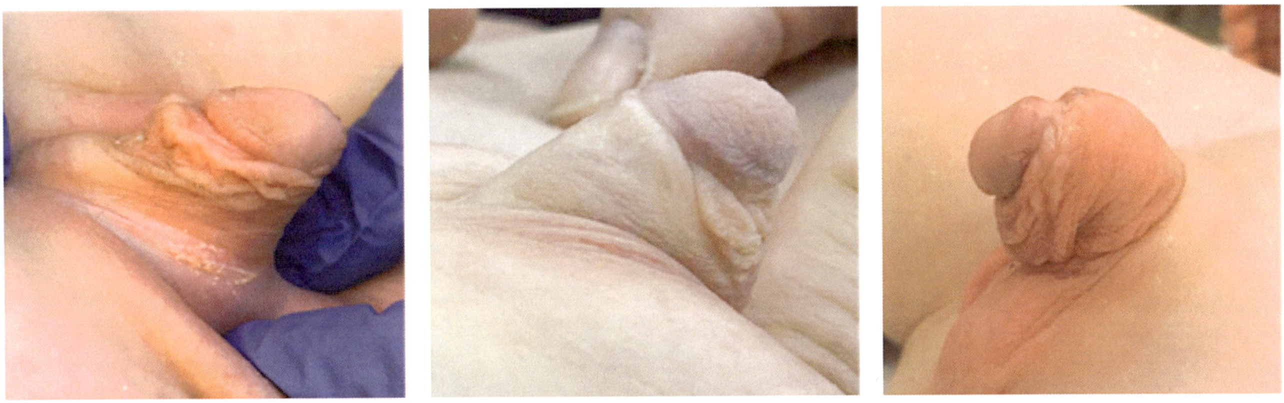

Figure 7. Typical appearance of recurrent VC in 3 prepubertal boys.
Each of these boys had recurrent VC which was more than 30°. Note the "hunched over" appearance. There was resistance to lifting the glans cephalad, and the penis immediately returned to this position when it was released. Some reviewers seeing these photographs protested that the curvature did not look significant to them, commenting that they would be satisfied with these postoperative results from a proximal hypospadias repair. However, when this VC is not corrected it only becomes more obvious during puberty, when it can no longer be denied.We have already mentioned above that 20° VC is sufficient to cause sexual dysfunction and dissatisfaction with the penis.

Ventral Penile Skin

After straightening curvature, making a normal penis from hypospadias next requires redistributing the penile skin to cover the shaft symmetrically. Most patients have some degree of ventral skin deficiency, and those with proximal hypospadias often have little or no penile skin ventrally. The lack of skin not only affects aesthetics, but can also contribute to complications such as fistulas and glans dehiscence from tension exerted on healing wounds by short skin. Furthermore, there is no other skin quite like penis skin, which is both more thin and elastic than that in other locations, and typically does not grow hair at puberty.

Of the basic components of hypospadias – penile curvature, deficient ventral skin, and the abnormally located meatus – the skin abnormalities receive the least attention. Surgeons know that the ventral skin deficiency of a distal hypospadias can be filled by incising down the hooded foreskin and rotating it to the underside when the desired outcome is circumcision. However, few are practiced in reconstructing the foreskin to give a natural, unoperated appearance when the family prefers that outcome.

The challenge of covering the ventral shaft with the appropriate length of penile skin is significantly greater in proximal hypospadias. Here, too, most surgeons simply cut the dorsal foreskin into 2 flaps to move ventrally, which is acceptable but then requires harvesting oral mucosa to create the urethroplasty graft. Meanwhile, surgeons who still use skin flaps for the urethroplasty typically emphasize the neourethra over penile shaft coverage, which can leave dorsal and ventral deficiencies. Ventral skin deficits are often filled using scrotal flaps, but men complain these are unsightly, difficult to keep shaved, and cause discomfort for their sexual partners during intercourse. Dorsal skin deficiencies may require Heineke-Mikulicz skin lengthening or skin grafting, which gives an unsightly appearance.

Since the goal of hypospadias repair is to create a normal penis, the end result must include penile skin covering the shaft symmetrically.

STAC repair dramatically increases ventral penile skin while preserving the foreskin to provide the urethroplasty graft at the 2nd stage.

In STAC, the ventral penile skin deficiency is resolved by 2 key maneuvers. First, the available ventral skin is lengthened by oblique incisions towards skin humps to gain additional skin, as shown in Figure 8. Second, the skin at the penoscrotal junction is pexed to the corpora at 3 and 9 o'clock (Figure 9) to provide fixed points for the skin to stretch against during spontaneous postoperative erections. We were amazed at the increased length and improved health of the ventral shaft skin when we began STAC repairs (Figure 10), which has nearly ended need for scrotal flaps, Cecil maneuvers, or external penile skin grafts.

While these same maneuvers can also be done at the first stage of a 2-stage graft repair, placing the urethroplasty graft further stresses the ventral skin. That skin already has a tenuous blood supply and deficient dartos, giving it a typical "thin" appearance, and the oblique cuts to make it longer can further impact its vascularity. As a result, scarring and contracture of both the skin and graft are more likely, which add to the inherent ventral skin deficiency and may require

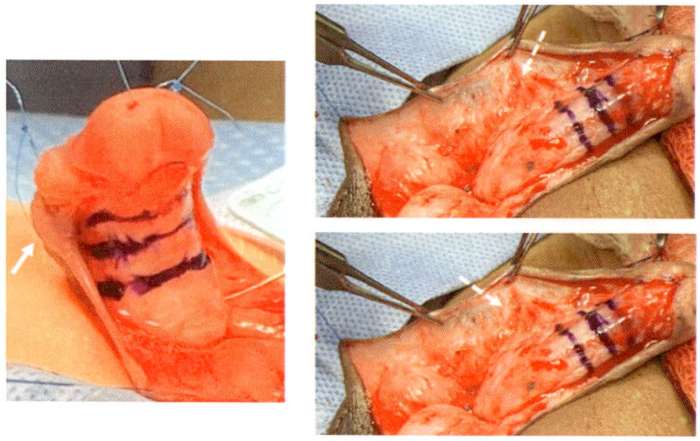

Figure 8. Lengthening ventral skin using oblique incisions towards skin humps.
A, arrow shows a skin hump, which is a respository of excess skin. Note that the ventral skin edge is already short, and will be even more so once the corporotomy incisions are made since those lengthen the shaft.
B,C, arrows show options for incising into the hump. Note the incisions are made obliquely, because horizontal cuts, especially when done bilaterally, make subsequent skin closure more difficult and tight.

patch or total urethroplasty regrafting. Delaying urethroplasty grafting to the next operation gives the skin time to revascularize and better support the graft.

Adequate foreskin to create the neourethra is ensured by prepucioplasty during STAC (Figure 11), which stretches the foreskin during postoperative erections. This is done in the same way as foreskin repair when families prefer a natural final appearance rather than circumcision. Incisions are made towards the corners of the dorsal prepuce, and then the inner and outer layers are separately approximated with interrupted subepithelial 7-0 Vicryl.

Urethroplasty

Only after correcting penile curvature and ventral shaft skin deficiency can attention turn to the urethroplasty. We read some operative notes indicating the surgeon began with the urethroplasty and only after completing it checked an artificial erection. If that is done, the surgeon will almost certainly plicate whatever degree of curvature exists, making the entire repair more likely to fail if the bending is 30° or more.

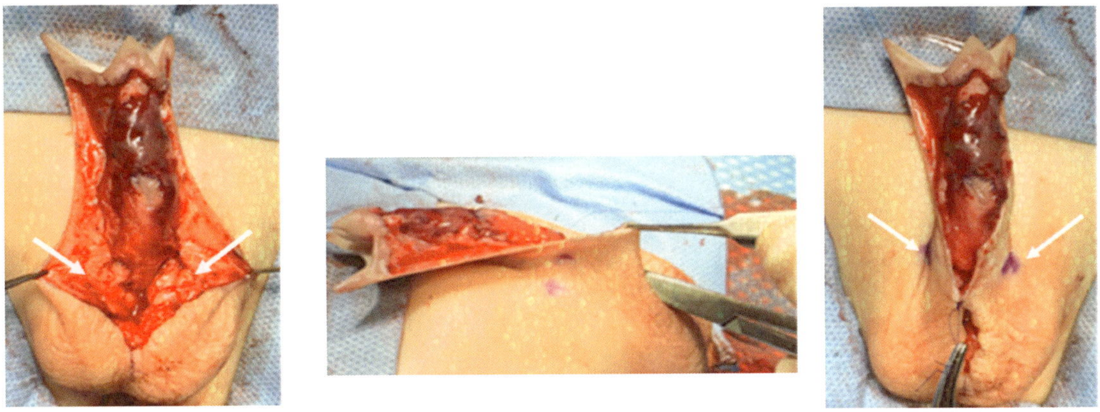

Figure 9. Pexing the penoscrotal junction to the corpora.
A, arrows indicate where the skin will be sewn to the corpora. B, the needle on a 5-0 PDS is catching the skin under the blue mark. C, finished appearance. This maneuver is very important to provide fixed points so that the shaft skin will stretch during spontaneous postoperative erections. Lengthening the ventral shaft skin and pexing it to the corpora at the penoscrotal junction have ensured there is sufficient penile skin at the subsequent stages to eventually close over the neourethra without requiring additional skin or scrotal flaps, or skin grafts.

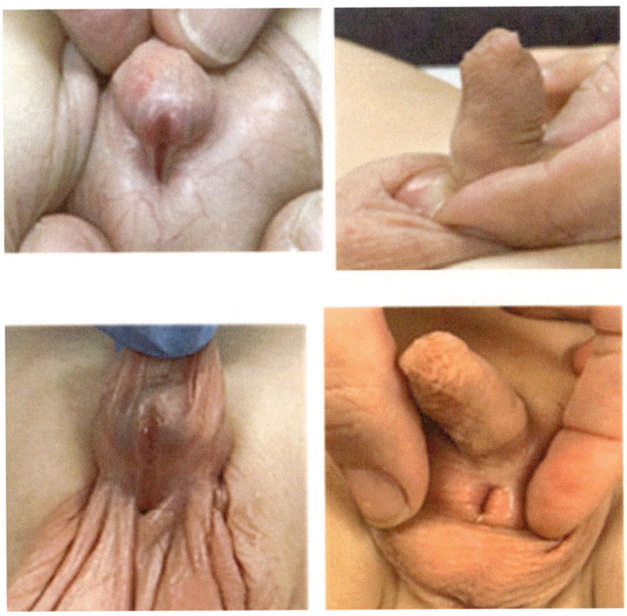

Figure 10. Increased ventral penile skin length achieved by STAC repair.
Dramatic increase in both the length and visual health of ventral penile skin achieved by STAC repair. Note that the penile skin in both patients is now symmetric circumferentially.

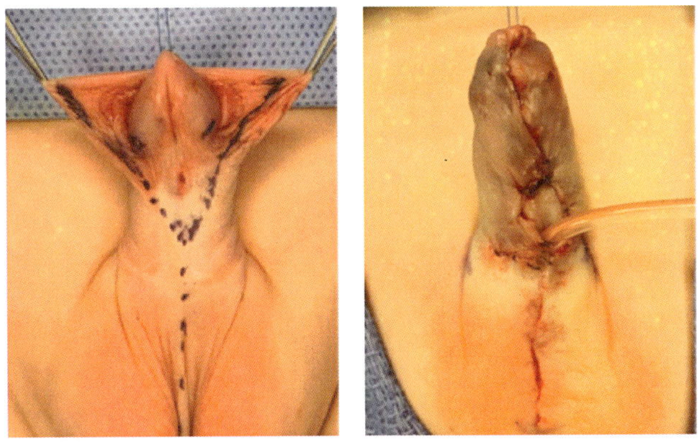

Figure 11. Prepucioplasty.
The steps in foreskin reconstruction are the same during a STAC 1 repair whether it is for the ultimate appearance with foreskin reconstruction, or with a cirucumcision. It is done during STAC 1 to stretch the foreskin and ensure sufficient skin in either case. In those wanting foreskin reconstruction, an oral graft is harvested during STAC 2. For those desiring a circumcised appearance, a neourethral prepucial graft is harvested at the STAC 2 repair. A, lines of incision extending to the corners of the foreskin. B, completed prepucioplasty in a STAC 1 repair.

The correct urethroplasty is determined by the extent of ventral curvature observed with artificial erection after freeing the ventral shaft skin, and measured using a goniometer or similar device.

TIP repairs hypospadias when VC is less than 30°

The penis of most boys with a distal hypospadiac meatus is straight, or has VC < 30° which can be straightened by a Heineke-Mikulicz dorsal plication while preserving the urethral plate. The key step in TIP repair is a midline relaxing incision made from the meatus to the end of the plate, extending down to the surface of the corpora, which ensures the neourethra will have a normal caliber.

Despite published evidence from thousands of patients that this incision does not stricture, some urologists still hesitate to incise the entire length of the plate or to make the incision deep, down to the underlying corpora. Ironically, failure to make the TIP incision correctly *increases* the risk for obstruction and related complications by creating a neourethra with an inadequate caliber.

Others believe surgeons must assess the "quality" of the urethral plate before deciding to use TIP. For example, two studies reported that pre-incision urethral plate width < 8mm contraindicates TIP repair (Holland and Smith, 2000; Sarhan et al, 2009), but in both the surgeons did not make the TIP incision down to the corpora. *This is the most common technical error in TIP repair.* Therefore, it was not the width of the plate which accounted for complications; it was inadequate incision of the plate, as seen in a photo from Sarhan et al (Figure 12).

We have not used any other technique for distal repair in 30 years and, as reviewed in Chapter 7, have not found any urethral plate "characteristic", such as its width or depth or "quality of its spongiosum", to predict outcomes or contraindicate its use. Surgeons can focus on performing the key steps of TIP in the best way rather than worrying whether TIP can be done—when the penis is straight or has less than 30° VC.

The contraindication to TIP repair is VC measuring 30° or more. Surgeons encountering VC in a hypospadias with a distal meatus often assume that the bending is mild and perform a dorsal plication. Although the penis is usually straight if artificial erection is repeated directly after plication placement, VC is likely to recur from postoperative erections and cause urethroplasty complications, as mentioned above. Curvature should be measured objectively, rather than eye-balled, and 3 ventral corporotomies done for straightening when VC is 30° or greater—regardless of a distal meatus.

The penis is straight in a minority of boys with a proximal meatus, and these, too, can have TIP repair. The procedure is similar to distal TIP, and the urethral plate should be deeply incised to the corpora throughout its length. A key difference in proximal TIP is that the first layer of the urethroplasty is sewn using

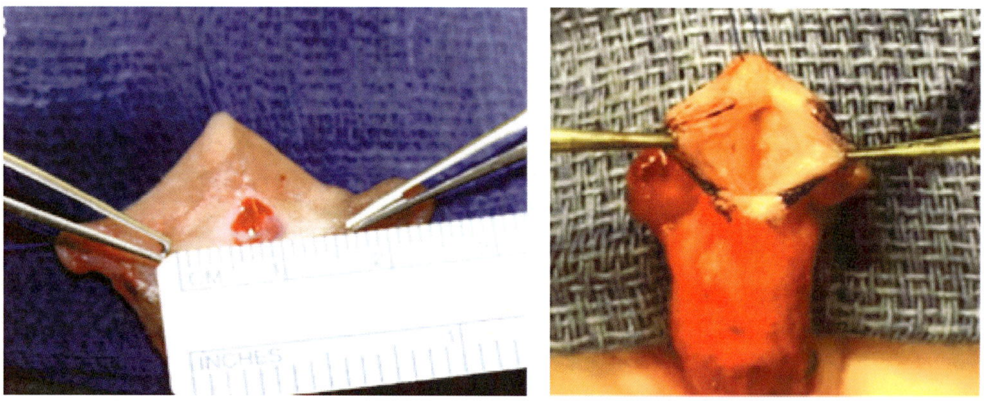

Figure 12. Inadequate vs correct TIP incision.
A, figure from Sarhan et al showing only a slight dorsal incision into the urethral plate, which minimally widened it. This is the most common technical error made by surgeons doing TIP repair. B, figure from Bush and Snodgrass, 2017, demonstrating the appearance of a properly incised urethral plate, which is obviously wider and will create a neourethra with a normal caliber.

interrupted subepithelial 7-0 Vicryl, followed by a second continuous layer of 7-0 or 6-0 PDS. The tubularization is then covered by a tunica vaginalis flap rather than dartos. We published that this method results in significantly fewer fistulas than 2-layer closure running the first and reinforcing it with some interrupted stitches in the second layer (Snodgrass & Bush, 2011). In fact, others have observed 5x more fistulas after this urethroplasty (Pippi-Salle et al, 2016; Braga, 2021).

The contraindication to proximal TIP is also VC 30° or more. Since the majority of patients with a proximal meatus have more than 30° of curvature, TIP is not often done. We emphasize that Snodgrass rarely does a "Long Snodgrass" proximal TIP repair anymore.

STAC repairs all severities of proximal hypospadias with ≥ 30° VC into a normal penis.

This is a powerful statement during a time when many surgeons have given up hope for successfully repairing severe hypospadias. Ironically, their nihilism arose largely from 3 reports on Byars flap repairs from Texas Children's, Boston Children's, and CHOP, whose complication rates of 50% or more convinced many to settle for changing proximal into distal hypospadias.

However, the key problems with those Byars flap repairs were almost certainly inadequate correction of VC and the fact that proximal flap repairs have greater complication rates than grafts despite both using the same foreskin (Snodgrass & Bush, 2017). In other words, technical factors, and not the anatomy of the patient, explain the high rate of complications.

STAC evolved through the lineage of staged graft repairs discussed in Chapter 1. We added 3 corporotomies to straighten the penis, improved the 2-layer urethroplasty by interrupting the first and running the second, then covered the neourethra with a tunica vaginalis flap instead of dartos, and added a more

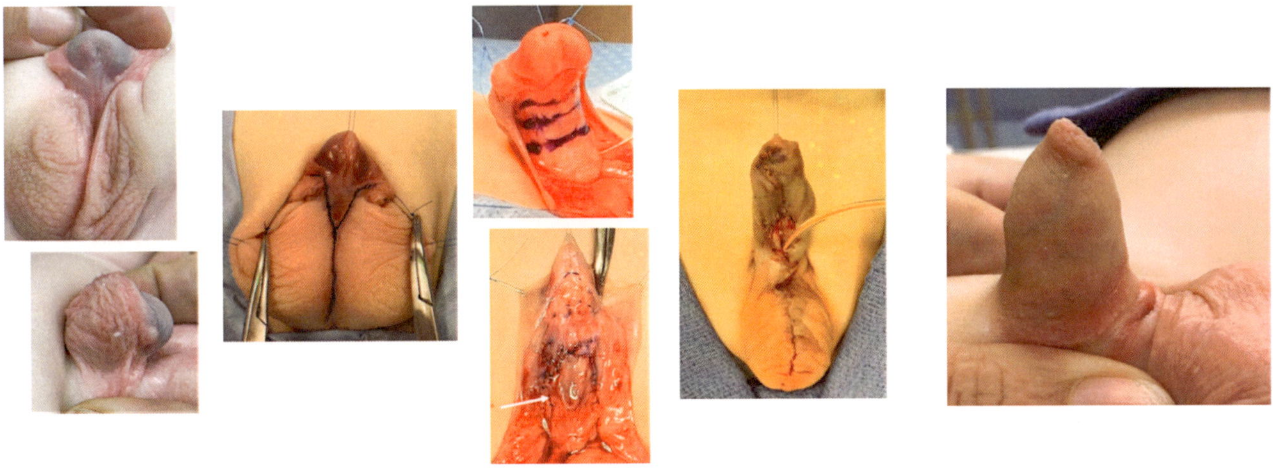

Figure 13. STAC repair: 1st stage.
A,B show a scrotal hypospadias with VC, no ventral penile shaft skin, and penoscrotal transposition. The lines for incision are marked in C. Note that the penis will *not* be degloved dorsally. After ventral dartos is released and artificial erection confirms VC greater than 30°, the urethral plate is transected at the corona and then dissected proximally along with the native urethra into the scrotum. This exposes the ventral corporal surface where lines for the 3 corporotomies have been marked in D across the arc of greatest curvature. Next, after those incisions are made just through the tunica albuginea, they are covered with a dartos flap as shown in E, and the urethra is advanced back distally to end in a proximal urethrostomy indicated by the arrow. The ventral shaft skin is lengthened by short oblique incisions as shown above in Figure 8, and then secured at the penoscrotal junction to the corpora at 3 and 9 o'clock as seen in Figure 9 above. Adjacent skin is then sewn to the urethrostomy. The foreskin is *not* divided into Byars flaps, but instead reconstructed around the glans to give the final result seen in F. G, the appearance of the penis in the same patient 6 months later. It is straight with symmetric, supple shaft skin and sufficient foreskin to now begin the STAC 2 graft harvest. Note the dramatic difference in the preoperative and postoperative appearance of this penis with severe hypospadias.

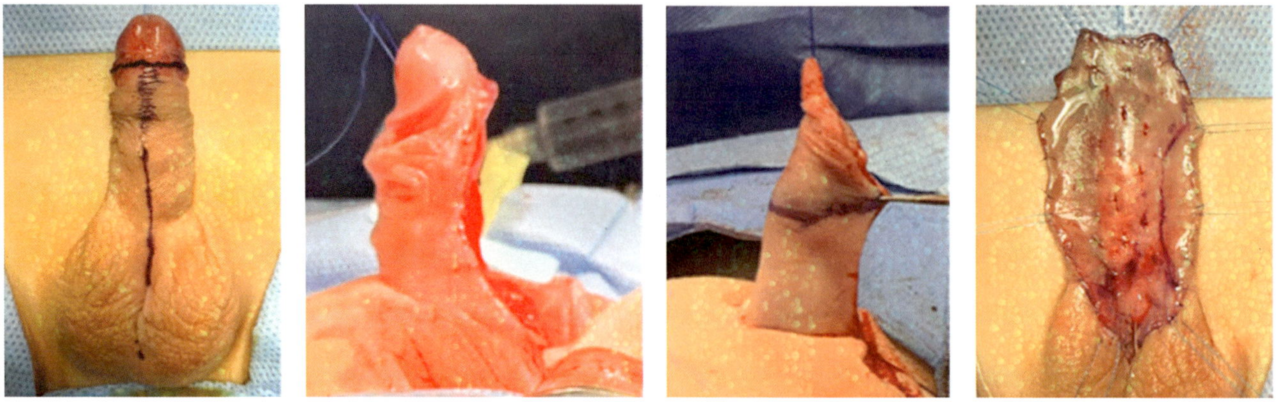

Figure 14. STAC 2 foreskin grafting.
A, the foreskin is retracted and a skin incision is made down the median raphe and around the meatus. The skin is opened, preserving its underlying dartos while excising remaining dartos on the tunica albuginea of the corpora. Care is taken to avoid small corporotomies which make it difficult to obtain a firm artificial erection. B, an erection test is always done to confirm successful straightening before proceeding with urethroplasty grafting. C, the foreskin graft is outlined around the corona, taking care not to shorten the penile shaft skin. D, the glans is opened and the graft sewn from the distal end of the glans and along the skin edges towards the buttonholed meatus. Finally, the graft is quilted at 5mm intervals to the corpora.

extensive glans wings dissection to Bracka's method to create the 2-stage STAG procedure. Then we learned that urethroplasty grafts placed onto corporal incisions are more likely to scar or contract than those sewn onto an intact, smooth corporal surface. And when we stopped placing grafts over corporotomies but observed that some grafts still scarred and contracted, we realized that good take also requires healthy ventral skin sewn to the margins to help revascularization. Consequently, we divided the first stage of STAG (STraighten And Graft) into its 2 main components, straightening the VC and reallocating the skin to cover the ventral shaft in the first operation named STAC (STraighten And Close), and then placing the urethroplasty graft at the second operation once the corporal incisions and relocated ventral penile shaft skin healed (STAC 2). These urethroplasty grafts are far healthier with less scarring and contracture than we observed after STAG (Snodgrass and Bush, 2024), making the final stage (STAC 3) tubularization easier with fewer complications than occur after other graft or flap repairs. STAC and STAG are described in Chapter 8. Key steps in STAC are shown in Figures 13-15.

In nearly all cases, after STAC 1 the penis is straight and has symmetric penile skin around the shaft, needing only urethroplasty to extend the meatus to the tip of the glans to finish making the penis normal. Urethroplasty is best done using a foreskin graft, meaning it is a 2-step process.

Key steps in the 2nd stage (STAC 2) are shown in Figure 14. The initial incision is made ventrally down the median raphe from the corona and encircling the meatus. The skin is opened preserving its dartos, while dartos remaining on the surface of the corpora is excised. Artificial erection is *always* done next to confirm the penis is straight. Then the circumcision line is marked approximately 2mm below the corona and the graft is harvested, taking care not to inadvertently shorten the shaft skin. The graft is sewn from the tip of the widely opened glans, then along the ventral skin perimeter, and to the meatus. It is additionally quilted to the corpora.

Successful graft take occurs in nearly 95% of cases. The final stage (STAC 3) tubularizes this now well-vascularized neourethral plate, as shown in Figure 15.

No other method so reliably makes a normal penis from severe hypospadias as does STAC. Some representative before and after pictures are shown in Figure 16. Every boy born with hypospadias grows into a man who wants his penis to be normal. This must be the goal of every surgeon who chooses to repair hypospadias.

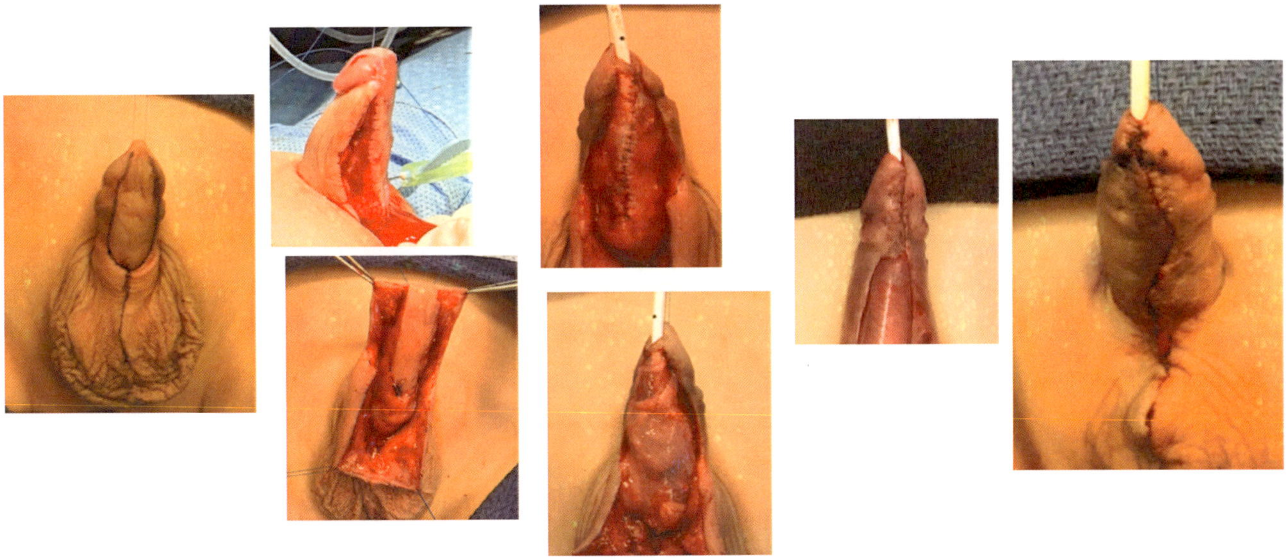

Figure 15. STAC 3 tubularization of the neourethral plate.
A, lines for incision are maked along the glans wings, continuing through the junction of the graft and shaft skin, and a short distance down the scrotum. B, the ventral skin is released and artificial erection done once more. C, after confirming the graft is healthy and the penis is straight, the glans wings are developed and dissected widely. D, the neourethra is sewn in 2-layers, the 1st using interrupted subepithelial 7-0 Vicryl and the 2nd with a continuous 6-0 or 7-0 PDS. E, a tunica vaginalis flap is created to cover the neourethra. F, glansplasty is done using 3 interrupted subepithelial 6-0 Vicryl stitches as in TIP repair. No stitches are placed through the glans surface. G, the completed repair after skin closure using subepithelial stitches. The meatus should *always* be in the normal location at the tip of the glans.

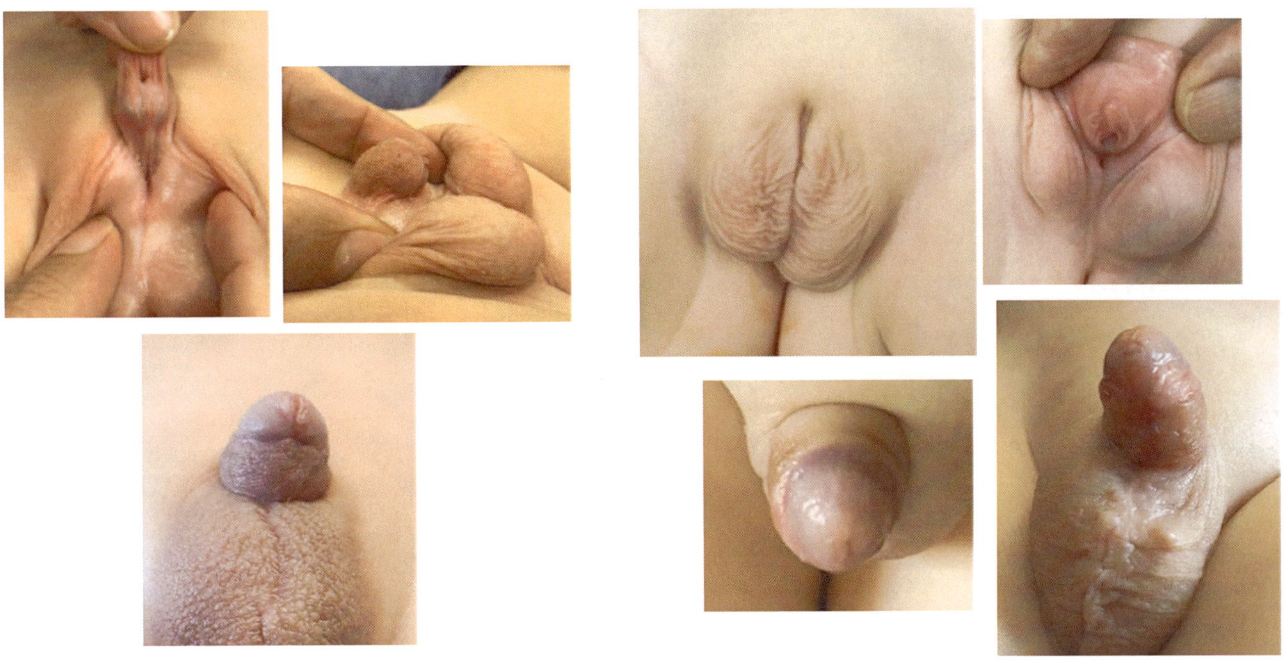

Figure 16. What STAC achieves.
These pictures show severe hypospadias in 2 boys and their final, normal penis.

Complications, and Getting Better

Most urethroplasty complications result from mistakes that the surgeon made.

How the surgeon performs the key steps in a hypospadias repair largely determines if complications will occur afterwards. For example, it is well-known that 2-layer urethroplasty covered with a barrier flap decreases the risk for fistulas, and wide mobilization of glans wings helps insure a tension-free approximation to reduce glans dehiscence. Less well recognized is the role that persistent or recurrent VC plays in these complications. As mentioned above, VC is the most consistent finding underlying urethroplasty complications, probably because spontaneous erections create tension on the bent ventral surface that is transmitted to the repair.

The operative notes we read rarely describe artificial erections during 2nd procedures of staged repairs to confirm the penis is straight before completing the urethroplasty. Similarly, these reports almost never mention artificial erection in reoperations, even when done for recurrent fistulas or dehiscences – in some cases despite parents informing the surgeon that the penis appears bent.

The good news is that we can all improve results and reduce complications by doing the best operations in the best way known. When we realize that recurrent curvature, meatal stenosis, and fistulas we encounter postoperatively happen because of mistakes we made, we view these complications differently. We are also motivated to then tally our personal outcomes and review how we do repairs step by step, looking for ways to do them better.

The risk for complications *doubles* when a reoperation is needed, and increases to nearly 50% after several unsuccessful repairs.

The importance of doing the right operation in the right way the first time is emphasized by the fact that complications increase when repairs have to be redone (Snodgrass and Bush, 2017b). This increased risk potentially relates to several factors, including persistent or recurrent VC and short, scarred penile skin, both of which can exert tension on the repair. But the risk remains high even when the penis is straight and the skin is adequate - indicating that surgery decreases tissue vascularity, particularly towards the end of the penis well away from the entrance of its blood supply at the base.

Therefore, surgeons performing reoperations must consider ways to improve wound healing in addition to identifying and correcting technical issues that contributed to the complication. A perfectly executed reoperation will fail if the tissues are unable to heal properly. Some factors known to impair wound healing include anemia, malnutrition, obesity, diabetes, and smoking which should all be considered but are not usually found in boys undergoing hypospadias repair.

Researching for ways to improve penile vascularity after failed repairs led us to hyperbaric oxygen therapy, and a trial comparing paired oral graft measurements in patients treated with HBOT versus others who were not. We found that perioperative HBOT significantly improved graft take (Bush & Snodgrass, 2019, Ahmed et al, 2024).

Hyperbaric oxygen improves tissue vascularity and promotes wound healing.

We also observed that treatment subjectively decreases skin and subcutaneous scarring. These benefits are difficult to prove objectively, but are apparent to surgeons otherwise accustomed to contracted, rigid tissues that only become worse with successive operations. Consequently, objective and subjective findings have made HBOT an integral component of our salvage repairs, and is described in Chapter 18.

Hypospadias repair harms more children than any other surgery done by pediatric urologists.

Even though it is a common birth defect, hypospadias occurs in only ½ % of newborn boys, and proximal hypospadias in only 1/10th of those. According to data collected by the American Board of Urology, the median number of distal repairs performed each year by certified pediatric urologists is 12, while the median number of proximal repairs is only 2 (Kogan and Feustel, 2011). Given that hypospadias surgery is both complex and technically demanding, this small experience increases the likelihood that surgical mistakes will be made.

Although distal TIP repairs can be done with less than 10% complications, many surgeons average more. And the results of proximal surgeries are so discouraging that many pediatric urologists question if the goal to make the penis normal can be achieved. While complications are distressing to parents and disappointing to surgeons, pediatric specialists may not fully realize the impact that poorly corrected hypospadias has on the boy grown into a man living every day with the consequences of his birth defect. Every man wants a normal penis, and every surgeon who decides to repair hypospadias must commit to achieving that.

We left the university confident that we knew how to manage all forms of primary and reoperative cases, but when our practice was only hypospadias we realized how many technical facts and nuances we still had to learn. Rather than write another compendium of all things related to hypospadias, this book shares those many surgical lessons to help others avoid our mistakes.

While still at the university, we realized that the mistakes we taught fellows not only harmed our patients, but their future ones as well. Chapter 25 discusses results of hypospadias surgery done by recent fellowship graduates and examines the topic of a learning curve. The final chapter ends this book with the answer to the most important question for us all: How do we get better?

References

Ahmed Hazem, Bush N, Snodgrass W: An objective analysis of over 600 paired graft measurements: prepucial vs oral results. ESPU abstract, 2024

Braga L: personal communication, 2021

Bush N and Snodgrass W: Complaints of men with uncorrected hypospadias: functional and aesthetic concerns. *Res Rep Urol 15:425, 2023*

Bush NC and Snodgrass W: Hyperbaric oxygen therapy improves oral graft take in hypospadias staged tubularized autograft reoperations. *J Urol* 202: 1, 2019

Holland AJA and Smith GHH: Effect of the depth and width of the urethral plate on tubularized incised plate urethroplasty. *J Urol* 164: 489, 2000

Kogan BA and Feustel PJ: What can we learn from pediatric urology certification logs? *Urology* 78: 147, 2011

Menon V, Breyer B, Copp HL, Baskin L, Disandro M, Schlomer BJ: Do adult men with untreated ventral penile curvature have adverse outcomes? *J Pediatr Urol* 12: 31, 2016

Pippi Salle JL, Sayed S, Salle A, Bagli D, Farhat W, Koyle M, Lorenzo AJ : Proximal hypospadias: a persistent challenge. Single institution outcome analysis of three surgical techniques over a 10-year period. *J Pediatr Urol* 12: 28, 2016

Poulsen J and Kirkeby HJ: Treatment of penile curvature – a retrospective study of 175 patients operated with plication of the tunica albuginea or with the Nesbit procedure. *Br J Urol* 75: 370, 1995

Sarhan O, Saad M, Helmy T, Hafez A. Effect of suturing technique and urethral plate characteristics on complication rate following hypospadias repair: a prospective randomized study. *J Urol* 2009; 182: 682.

Snodgrass W and Bush N: Efficacy of three corporotomies to straighten hypospadias with ventral curvature. SPU abstract, 2024

Snodgrass W and Bush N: Tubularized incised plate proximal hypospadias repair: continued evolution and extended applications. *J Pediatr Urol* 7: 2, 2011

Snodgrass W and Bush N: Staged tubularized autograft repair for primary proximal hypospadias with 30-degree or greater ventral curvature. *J Urol* 198: 680, 2017

Snodgrass W and Bush NC: Re-operative urethroplasty after failed hypospadias repair: how prior surgery impacts risk for additional complications. *J Pediatr Urol* 13: 289, 2017 (b)

Snodgrass W and Bush NC: Persistent or recurrent ventral curvature after failed proximal hypospadias repair. *J Pediatr Urol* 15: 344, 2019

Snodgrass W and Bush NC: Graft and skin complications in 342 primary proximal hypospadias patients: STAG vs STAC repairs. ESPU abstract, 2024.

Stojanovic B, Bizic M, Majstorovic M, Kojovic V, and Djordjevic M: Penile curvature incidence in hypospadias: can it be determined? *Adv Urol,* 2011

Yachia D: Modified corporoplasty for the treatment of penile curvature. *J Urol* 143: 80, 1990

Chapter 1

Milestones in Hypospadias Surgery

Hypospadias surgery began with the most difficult cases. The earliest repairs were done in the late 1800s, after advances in anesthesia and antisepsis made elective operations feasible. It was natural for surgeons to first attempt correction of proximal hypospadias, given the impact of the malformation on both urination and sexual intercourse. Surgery for distal hypospadias lagged behind, the lesser deformity generally not considered sufficiently bothersome to warrant the risks of repair.

Straightening Ventral Curvature

Chordee Excision

The focus on proximal hypospadias meant that most patients had VC. The first surgeons understood this curvature to result from "fibrous bands" on the surface of the corpora restricting expansion during erections. To make the penis straight, they cut across the most bent region and then developed distal and proximal skin flaps to expose the ventral surface and strip tissues off the surface of the corpora (Figure 1). This procedure was variously attributed to two French surgeons, Etienne-Frederick Boisson and Simon-Emmanuel Duplay.

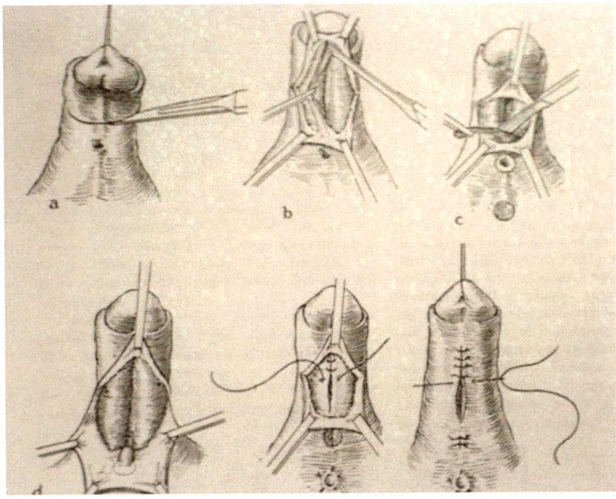

Figure 1. Excising "fibrous bands" thought to restrict expansion of the corpora.
A transverse skin incision was made through the most bent region across what is now known as the urethral plate. Then subcutaneous tissues were excised distally to the glans and proximally to the meatus until the surface of the corpora was completely stripped clean. Finally, the skin was closed longitudinally, with urethroplasty delayed for another operation.

These presumed contracted bands of tissue became known as "chordee" in the 1930s, when an American urologist stated that "all hypospadias are associated with some degree of congenital chordee" (Smith, 1938). Later, this chordee was described as "dysgenetic corpus spongiosum" and depicted as a fan of fibrous tissue extending from the meatus to the glans (Figure 2). It was widely believed that penile straightening was routinely accomplished by a meticulous and complete excision of these chordee tissues (Creevy, 1958). However, the fact that curvature often persisted was a reason for delaying urethroplasty until straight natural erections could be verified postoperatively (Culp, 1958).

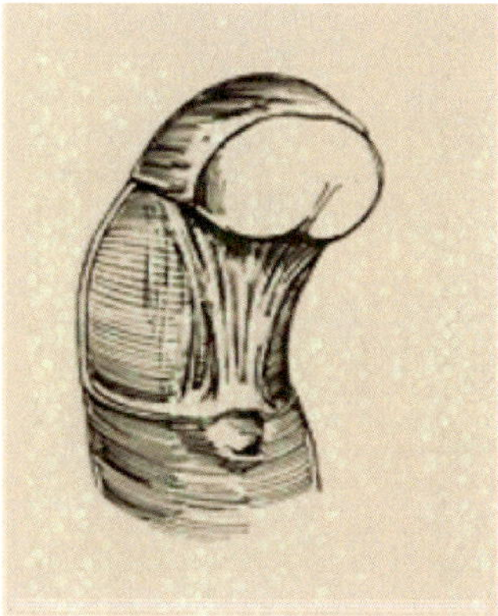

Figure 2. "Chordee."
The "fibrous bands" that the first surgeons described restricting the surface of the corpora were further defined as "dysgenetic corpus spongiosum" by later surgeons in the 1940s and 50s. The underlying concept remained the same, that VC could be straightened by meticulous dissection of tissues overlying the tunica albuginea.

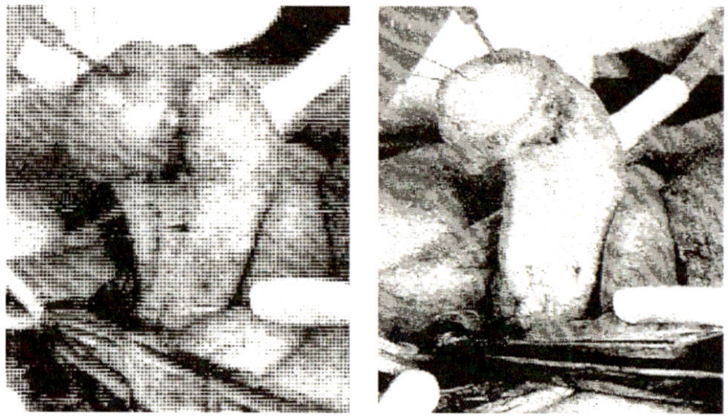

Figure 3. Persistent VC after excision of chordee, including the urethral plate.
A, this grainy picture taken from Baskin et al, 1994 shows VC after the penis was degloved preserving the urethral plate. B, similar VC persists after the urethral plate was excised. Because the penis remained bent after excising the urethral plate, Duckett thought it better to preserve the plate for urethroplasty and straighten the corpora using plications.

Artificial erection was described by Gittes and McLaughlin in 1974, and for the first time, intraoperative assessment could be done to determine if chordee excision made the penis straight. Most often it did not. John Duckett found that chordee excision, including removal of the urethral plate, did not straighten curvature that persisted after degloving (Figure 3). Rather than *external* tissues restricting the corpora, it was the *tunica albuginea sheath* enclosing the erectile tissues which developed shorter on the ventral surface and caused erections to bend. Since excision of tissues *on* the corpora did not affect this "corporal disproportion", Duckett advised surgeons to preserve the urethral plate and correct VC by dorsal plication into the tunica to shorten the longer side of the corpora (Baskin and Duckett, 1994).

Dorsal Plication

Reed Nesbit agreed with the prevailing wisdom that penile curvature was due to fibrous chordee—until he encountered a college student complaining that his penis was bent sideways. Nesbit degloved, expecting to find chordee on that side causing this man's lateral curvature, but, despite a thorough inspection, he could not find fibrous tissues constricting the corpora. Nesbit imagined two solutions, to shorten the longer side or to lengthen the shorter side of the corpora. He chose to plicate the tunica albuginea with a suture plication on the side opposite the bend as the most expedient course. While initially successful, within a few months the curvature recurred. So he reoperated and next excised transverse ellipses of tunica albuginea and then sewed the defects closed. This time the penis remained straight at last follow up a year later (Nesbit, 1965).

Subsequently, another young man presented with ventral curvature, and Nesbit again could not find tethering fibrous bands. He straightened the penis by excising parallel rows of tunica albuginea on either side of the midline, which he then closed using "heavy" silk (Figure 4).

As mentioned above, when artificial erection showed the penis was still bent after thorough chordee excision, Duckett realized VC was due to corporal disproportion - the tunica albuginea forming shorter on the ventral than the dorsal surface. At a time when he was transitioning from transverse island to onlay flap urethroplasties, he was motivated to preserve the urethral plate and so he, like Nesbit, chose to shorten the longer side.

However, rather than excise ellipses of tunica albuginea, Duckett elevated the neurovascular bundle on either side and then made 2 parallel transverse

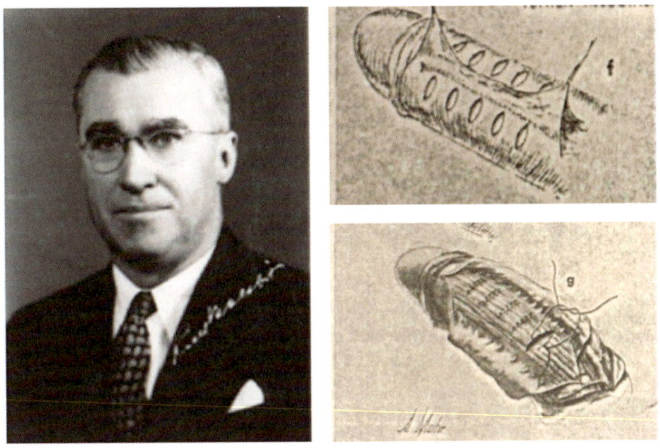

Figure 4. Nesbit plications.
Nesbit (pictured here in 1954) excised ellipses of tunica albuginea on either side of the midline and then closed the defects with silk to straighten VC.

incisions under each of them 4-6mm long and approximately 8mm apart in the area opposite the bending. Next, he sewed the incisions together, ducking the intervening tunica (Figure 5).

Duckett's report included photographs of 2 proximal hypospadias cases. One had approximately 45° VC that he straightened by this Tunica Albuginea Plication (TAP) procedure while preserving the urethral plate, while the other had bending of 90° in which he excised the plate and also did a TAP procedure. However, he subsequently speculated that the urethral plate could be kept intact and plication done in "even the most severe cases" (Baskin and Duckett, 1994). Two years later he went further and said it was a "rare case" that needed ventral lengthening (Baskin et al, 1996).

After completing fellowship training with Duckett, Larry Baskin moved to San Francisco. There he watched Tom Lue correct curvature from Peyronie's disease by plicating in 2 rows near the neurovascular bundles *without incising* the tunica albuginea. When anatomic studies of fetal penises showed no nerves running dorsally at 12 o'clock, Baskin recommended a single row of plications into the intact tunica in the midline, as seen in Figure 6, to avoid potential damage from operating near or under the neurovascular bundles (Baskin et al, 1998).

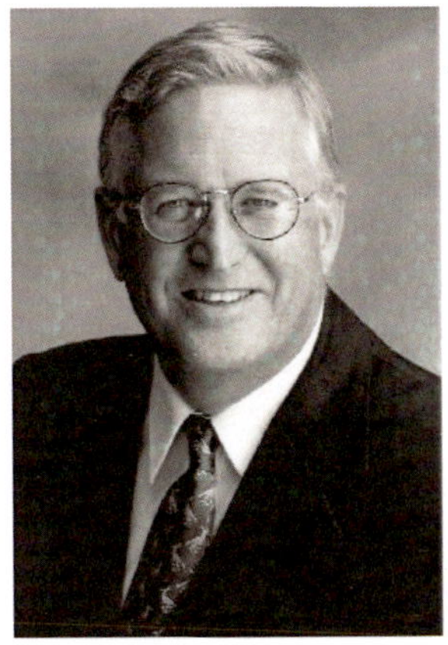

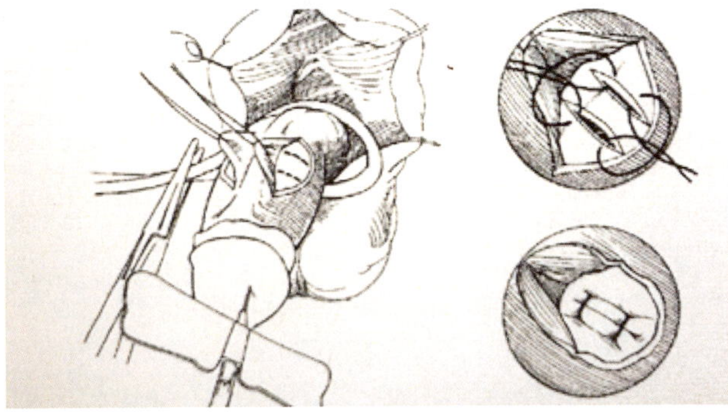

Figure 5. Duckett Tunica Albuginea Plication (TAP).
John Duckett raised the neurovascular bundles and made a pair of transverse incisions under them 4mm apart opposite the bent region. Then he sewed the incisions together, ducking down the strip of tunica between them.

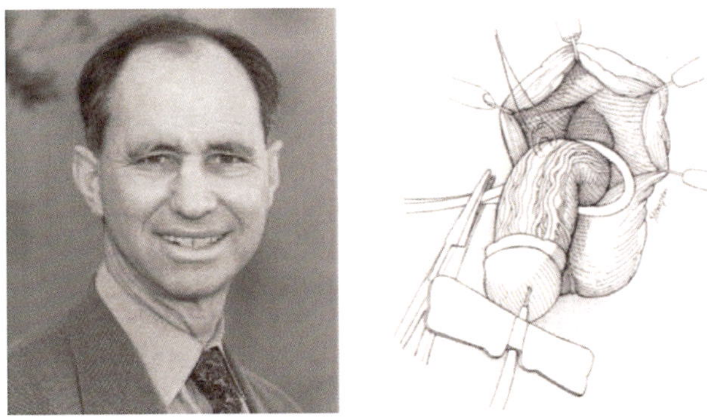

Figure 6. Baskin plication.
Baskin placed 1 or more plication stitches directly into the midline tunica albuginea without incising it.

Even though the first Nesbit plication done by suture plication without incision or excision of the tunica albuginea failed, and a subsequent article warned there was significantly more recurrent curvature after simple plication versus plication with excision of tunica ellipses (Poulsen and Kirkeby, 1995), Baskin's method was rapidly adopted by surgeons worldwide.

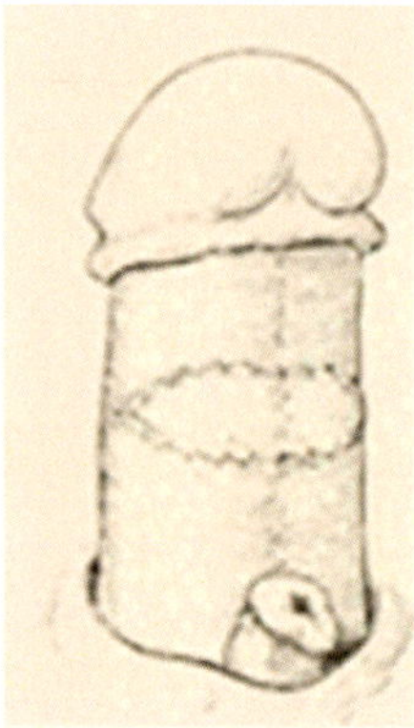

Figure 7. Single corporotomy with corporal graft. A transverse incision was made through the tunica albuginea at the point of maximum curvature, and then the resulting corporal defect was closed using a dermal graft.

The influence of Duckett and Baskin was evident in a survey of American pediatric urologists in 1999. Shown drawings with VC ranging to a maximum of 50°, most answered they used plications for straightening while preserving the urethral plate (Bologna et al, 1999).

Single Corporotomy with Corporal Grafting

When bending caused by Peyronie's disease was judged too severe for plication, surgeons excised the plaque and then filled the corporal defect with fat grafts. Charles Devine Jr and Charles Horton, the urologist-plastic surgeon team, thought these were not sufficiently strong to contain erections, and so they experimented with fascia, and arteries and veins, in animals before deciding that dermis best closed the corporotomy (Devine and Horton, 1977).

It was a natural progression to make a ventral corporotomy with dermal grafting to straighten VC in hypospadias patients, as illustrated in Figure 7.

However, dermal grafts require another skin incision to harvest. Surgeons subsequently tried tunica vaginalis grafts and flaps, and biomaterials such as SIS (small intestinal submucosa), to bridge the corporotomy.

3 Corporotomies without Corporal Grafting

During residency, Warren Snodgrass learned to straighten nearly all curvature using dorsal plications as Duckett recommended. When he encountered patients with proximal hypospadias and VC that he thought was too severe for plication, Snodgrass initially used a single corporotomy with dermal grafting for straightening.

However, when he stopped doing flap urethroplasties and moved to staged graft repairs he needed an alternative means to straighten severe VC, since he could not place a urethroplasty graft onto a dermal corporal graft. Snodgrass recalled hearing of "fairy cuts" done by Devine and Horton, but could not find either a description or illustration of their multiple superficial incisions into the tunica albuginea.

Snodgrass decided to incise the corporal sheath across the point of greatest curvature, and then made a second parallel incision 4mm below and a third 4 mm distal to the first (Figure 8). He left these open to heal spontaneously. Snodgrass originally referred to these as fairy cuts in recognition of Devine and Horton's earlier inspiration, but found that name confused surgeons to believe that his incisions were

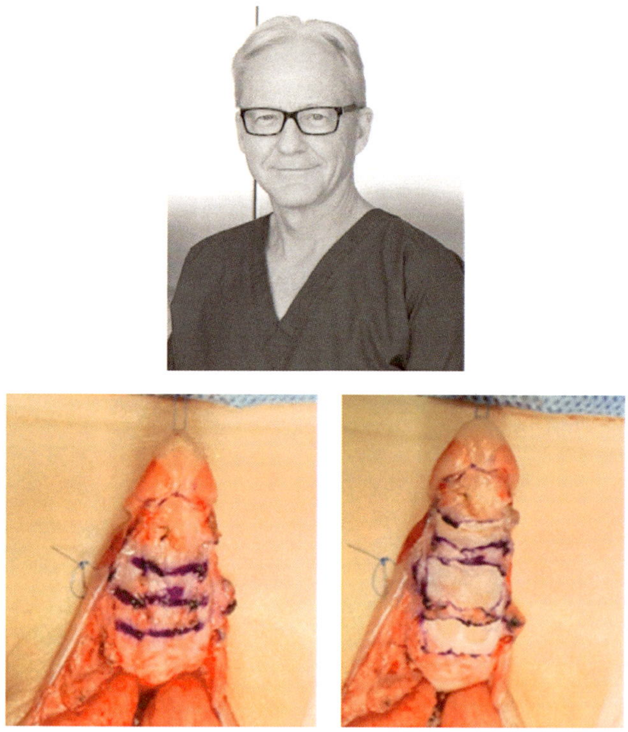

Figure 8. 3 corporotomies without corporal grafting. Snodgrass, as he appeared in 2020. B, the corporal incisions are made across the arc of curvature, with the middle one at the point of maximum bending. C, each extends through the tunica albuginea.

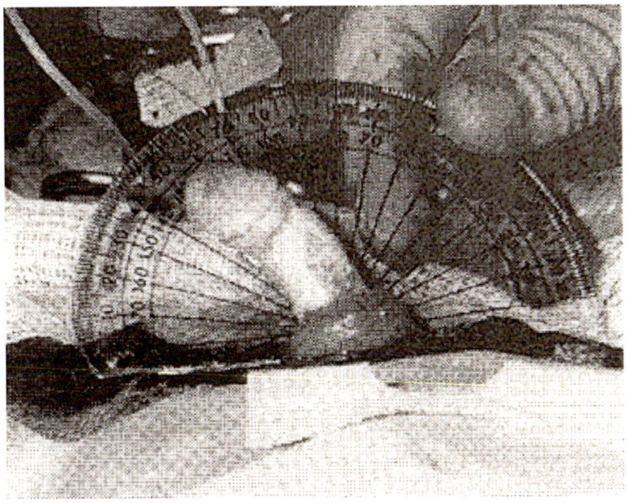

Figure 9. Using a protractor to measure VC.

very superficial. Subsequently, he instead referred to "3 corporotomies without corporal grafting" and emphasized that the incisions went through the tunica albuginea.

Measuring Ventral Curvature

Successful hypospadias repair requires durable straightening of the bent penis. Because the means for straightening vary according to the extent of VC, surgeons should measure it objectively - both to make correct choices and to accurately share their observations with others. Nevertheless, 25 years after Gittes and McLaughlin described artificial erection, nearly all surgeons estimated it visually. In their report on surgical preferences for straightening VC, Bologna et al (1999) lamented such terms as "significant" chordee and encouraged protractors be used for accurate numerical assessment. They argued that advances in the understanding and management of VC required objective measurements (Figure 9).

However, few surgeons transitioned from "eyeballing" curvature to measuring it. In 2014, Nicol Bush happened upon a goniometer, an orthopedic instrument used to measure angles, and realized it could be used to determine the degree of penile curvature accurately (Figure 10). She quickly realized that we were underestimating curvature ranging from 25 to 45 degrees. We describe how to use the goniometer in Chapter 3.

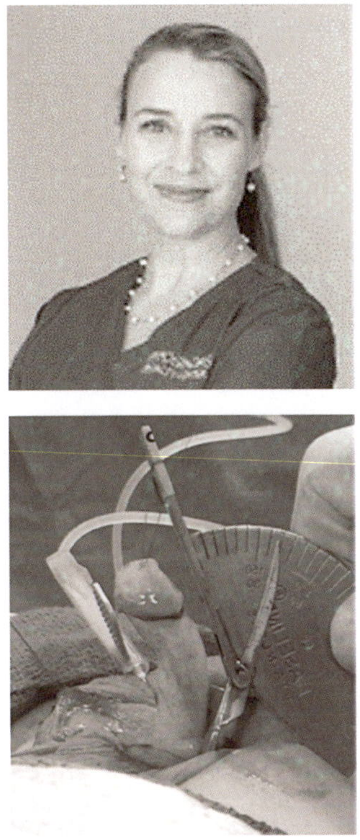

Figure 10. Measuring ventral curvature using a goniometer.
A, Nicol Bush. B, goniometer being used to objectively measure VC. These orthopedic instruments are readily available, easily adapted to the prepubertal penis, and accurate for measuring the degree of bending.

A Summary of Current Practice

Even though artificial erection was described in the early 1970s, and Duckett subsequently published that this test proved chordee excision did not straighten the penis, many surgeons today still understand VC as resulting from chordee and still perform chordee excision to correct it. We reviewed operative records in patients presenting with urethroplasty complications after proximal hypospadias repairs done by other pediatric urologists and found chordee excision was the 2nd most common straightening maneuver done, after dorsal plication. Of these, 83% had persistent VC that averaged 50° (Snodgrass & Bush, 2019). As discussed in chapter 2, it cannot be overemphasized that there is no "chordee", and that the most extensive ventral dissection stripping away all tissues from the surface of the corpora usually does *not* make the penis straight – because VC that persists after degloving is almost always due to an intrinsic malformation of the sheath enclosing the corpora rather than a fibrous constriction on its surface.

The most common means pediatric urologists use today to straighten VC that persists after degloving is dorsal plication, which Duckett championed to preserve the urethral plate for urethroplasty. Initially he limited plications to lesser degrees of VC, but subsequently declared they could be used for nearly all cases. It is easy to do, and repeat artificial erection most often shows the penis to be straight. However, plications on the dorsal side of the corpora do not release the tension that develops on the ventral side during erections. Consequently, as discussed in Chapter 2, recurrent VC is common because that ventral tension overcomes the dorsal plication stitch(es). We found that 70% of patients in our series who had dorsal plication by either the Baskin technique or with tunica incision or excision developed recurrent VC which averaged 40°.

Only 25% of patients in our series with complications after proximal repairs initially had ventral lengthening, which was done in most using a single corporotomy with a corporal graft. One of every 3 of these had recurrent VC averaging 50°. Two patients had 3 corporotomies without corporal grafting and neither of them developed recurrent VC (Snodgrass and Bush, 2019).

Every patient in our series with persistent or recurrent VC also developed a urethroplasty complication, which was the chief complaint.

Despite the importance of VC, no patient had objective measurement of their bending recorded in the operative notes, and only a third had an estimated numerical value recorded. Furthermore, only half had a repeat artificial erection after straightening to confirm success immediately after suture placement. Furthermore, although not mentioned in our report, exceptionally few had another artificial erection during a planned 2nd stage operation. Similarly, artificial erection was rarely reported during reoperations for complications, in some cases despite the surgeon being told by the parents that they suspected recurrent VC.

Together these observations indicate there is ongoing confusion regarding the etiology of VC and the best means to correct it. They also suggest that most surgeons consider whatever means they used to correct VC was sufficiently successful that there was no need to confirm the penis was straight at 2nd stages or during reoperations, irrespective of the initial extent of curvature. The fact that nearly 85% of patients evaluated for urethoplasty complications had persistent or recurrent VC despite prior correction by pediatric urologists is deeply concerning.

Urethroplasty

There are four basic methods to create the neourethra: flaps, grafts, urethral advancements, and urethral plate tubularizations. Key evolutionary procedures for each of these are shown in Figure 11. A review of these operations shows how standard maneuvers were described, and then largely forgotten until they were re-discovered by another surgeon and re-named for him, generations later. Although authors commonly write that there are more than 200 hypospadias repairs, in fact there is much less complexity than this statement implies.

Flaps

From the beginning most surgeons considered flaps the best way to create a neourethra, and most of the evolution of hypospadias urethroplasty follows innovations to relocate prepucial and penile shaft skin while still attached to the penis. The reasoning seemed obvious, that a flap of skin mobilized in continuity with its blood supply would perform better than a graft taken from the same skin that then must reestablish vascularity. Only recently have results from flap and graft repairs shown that grafts have significantly better outcomes for proximal hypospadias (Snodgrass and Bush, 2017).

Prepucial Tubes

Convinced by the presumed superiority of flaps, urologists experimented with various ways to either roll a tube entirely from a skin flap or combine a rectangular skin flap with the urethral plate to make the neourethra. Inspired by the skin flaps that Karl Thiersch used to repair epispadias, Weller Van Hook, the Chief of Surgery at Northwestern Medical School in Chicago, devised the first prepucial pedicle flap, a rolled skin tube which he moved ventrally and tunneled from the tip of the glans to the penoscrotal meatus

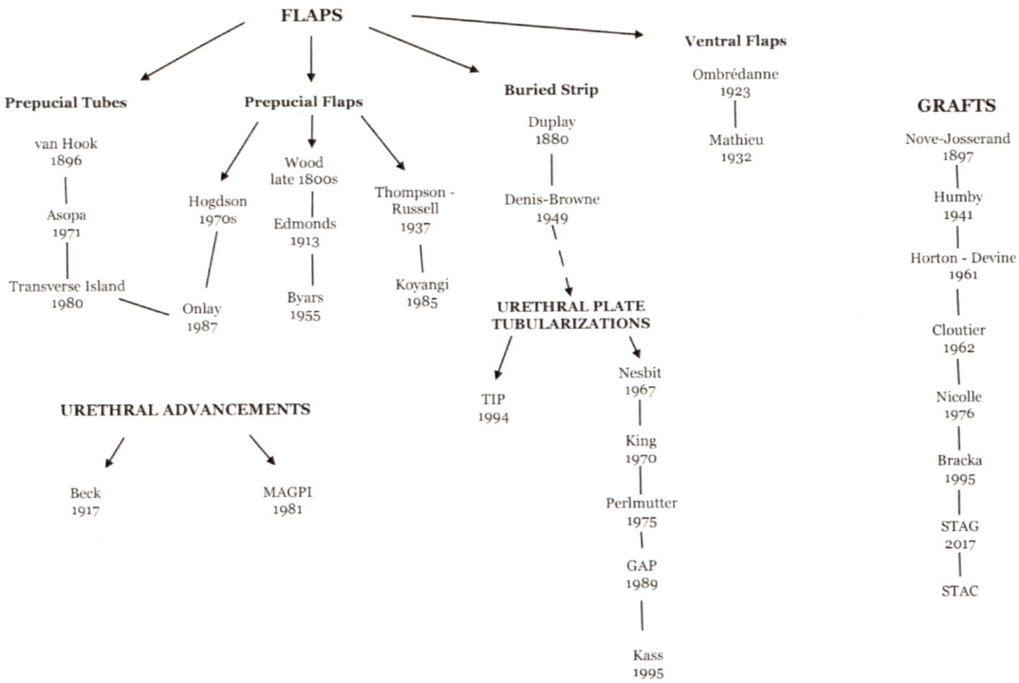

Figure 11. Genealogy of Hypospadias Urethroplasties.

(Figure 12). He reported that the proximal junction obliterated, however, and he tried 3 more local flap repairs to establish continuity. Then a 5th operation was needed to close a large fistula at the penoscrotal junction. These 5 procedures were accomplished in 6 months' time, and 2 new fistulas remained when he published his report. Nevertheless, the surgeon described the penis as having "an extremely good appearance, exactly like a normally developed organ", except, presumedly, for the scars and fistulas on the ventral side (Van Hook, 1896).

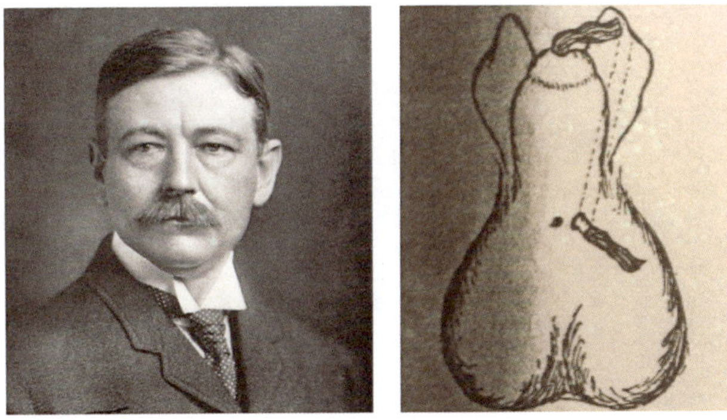

Figure 12. The first tubularized prepucial pedicle flap. Weller Van Hook tubularized a portion of the foreskin in situ, shown by the dotted lines, and then swung the entire flap ventrally and tunneled it from the penoscrotal meatus to the glans tip.

Nearly 100 years later, Hari Asopa also tubularized a strip of prepuce in situ and transferred it ventrally to connect to the native urethra and extend into the glans, as shown in Figure 13 (Asopa et al, 1971). Similar to Van Hook's diagram above, Asopa did not tunnel the neourethra under the skin.

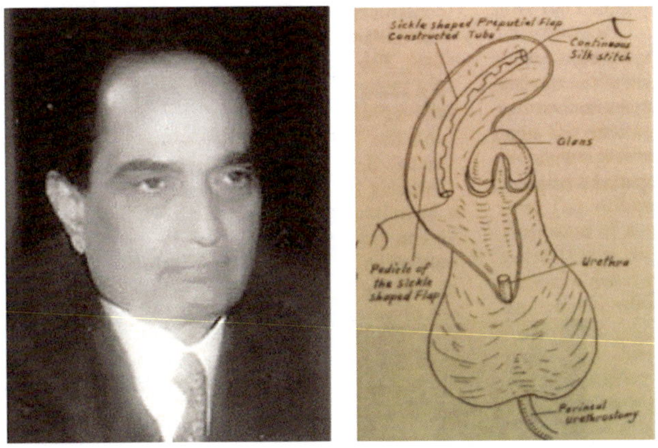

Figure 13. Asopa's tubed prepucial flap.

Norman Hodgson transferred the foreskin ventrally via a buttonhole and then created the neourethra from vertical flaps made 3 different ways. The Hodgson I tubularized the inner prepuce and used the outer prepuce to cover the ventral penile shaft. In the Hodgson II operation, the outer prepuce was sewn to the urethral groove tissues (later known as the urethral plate) in a forerunner of the onlay flap (Figure

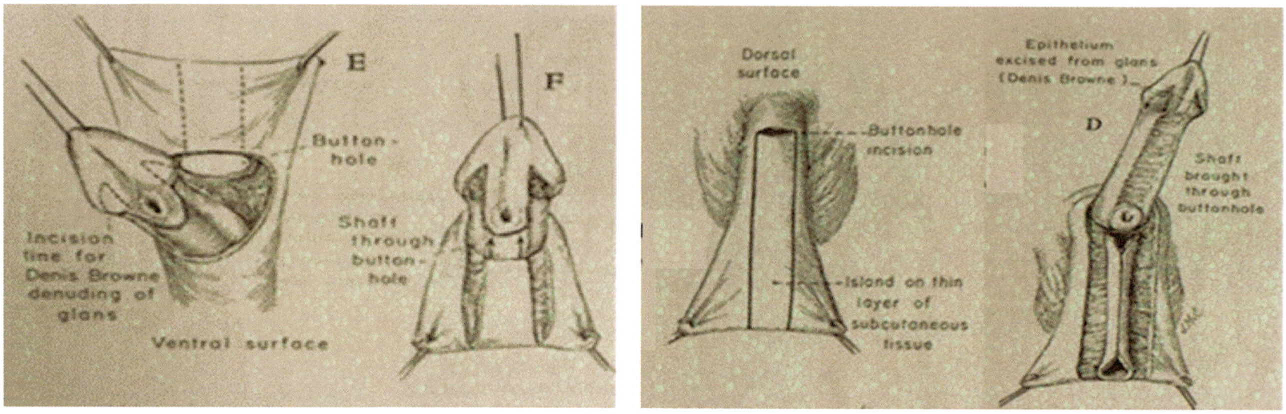

Figure 14. The Hodgson II and III repairs.
A, the Hodgson II used a vertical prepucial flap sewn to the urethral groove to make the neourethra, in a manner similar to the onlay flap described by Duckett over a decade later. B, the Hodgson III was a single stage prepucial and shaft skin flap repair for proximal hypospadias.

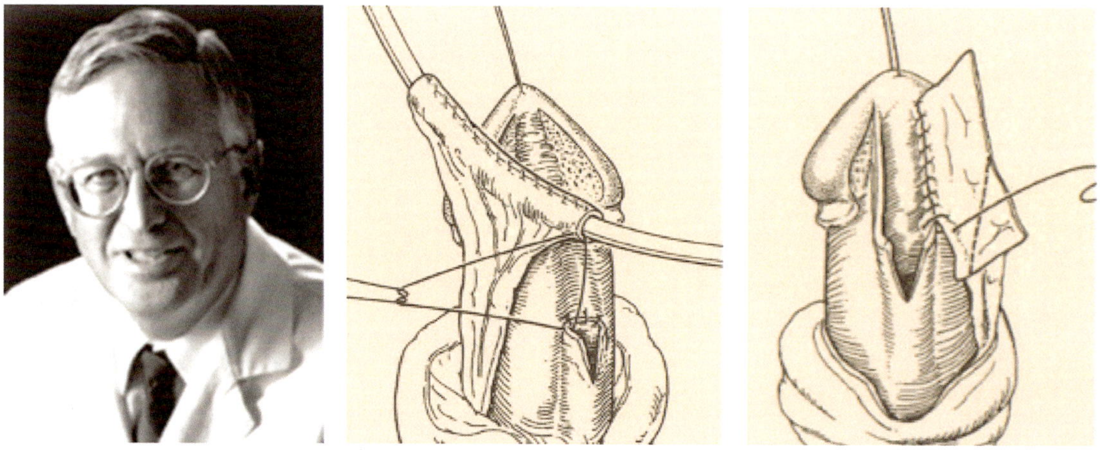

Figure 15. Duckett prepucial flaps.
A, John Duckett. B, transverse island flap. C, onlay flap

14A). Both these procedures were designed for distal hypospadias repairs. The Hodgson III transferred the prepuce and dorsal shaft skin ventrally through a buttonhole, and then rolled a long neourethra for proximal hypospadias as seen in Figure 14B (Hodgson, 1975).

Duckett improved these designs by dissecting the prepucial flap along with dartos away from the dorsal shaft skin, as shown in Figure 15B (Duckett, 1980). This increased mobility to move the neourethra ventrally without a broad skin pedicle, which also simplified shaft skin management compared to the Van Hook and Asopa repairs. His "transverse island", named for the fact that the tube was made transversely across the prepuce rather than vertically as Hodgson described, rapidly gained popularity. A few years later, Duckett modified his own procedure by leaving the foreskin as a rectangular flap that he sewed onto the urethral plate to form the neourethra, a procedure he named the "onlay" prepucial flap (Figure 15C) (Elder et al, 1987).

Split Prepucial Flaps

Arthur Edmunds, a surgeon in London, was also inspired by Thiersch's approach to move skin flaps ventrally to make the neourethra, but in a fashion which

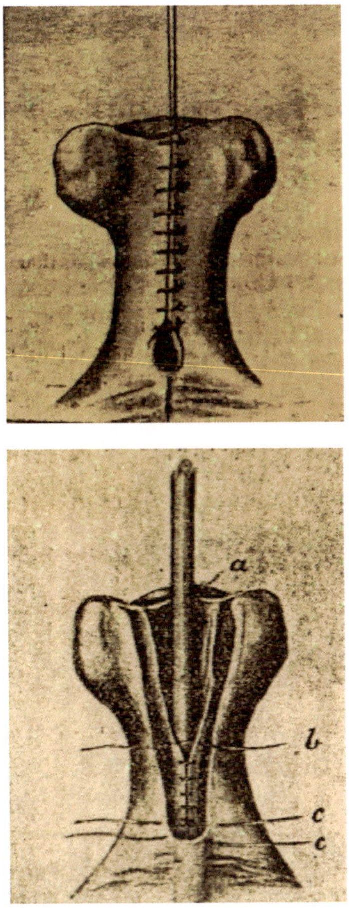

Figure 16. Edmunds' prepucial flap.
A, after excising fibrous bands for penile straightening, the split prepuce was re-approximated ventrally up the midline. B, when that healed, parallel incisions on either side of the midline created a flap to form the neourethra.

modern readers would recognize as Byars flaps (Figure 16). His multistage urethroplasty began by making a buttonhole in the prepuce dorsally. 3 months later, he excised fibrous bands ventrally for penile straightening and then split the buttonhole to make 2 flaps which he transferred to fill the ventral skin defect. A third operation used a U-shaped incision to create a urethroplasty flap that was tubularized over a catheter. The overlying skin was closed directly over the neourethra without a barrier layer, using horsehair stitches (Edmunds, 1913).

A plastic surgeon at Barnes Hospital in St Louis, Louis Byars, described a 2-stage repair that began with chordee excision and then divided the foreskin longitudinally, transposed it ventrally, and reapproximated

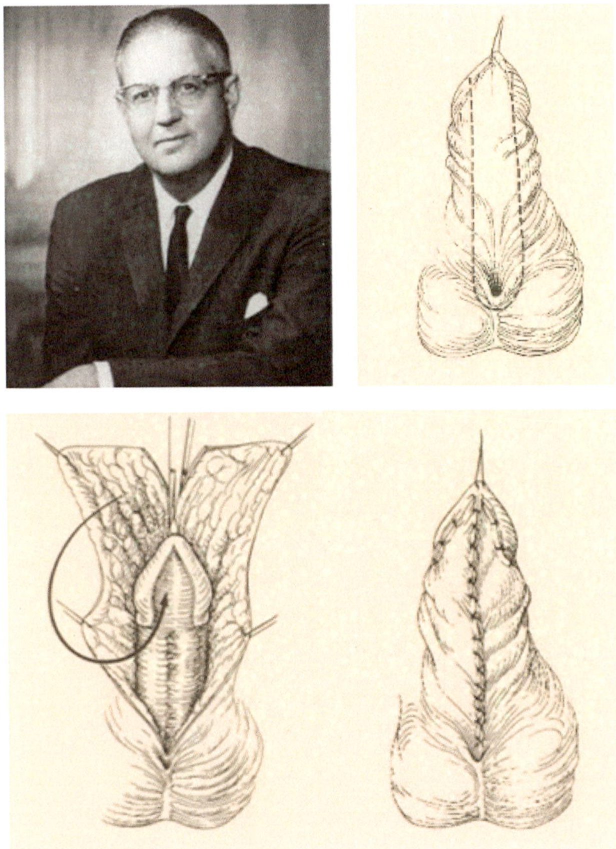

Figure 17. Byars flap urethroplasty.
A, Louis Byars. B, the first stage included chordee excision and ventral transfer of flaps made by splitting the dorsal foreskin. C, a skin flap was tubularized at a second operation. Although this diagram shows the neourethra extending to the tip of the glans, Byars left the neomeatus lower, "near enough to the normal location to be acceptable" (Byars, 1955).

the flaps in the midline, all in a manner reminiscent of Edmunds, although done in one step rather than two (Figure 17). Similarly, after healing, a long U incision created the urethroplasty flap to tubularize over a catheter (Byars, 1955).

The Thompson-Russell procedure had similarities to these other prepucial flaps, but was done in 1 stage (Thompson, 1937). The foreskin was moved ventrally via a buttonhole, which was immediately closed again. Then the transposed strip was tubularized (Figure 18). Years later, the Koyanagi repair followed the same general steps to move the foreskin ventrally and create the tubularized neourethra, also in a single operation (Figure 19).

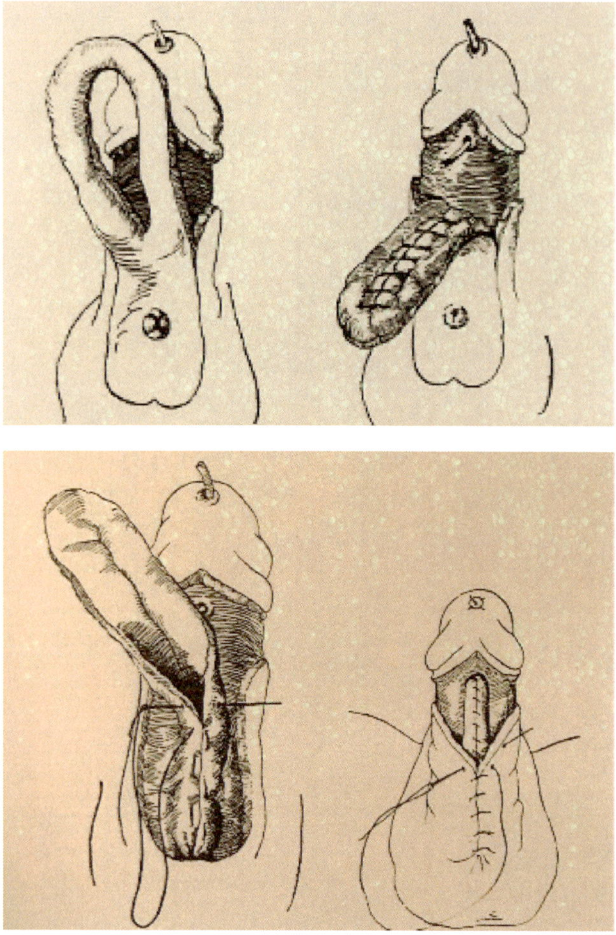

Figure 18. Thompson-Russell prepucial flap repair. Rather than buttonhole the foreskin and then split it into halves to move ventrally as Edmunds described, the Thompson-Russell procedure kept the buttonhole intact and moved the flap in one piece over the glans. Then the buttonhole was closed and the entire flap tubularized. The neourethra was brought to the tip of the glans through a tunnel to complete the operation in 1 stage.

Buried Strip

After excising ventral fibrous tissues to straighten the penis, Duplay closed the skin edges longitudinally without adding skin from prepucial flaps. Consequently, there was not enough ventral skin at the next operation to make the neourethra and close shaft skin over it. He initially solved this problem with a relaxing incision running down the dorsal midline from near the corona to the penopubic junction. This left an unsightly scar, and likely did not reliably relieve tension on the ventral wound closure. Six years later he modified the procedure, making the incisions for his neourethra less wide so that he could close the ventral shaft skin. However, now the caliber of the neourethra

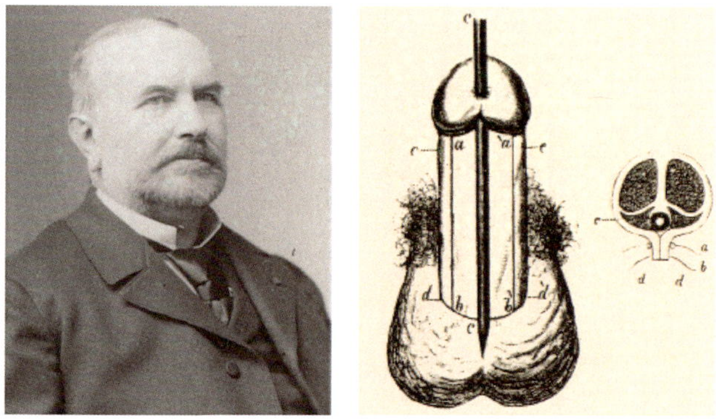

Figure 20. Duplay's buried strip urethroplasty.
In his second method, Simon Duplay sized the width of the skin strip for the neourethra making certain there was enough shaft skin to close the wound over it. That left too narrow a strip to tubularize into the urethra, and so he placed a catheter onto the strip and then closed the shaft skin over it, relying on healing around the catheter to complete the neourethra.

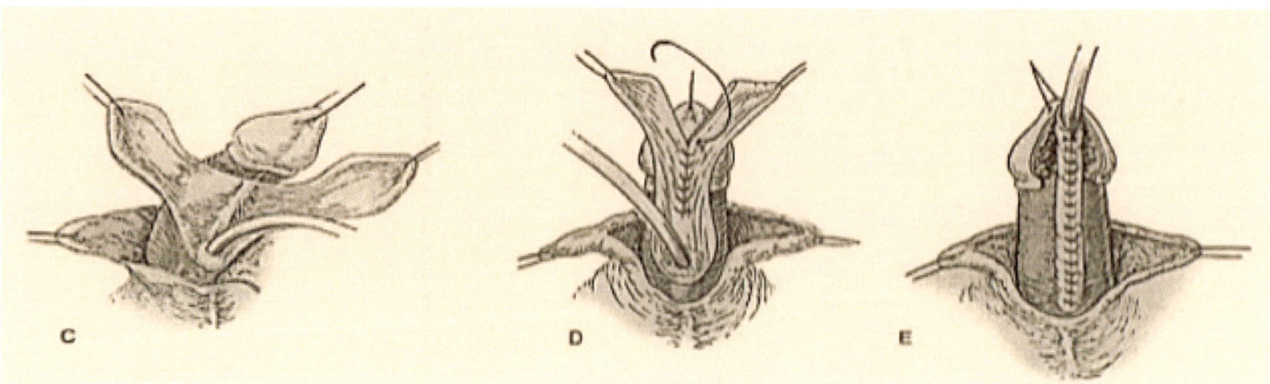

Figure 19. Koyanagi repair.
This one-stage repair divides the foreskin into 2 halves, moves them ventrally, and then re-unites them. The strip is then tubularized.

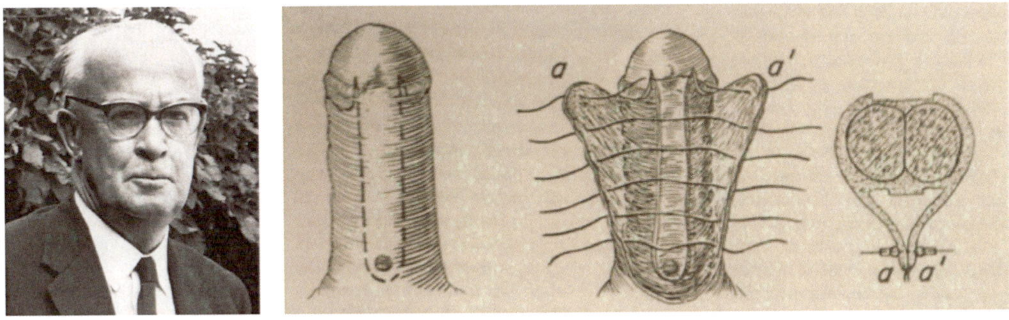

Figure 21. Browne's buried strip urethroplasty.
Shaft skin was closed over a catheter lying on a strip of skin. That strip was the dorsal wall of the neourethra, while the ventral wall developed by epithelialization over the catheter.

was too small. So he simply laid a catheter in the middle of the skin strip and then closed the shaft skin over this incompletely tubularized neourethra on the presumption it would complete ventral tubularization spontaneously (Figure 20) (Beck, 1917).

Sir Denis Browne, the first surgeon to limit his practice to pediatric urology, published a quite similar operation to Duplay's second method in 1949. He also closed the shaft skin over a "buried strip" that formed itself into the neourethra (Figure 21). Critics found little difference in his technique and that of Duplay's, described over 50 years earlier.

The buried strip inspired another procedure that the author named a reversed Denis-Browne (Orkiszewski, 1987). He used this method in reoperations when available ventral shaft skin was too narrow to tubularize a strip into a neourethra. Midline incision of the skin strip allowed it to be tubularized. He did not apply this method to primary repairs.

Ventral Shaft Skin Flaps

Flaps raised from the ventral penile shaft were used to repair distal to midshaft hypospadias. The first was devised by Louis Ombredanne, the head of pediatric surgery at the Hospital Necker in Paris. He fashioned a meatal-based flap which he elevated towards the glans tip with a purse-string suture. The dorsal shaft skin was button-holed and transferred ventrally to cover the shaft. The finished repair was suspended from an apparatus to reduce edema (Figure 22).

Another French surgeon, Paul Mathieu, refined the Ombredanne operation to become one of the most popular distal hypospadias repairs from the 1930s into modern times. Rather than draw the ventral flap distally with a purse string, he sewed its edges to the border of the glans groove. His article included the first illustration of glansplasty, using glans wings to enclose the neourethra, rather than perforating the glans and tunneling the neourethra (Mathieu, 1932).

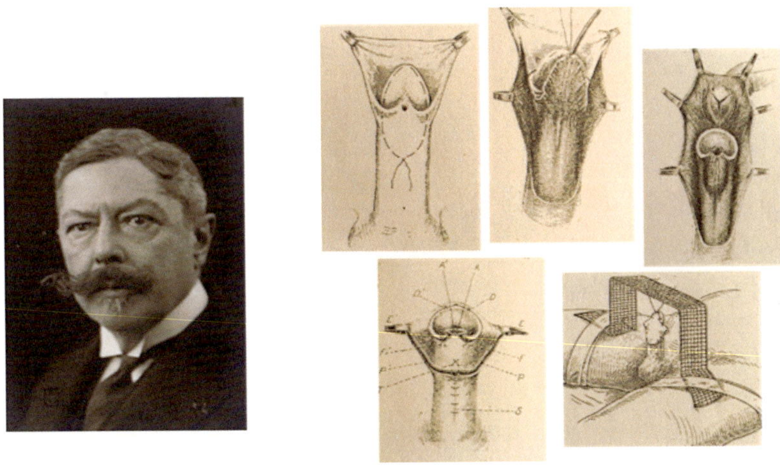

Figure 22. Ombredanne ventral skin flap.

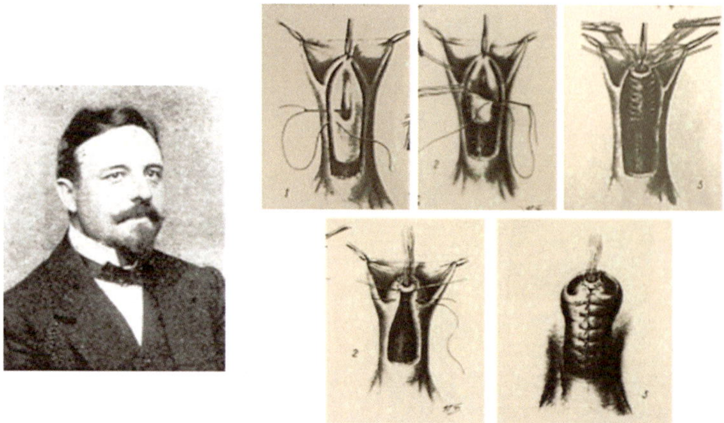

Figure 23. Mathieu flip-flap.
A ventral skin flap was flipped up to sew to incisions made along the urethral groove. Glans flaps were closed around the neourethra, leaving a round meatus.

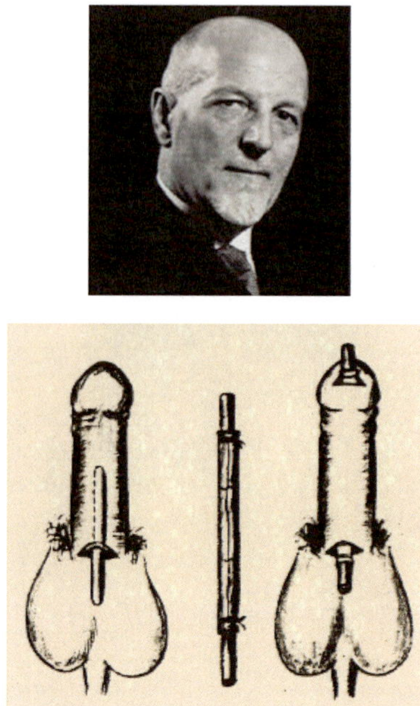

Figure 24. Nove-Josserand partial-thickness skin graft urethroplasty.

This repair is commonly referred to as the flip-flap, highlighting the key step in the urethroplasty which lifts a ventral flap distally. Note that the neomeatus is drawn round, rather than as a vertical slit, which accurately depicts the usual appearance postoperatively (Figure 23). Although still used by some, the Mathieu repair has mostly been replaced by TIP urethroplasty, which makes a more normal-appearing slit meatus.

Grafts

The first graft urethroplasties were reported by Gabriel Nove-Josserand, a French surgeon working in Lyon. He cut a partial-thickness skin graft from the thigh, wrapped it around a trocar, and then tunneled it from the meatus to the glans tip, as shown in Figure 24 (Nove-Josserand, 1914). However, split-thickness grafts have a tendency to contract, and his first neourethra shriveled and then obliterated.

There does not appear to have been much enthusiasm for graft hypospadias repairs for many years after that experience, and, in fact, Nove-Josserand abandoned his own method in favor of Ombredanne's flap repair. Then, in the early 1940s, a British surgeon at Great Ormand Street published results using grafts tubularized around a catheter. The glans was widely opened, rather than perforated, to bring the meatus to the tip. In the first 2 cases Graham Humby harvested split-thickness grafts, but both contracted and so he changed to full-thickness grafts. His 3rd case is the most relevant today. The patient had penoscrotal hypospadias and suffered many prior failed repairs leaving his penis scarred and contracted. Humby harvested the graft from the lower lip and tubularized it. On the 6th day the wound dehisced, and the entire ventral surface of the neourethra was lost. However, the dorsal side of the graft, against the corpora, took "perfectly", and he was subsequently able to tubularize this remaining portion successfully (Humby, 1941).

Although Humby did not recognize the lesson, this case showed the benefit of staging graft repairs by first placing the graft flat onto the corpora to facilitate neovascularization, which is much less reliable when new vessels have to grow around a tube. When that process is complete, the revascularized graft is tubularized at a 2nd stage.

Humby did, however, recognize another principle which was then forgotten. He wrote that the scarred penile skin also contributed to graft failure in his 3rd case because it could not provide the vascularity the graft needed. This important observation later became one of the reasons for STAC repair.

Devine and Horton also described repairing proximal hypospadias in 1 stage using a tubed full-thickness

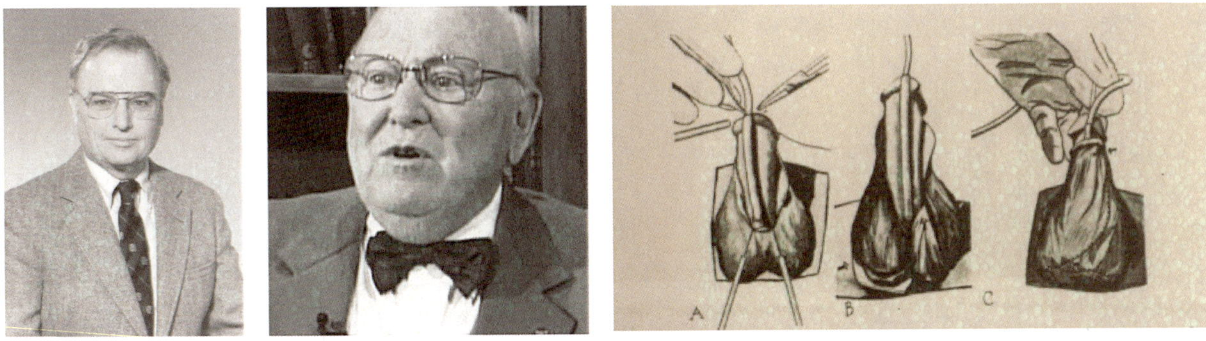

Figure 25. 1 stage full-thickness prepucial graft urethroplasty by Devine and Horton.
A, Charles Devine Jr and B, Charles Horton. C, Their tubed prepucial graft was covered by a scrotal flap, with a second scrotal flap mobilized to close the defect left from the first.

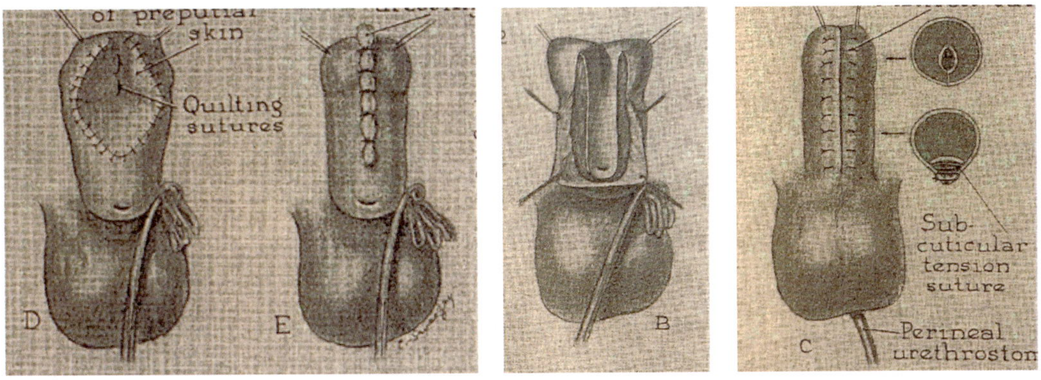

Figure 26. Cloutier's 2-stage full-thickness prepucial graft repair.
A, during the first stage the glans was opened widely and a prepucial graft placed. A tie-over bandage provided gentle compression to the graft to help it take. B, at the second stage Cloutier used the Denis-Browne method to make the neourethra by cutting a strip of skin, placing a catheter onto it, and then closing the shaft skin without stitching the urethra into a tube.

---

graft. After experimenting with inner arm and groin donor sites, they settled on prepucial grafts as a more pliable tissue. They covered the implanted graft and ventral penile shaft with a large scrotal flap, and then used a second scrotal flap to help fill the defect left by the first one (Figure 25) (Devine and Horton, 1961).

Apparently the first surgeon to publish a full-thickness graft urethroplasty done in 2 stages was the plastic surgeon A MacLeod Cloutier, in Montreal. He did chordee excision and then split open the glans and grafted prepucial skin. A tie-over bandage helped secure the graft (Figure 26).

The neourethra was created at a 2nd stage done 3 or more months later. Cloutier used Denis-Browne's method for this step, closing the shaft skin over a buried skin strip rather than tubularizing the prepucial skin strip (Cloutier, 1962).

Frederick Villeneuve Nicolle, a British plastic surgeon who trained under Cloutier, refined his mentor's technique by directly tubularizing the neourethra at the second stage (Nicolle, 1976). Nicolle published his method after moving away to London, providing the first example of the modern staged graft repair. A few years later, Aivar Bracka, another British plastic surgeon, developed the same technique as Nicolle (Figure 27), adding a dartos barrier layer over the neourethra at the 2nd stage. Bracka said he was not aware of Nicolle's earlier work and subsequently credited him in the evolution of the staged graft repair (Bracka, 1995). Bracka maintained the Nicolle operation did not gain a larger following because other plastic surgeons thought his results were too good to be true and suspected he manipulated his data to achieve them (Bracka, 2011).

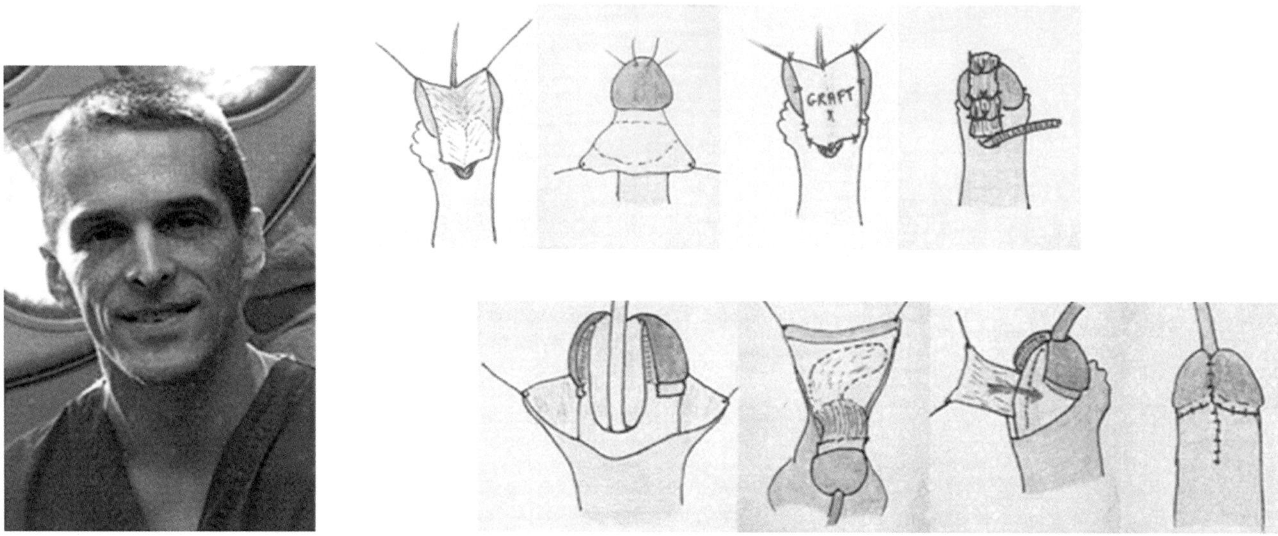

Figure 27. Bracka's 2-stage graft repair.
In the first stage the glans was opened widely and a foreskin graft harvested and sewn into it. A tie-over bandage added gentle compression. The revascularized graft was tubularized during the 2nd stage, and then covered by a dartos flap taken from under the dorsal shaft skin. Glansplasty and skin closure completed the repair.

Throughout the development of graft repairs, penile straightening was done by chordee excision. Like his predecessors, Bracka considered the penis straight after the urethral plate was excised and the surface of the ventral corpora cleared of overlying tissues. If there was residual curvature he recommended dorsal Nesbit plication during the 2nd stage. However, WS does not recall seeing Bracka ever do either an artificial erection or a dorsal plication, and no data is available in a consecutive series of Bracka's repairs.

Snodgrass used Bracka's operation in primary proximal repairs when there was too much curvature for dorsal plication and TIP urethroplasty. Converting from Byars flaps, which all developed complications in his hands, to prepucial grafts, WS also revised his straightening method. As discussed above, rather than make a single ventral corporotomy closed with a dermal graft, Snodgrass cut 3 parallel corporotomies and did not graft these incisions so that he could place a urethroplasty graft over them during the same stage. He also mobilized the urethra to the external sphincter to bring the proximal urethrostomy out of the scrotum and reduce the length of urethroplasty graft that was needed.

Later, he and Bush learned that urethroplasty grafts placed onto intact corpora take better than those placed over corporotomy incisions. Consequently, they preserved the urethral plate in continuity with the native urethra as they dissected back to the sphincter, and then advanced the urethral plate/urethra over the incisions whenever possible so that the graft would lie on a smooth corporal surface.

Snodgrass also used tunica vaginalis to cover the neourethra at the 2nd stage, finding it decreased fistulas compared to a dartos flap. To distinguish this repair from Bracka's, Bush named it the STAG, which originally meant **S**taged **T**ubularized **A**uto**G**raft (Snodgrass and Bush, 2017). Today STAG is better understood as **ST**raighten **A**nd **G**raft.

When the urethra did not reach past the corporotomies and graft would have to be placed onto them, Snodgrass and Bush decided to instead cover the corporal incisions with a dartos flap and then close the shaft skin without placing a urethroplasty graft. 6 months later when the corporotomy incisions were healed, a midline skin incision was made from glans tip to either side of the proximal urethrostomy and a prepucial graft sewn onto the now-smooth corporal surface. Rather than straighten and graft at the first operation, they **ST**raightened **A**nd **C**losed (STAC), delaying grafting to the next stage and tubularization of the neourethra to a final, third operation.

STAC quickly replaced STAG repairs, because it allows both the corporotomies and the reconfigured shaft skin to heal before a urethroplasty graft is placed, which increases the likelihood for supple ventral penile skin and a healthy graft (Snodgrass and Bush, 2024). In fact, the surgeons considered STAC a "gamechanger" for repairing severe hypospadias. STAC is described and illustrated in Chapter 8.

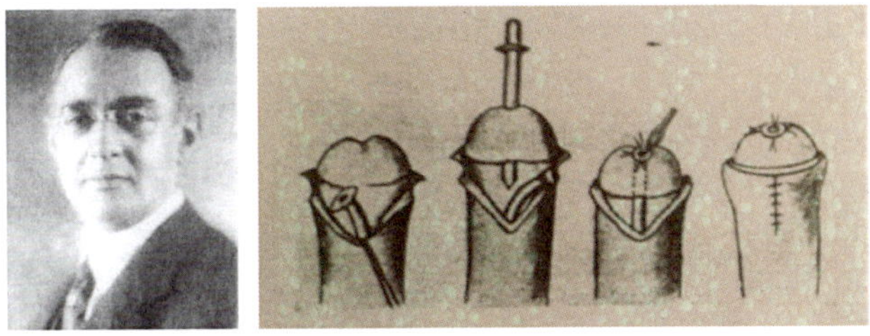

Figure 28. Beck's urethral advancement.

Urethral Advancement

One of the first repairs for distal hypospadias was Carl Beck's urethral advancement (Figure 28). The urethra was dissected proximally and then brought to the tip of the glans via a tunnel made by a trocar (Beck, 1917). Over a half-century later Steven Koff used this same method, including tunneling through the glans. Koff also thought advancement was worthwhile in proximal repairs to move the meatus further distally and thereby reduce the length of the neourethra (Koff, 1981).

Paola Caione opened the glans rather than tunneling through it to perform urethral mobilization (Caione et al, 1991). Following that, many surgeons reported distal hypospadias repair using this method.

Meatal advancement *without* dissecting the distal urethra circumferentially was the basic principle of the MAGPI (meatal advancement and glanuloplasty) repair that Duckett published in 1981. He used a Heineke-Mikulicz maneuver to pull the dorsal wall of the meatus distally, further into the glans, and then closed the glans ventrally around it (Figure 29). Duckett reported the operation was applicable to most anterior hypospadias, including cases in which the meatus was as far as 1-2cm below the glans (Duckett,1981).

Duckett's enthusiasm led surgeons to use the MAGPI for anatomy to which it was not suited. His former fellow, David Gibbons, working with Edmond Gonzales Jr, subsequently defined "meatal variants" that were better managed by alternative techniques (Gibbons and Gonzales, 1983). Today MAGPI is not often used because of its limited applicability to specific anatomy that is not commonly found, and the tendency for the meatus to regress proximally. Nevertheless, the MAGPI is historically significant as the distal repair that helped overcome reticence to repair coronal hypospadias.

Urethral Plate Tubularization

The tissues extending from the hypospadias meatus distally into the glans were once considered fibrous chordee, comprising dysplastic urethra and corpus spongiosum. As described above, the prevailing

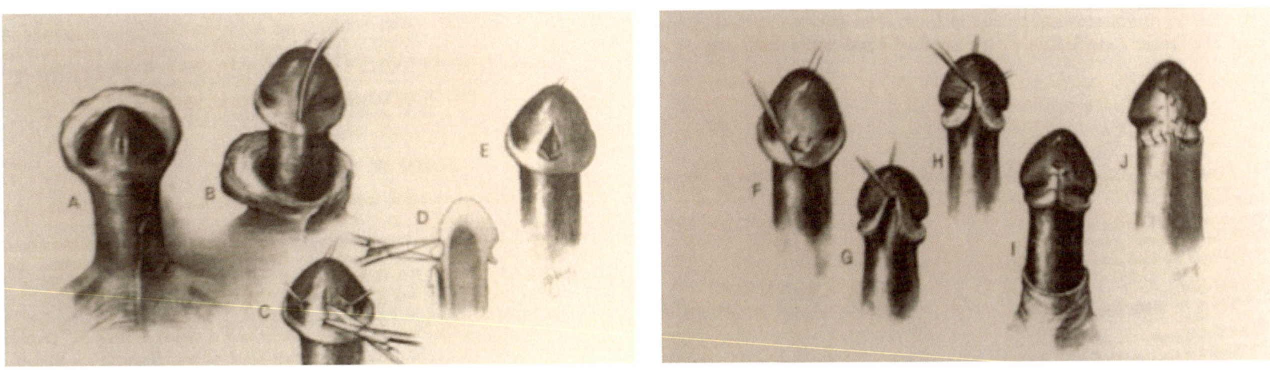

Figure 29. MAGPI.
This diagram is from Duckett's first article introducing the MAGPI. He wrote that he struggled to illustrate the key steps clearly, saying they were easier to demonstrate in person. In fact, he recommended surgeons who wanted to use the procedure first observe others who had already mastered it.

dogma was that these tissues restricted erection, causing ventral curvature. Therefore, most early hypospadias repairs included chordee excision which removed the urethral plate.

Duckett first used the term "urethral plate" (Elder et al, 1987). Then he challenged chordee excision when, using the newly described artificial erection, he observed that curvature usually persisted despite removing the plate (Hollowell et al, 1990).

Previously, these tissues were referred to simply as the skin distal to the meatus, or as the urethral or glans groove. Few publications mentioned using them for urethroplasty. Possibly the first of those was written by Nesbit in 1967. He recommended straightening the penis using dorsal plication, and then completing urethroplasty by either the "Thiersch-Duplay" or Denis-Browne technique. The complete tubularization of the urethral groove into the lower glans that he called a Thiersch-Duplay is seen in Figure 30. The ventral skin defect was filled by prepuce moved by a buttonhole (Nesbit, 1967).

In 1970 Lowell King, the first full-time pediatric urologist in the US, described the same repair. The patient was a boy with midshaft hypospadias who he considered noteworthy because there was no chordee. King said the urethroplasty was easily done in 1 stage by rolling the ventral skin, which included the urethral groove, from the meatus to the coronal sulcus. Following that case, he repeated this repair in others with a distal shaft meatus and "relatively mild chordee". After rolling the tube, he, like Nesbit, also brought the dorsal prepuce ventrally via a buttonhole to cover the penile shaft (Figure 31) (King,1970).

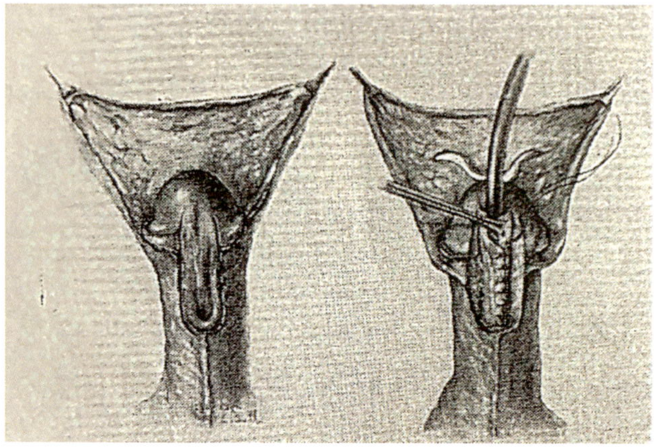

Figure 30. Nesbit urethral groove tubularization onto the lower glans.

King did not think it necessary to repair coronal hypospadias when the penis was straight. Five years after his article, Alan Perlmutter described a procedure to tubularized the glanular groove in coronal hypospadias (Perlmutter and Vatz, 1975). Although the urethroplasty extended the meatus to the normal location, glansplasty was not done. Instead, ventral shaft skin was advanced distally and sewn to the open glans wings (Figure 32).

Then, nearly 20 years later, Mark Zaontz described tubularization of a deep glans groove in what he called the GAP (glans approximation procedure). As seen in Figure 33, there was little glans wings mobilization and no barrier tissue interposed between the urethroplasty and glansplasty. These potentially increased risk for fistulas and glans dehiscence, although Zaontz reported that these rarely occurred (Zaontz, 1989).

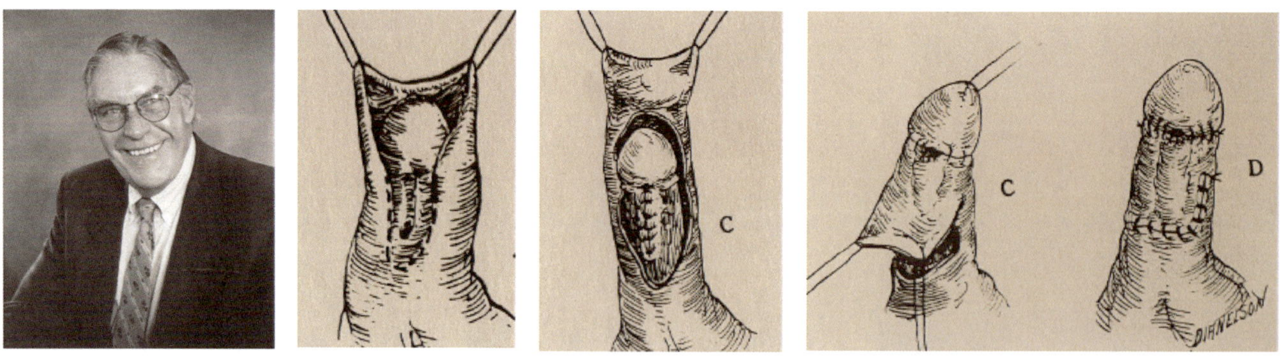

Figure 31. King's tubularized urethral groove. Note the urethroplasty ended at the corona.

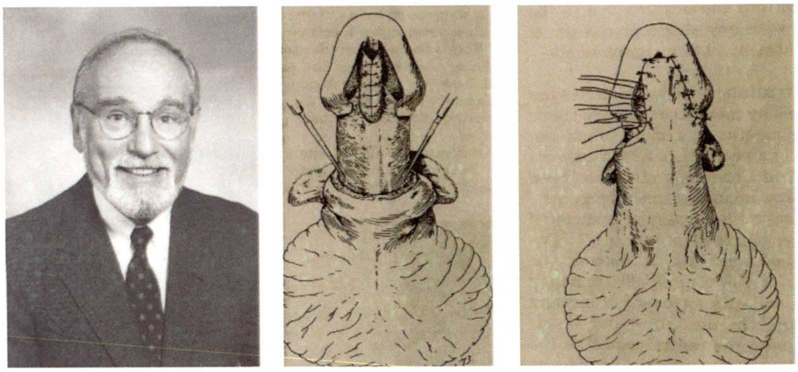

Figure 32. Tubularized glans groove without glansplasty.
Alan Perlmutter, the first pediatric urologist in Detroit, tubularized the urethral groove distally, but did not enclose it within glans wings.

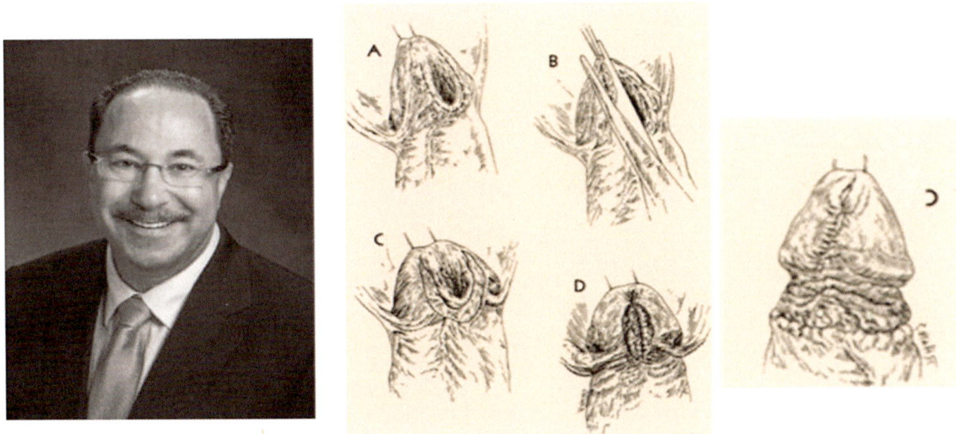

Figure 33. Glans Approximation Procedure.
When the urethral groove was deep, a U incision was made around its edges and the groove was tubularized. No barrier flap covered the neourethra, and minimal glans wings dissection was done.

Another urethral plate tubularization described one year after TIP repair by Evan Kass involved more extensive glans wings dissection and placed a dartos flap between the neourethra and glans closure (Figure 34). Dorsal incision of the urethral plate was not done (Van Horn and Kass, 1995), which limited this method to cases with a sufficiently wide and deep plate to make a normal caliber neourethra.

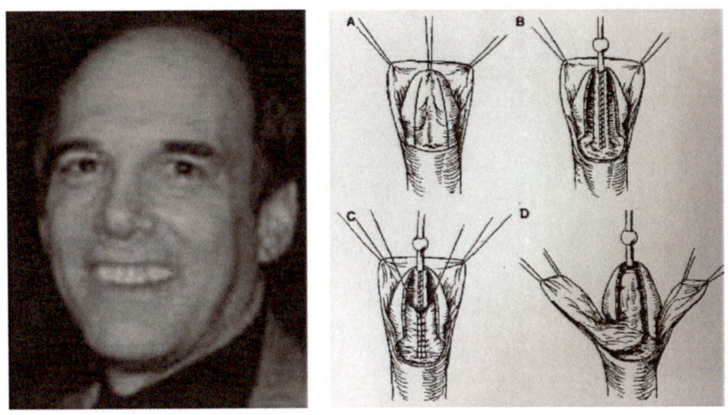

Figure 34. Tubularization of the (intact) urethral plate.
Evan Kass published this operation resembling TIP repair, but without urethral plate incision, in 1995.

The **T**ubularized **I**ncised **P**late (TIP) repair was published in 1994 (Snodgrass). This operation separated the glans wings from the urethral plate along their visible junction, and then deeply incised the plate to widen it (Figure 35). That TIP incision ensured the caliber of the urethra would be normal, making the repair effective whether there was a wide or narrow, flat

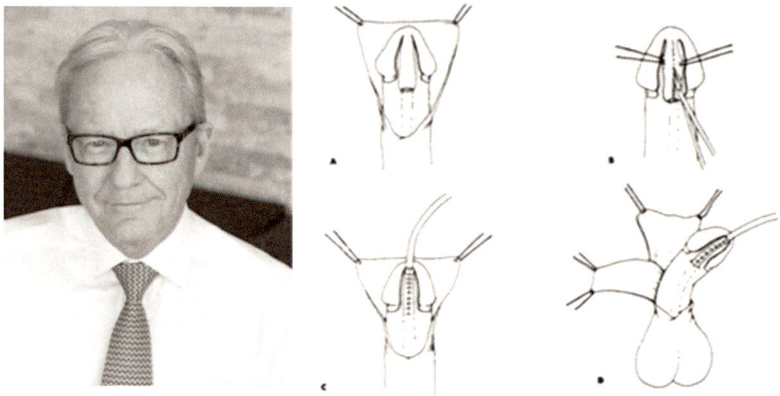

Figure 35. TIP repair.
This is the original diagram of the procedure. In C and D, the urethral plate is shown tubularized too far distally, a technical error that can result in iatrogenic meatal stenosis.

or more deeply grooved, urethral plate. The incision healed without meatal stenosis or urethral stricture.

Even though strictures after TIP are rarely encountered, some surgeons graft the plate incision with prepuce in a modification referred to as the G-TIP or "Snodgraft" procedure. Knowing that they are going to graft probably encourages some concerned for strictures to adequately incise the plate.

The ability to use TIP to repair the gamut of distal hypospadias anatomy and reliably create a normal appearing meatus led to its rapid acceptance worldwide, largely replacing the Mathieu, MAPGI and urethral advancement procedures.

The Evolution of Modern Decision-Making

Most hypospadias is distal with a straight penis. With urethral advancement, Mathieu, MAGPI and GAP, plus related repairs such as the Arap, M inverted V, and Mustarde techniques, a surgeon in the 1980s and 90s had to select the best repair to fit the anatomy of a given patient from a variety of techniques. As a result, Gibbons and Gonzales (1983) suggested MAGPI be avoided when there were "meatal variants" defined as a "fishmouth", "non-compliant", or "hypospastic". Zaontz (1989) recommended the GAP when the meatus was "non-compliant", "patulous" or "fishmouth" and the glans groove was "excessively deep".

While such characterizations were understood by the authors, different surgeons examining the same patient often reached different conclusions about the anatomy. Duckett started a postgraduate hypospadias course during the annual AUA congress, showing invited "experts" photographs of case after case to ask what repair they thought best fit the anatomy they saw. WS recalls how Gibbons covered the surgical drapes with drawings at the beginning of each distal repair as he analyzed the meatus to determine if it was satisfactory for a MAGPI or better suited for a Mathieu.

Viewed from this perspective, complications resulted from the surgeon choosing the wrong operation for the anatomy (Keating and Duckett, 1995).

TIP has the advantage of being applicable to any distal hypospadias, as long as any associated VC measures less than 30°. WS emphasized the TIP incision should always be made from the meatus to the end of the plate and extend down to the surface of the corpora. That makes the operation effective for any distal hypospadias anatomy.

This adaptability, combined with a low complication rate and the routine creation of a normal-appearing, slit meatus, explains TIP's widespread use. With more surgeons using the same technique for distal repairs, it became apparent that complications result less from choosing the wrong operation than from making technical errors while performing the right operation.

But then 2 articles questioned TIP when the pre-incision urethral plate width was <8mm, reporting that the midline plate relaxing incision did not result in an adequate diameter in this situation (Holland and Smith, 2000; Sarhan et al, 2009). However, their findings could be explained by inadequate TIP incision rather than a limitation of the anatomy. Details of these articles are reviewed in Chapter 7, but Smith (2014) later admitted that he did not incise the plate as deeply as Snodgrass after watching him do a TIP repair during a live-surgery workshop. The incision made by Sarhan et al was also not deep enough, as is immediately apparent in comparing photographs of the incised plates from their and our articles (Figure 36).

Consequently, it was not the anatomy which created the complications reported by Holland and Smith and Sarhan et al. It was the technical error of not incising the urethral plate to the underlying corpora. Today it is clear that most complications after hypospadias repair are the result of such technical errors, and failing to deeply incise the plate is the most common mistake made by surgeons doing TIP.

While Duckett worked to perfect his onlay and transverse island flap repairs for proximal cases, Bracka instead used grafts and found them applicable to the broad range of phenotypes comprising severe hypospadias. There was no need to choose between onlay and tubularized, Byars, or Koyanagi flaps when staged grafts were universally effective and created a normal-appearing glans and meatus which flaps most often did not.

But urologists remained convinced that flaps were superior to grafts. Then 3 major centers published results after flap repairs, with Texas Children's, Boston Children's, and CHOP admitting that complication rates were greater than surgeons generally thought. The transverse island that Duckett once wrote had 85% success was found by his successors to instead have 85% failures in their hands (Long et al, 2017). The Byars flaps once reported to have only 5% fistulas (Retik et al, 1994), instead were found to have the range of urethroplasty complications in from nearly 50% to 70% of patients (Stanasel et al, 2015; McNamara et al, 2015; Long et al, 2017), making the 2-stage repair into 3 stages or more in over two-thirds of cases (Stanasel et al, Long et al).

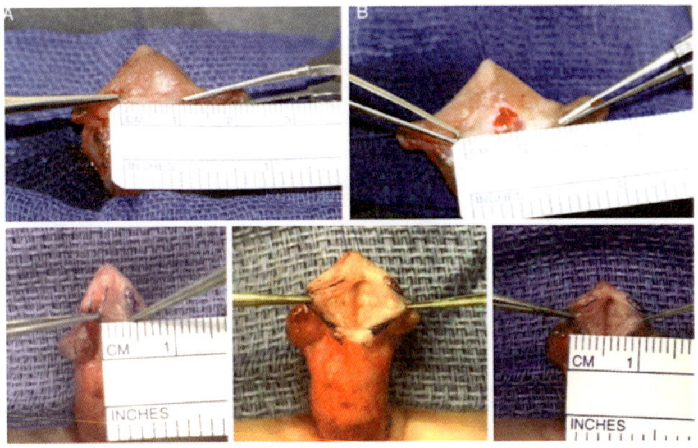

Figure 36. Inadequate vs correct TIP incision. A, appearance after TIP incision reported by Sarhan et al vs B, the appearance after TIP incision done by Snodgrass and Bush. An inadequate incision will not sufficiently widen the urethral plate, and thereby creates a small caliber neourethra more prone to complications. The TIP incision should *always* extend the length of the urethral plate and down to the surface of the underlying corpora.

In contrast, staged grafts had reported complications ranging from 23% to 33% after proximal repairs (Ferro et al, 2002; Castagnetti et al, 2013; Pippi-Salle et al, 2016; Snodgrass and Bush, 2017). STAG evolved from steps to better correct VC than the operation which Bracka taught. STAC was a logical refinement to allow corporotomies and realigned penile skin to heal before placing the urethroplasty graft.

Decision-Making Today

Our algorithm shows that it is the extent of VC, and not meatal location or "characteristics" of the urethral plate, which determines the correct urethroplasty technique. Today surgeons do not have to study the anatomy of the meatus and the urethral plate to decide which repair to use. Instead, they can focus on doing TIP or STAC repairs in the best ways known, adapting the steps to the anatomy encountered in each case.

Consequently, decision-making is greatly simplified compared to prior times. Surgeons should be wary of claims that urethral plate "quality" or its width or shape need to be considered in choosing the operative technique. We have not used any operation other than TIP to repair distal hypospadias in over 30 years. No other operation can repair the range of distal hypospadias phenotypes and create a normal-appearing glans and meatus with few complications like TIP does.

As discussed in Chapter 6, meta-analysis of TIP results shows that complication rates of approximately 5% have been achieved by surgeons worldwide (Pfistermuller et al, 2015). Those with more than 10% complications almost certainly are making technical errors which can be corrected to improve their outcomes.

Similarly, STAC can be used to repair any hypospadias with VC ≥ 30°. This procedure straightens the penis, lengthens the ventral shaft skin, and creates a neourethra with normal caliber ending in a normal-appearing glans and meatus. The earlier push to repair all hypospadias in a single operation has given way to the realization that reliably making a normal penis from severe hypospadias requires 3 procedures.

Therefore, surgeons can correct all hypospadias by tubularizing the incised urethral plate, or a substitute urethral plate made from grafts. The steps in these operations are similar, and so are easier to master.

After more than 100 years experimenting with flaps and grafts, hypospadias surgery has reached the milestone that this birth defect can be repaired using 2 basic and related techniques. Given that the median number of distal repairs done by certified pediatric urologists in the US is approximately 1 a month, and the median number of proximal repairs is only 2 a year (Kogan and Feustel, 2011), using TIP and STAC and performing their steps optimally is the best way to improve results for patients.

Quality Improvement

Even when a surgeon follows this algorithm, how can he or she be certain they are doing the operations in the best way and achieving the best results? What is best, and who decides?

The goal of hypospadias reconstructive surgery is to make the abnormal anatomy of this birth defect into a normal penis. That means the penis is straight, with a vertical meatus at the tip of the glans, no visible scars outside of the median raphe and circumcision line, and no lingering complications. These define success.

How often should surgeons achieve that goal? Based on published data, distal repairs should be successful in over 90% of cases. The TIP meta-analysis by Pfistermuller et al proves that surgeons can repair distal hypospadias with less than 10% complications. Proximal repairs should be successful in at least 75% of cases, with several studies reporting staged grafts can achieve the goal of a normal penis that often (Ferro et al, 2002; Castagnetti et al, 2013; Snodgrass and Bush, 2017). After closing a fistula or repairing a glans dehiscence, surgeons can accomplish repairing both distal and proximal hypospadias into a normal penis nearly 100% of the time.

For a surgeon to know if he or she is meeting these performance standards requires they review their own results. That is most reliably done prospectively, creating a simple spreadsheet recording the patient's name, primary vs redo surgery, degree of VC, TIP or STAC, and follow-up listing any complications. These data can be rapidly entered after surgery and clinic, and then tallied periodically to determine outcomes.

WS started a hypospadias database in 1999 which we still maintain more than 25 years later. Periodically reviewing his own results has proved the need to make technical changes to reduce his own complications. Most of these have been published and are discussed elsewhere in this book. For example, he was taught to tubularize prepucial flaps with a single continuous epithelial suture, which he then used in the first proximal TIP repairs. Despite covering the suture line with dartos, 33% of those initial patients developed fistulas. Simply changing to subepithelial suturing in 2 layers, the first interrupted and the second continuous, resulted in a decrease to 11% fistulas in the next series. Then he changed the coverage layer from dartos to tunica vaginalis and no fistulas occurred in the third group (Snodgrass and Bush, 2011).

Without this personal quality assessment, he might still be suturing proximal neourethras in a single layer covered with dartos, with 1 out of every 3 boys suffering as a result. WS refers to this process as the 3Ps, for ***P***rospective data recording, ***P***eriodic outcomes review, and ***P***ractice changes to improve results.

Institutions should also review results of the surgeons performing and teaching hypospadias repair to be certain that operations are being done, and taught to trainees, in the best known manner. Otherwise, technical errors a mentor teaches a fellow will cause complications in his or her future patients, too. This topic of teaching and learning curves is discussed further in Chapter 25.

It was a big step forward when those 3 proximal repair articles from Texas Children's, Boston Children's and CHOP published results that were not as good as surgeons thought them to be. So was the Dutch Hypospadias Study which reported that only 1 of every 5 surgeons at their major centers had 10% or less complications after distal repairs. In fact, the average was 20% and ranged up to 45% (Van der Toorn et al, 2015).

Finding more complications than they expected nearly always happens when surgeons review their own work, but by using the 3Ps we can improve our surgical technique and then verify those changes yield better results. It will be a future milestone in hypospadias surgery when this personal and institutional quality review is done routinely.

Wound Healing

Although most complications result from surgeon error and can be decreased by improving surgical technique, perfection doing an operation would still not eliminate them. Disturbances in wound healing play at least a supporting role in some postoperative complications. For example, approximately 5% of grafts contract regardless of the donor or recipient sites, for reasons which are unclear. Although we no longer place grafts onto corporotomy incisions, or when skin has to be relocated to fill a ventral deficiency, a few placed in what appear to be optimal conditions will still develop scars making tubularization more difficult. Are there other factors at play which surgeons can influence to improve healing?

The consistent observation that reoperations have more complications than similar primary repairs also points to issues with wound healing, in this case from decreased tissue vascularity. That is not surprising, given that the distal end of the penis, where most hypospadias surgery is focused, is furthest from the blood supply entering at the base. Currently the only known therapy to restore vascularity is hyperbaric oxygen, discussed in Chapter 18, which improves graft take in reoperations (Bush and Snodgrass, 2019).

Nutrition also impacts wound healing, but nutritional assessment for surgery is not well-defined currently. Similarly, a history of excessive scarring in the patient or relatives might predict increased risk for complications, as could eczema. Studies of these factors might someday lead to new milestones for improving results.

References

Asopa HS, Elhence IP, Atri SP and Bansal NK: One stage correction of penile hypospadias using a foreskin tube. *Int Surg* 55: 435, 1971

Backus LH and De Felice CA: Hypospadias – then and now. *Plast Reconstr Surg* 25: 146, 1960

Baskin LS and Duckett JW: Dorsal tunica albuginea plication for hypospadias curvature. *J Urol* 151: 1668, 1994

Baskin LS, Duckett JW and Lue TF: Penile curvature. *Urology* 48: 347, 1996

Baskin LS, Erol A, Li YW, and Cunha GR: Anatomic studies of hypospadias. *J Urol* 160: 1108, 1998

Beck C: Hypospadias and its treatment. *SGO* 24: 511, 1917

Bologna RA, Noah TA, Nasralla PF, McMahon DR: Chordee: varied opinions and treatments as documented in a survey of the American Academy of Pediatrics, Section on Urology. *Urology* 53: 608, 1999

Bracka A: A versatile two-stage hypospadias repair. *Br J Plast Surg* 48: 345, 1995

Bracka A: personal communication, 2010

Browne D: An operation for hypospadias. *Post-Grad M J* 25: 367, 1949

Bush NC and Snodgrass W: Pre-incision urethral plate width does not impact short-term tubularized incised plate urethroplasty outcomes. J Pediatr Urol 13: 625, 2017

Bush NC and Snodgrass W: Hyperbaric oxygen therapy improves oral graft take in hypospadias staged tubularized autograft reoperations. *J Urol* 202: 1, 2019

Byars LT: A technique for consistently satisfactory repair of hypospadias. *Surg Gynecol Obstet* 100: 184, 1955

Caione P, Capozza N, De Gennaro M, Creti G, Zaccara A, Lais A: Distal hypospadias repair by urethral sliding advancement and Y-V glanuloplasty. *J Urol* 146: 644, 1991

Castagnetti M, Zhapa E, Rigamonti W: Primary severe hypospadias: comparison of reoperative rates and parental perception of urinary symptoms and cosmetic outcomes among 4 repairs. *J Urol* 189:1508, 2013

Cloutier AM: A method for hypospadias repair. *Plast Reconstr Surg* 30: 368, 1962

Creevy CD: The correction of hypospadias: a review. *Urol Surg* 8:2, 1958

Devine CJ Jr and Horton CE: A one stage hypospadias repair. *J Urol* 85: 166, 1961

Devine CJ, Jr and Horton CE, Jr: Hypospadias repair. *J Urol* 118: 188, 1977

Duckett JW: Transverse preputial island flap technique for repair of severe hypospadias. *Urol Clin North Am* 7: 423, 1980

Duckett JW: MAGPI (meatal advancement and glanuloplasty). A procedure for subcoronal hypospadias. *Urol Clin North Am* 8: 513, 1981

Edmunds A: An operation for hypospadias. *The Lancet*, February 15: 447, 1913

Elder JS, Duckett JW, and Snyder HM: Onlay island flap in the repair of mid and distally penile hypospadias without chordee. *J Urol* 138: 376, 1987

Ferro F, Zaccara A, Spagnoli A, Lucchetti MC, Capitanucci L, Villa M: Skin graft for 2-stage treatment of severe hypospadias: back to the future? *J Urol* 168: 1730, 2002

Gibbons MD and Gonzales ET, Jr: The subcoronal meatus. *J Urol* 130: 739, 1983

Gittes RF and McLaughlin AP: Injection technique to induce penile erection. *Urology* 4: 473, 1974

Hodgson NB: Hypospadias. In Glenn J and Boyce W (Eds): **Urologic Surgery**. Philadelphia, JP Lippincott, 1975, p 656

Holland AJA, Smith GHH. Effect of the depth and width of the urethral plate on tubularized incised plate urethroplasty. *J Urol* ;164:489, 2000

Hollowell JG, Keating MA, Snyder HM, III, and Duckett JW: Preservation of the urethral plate in hypospadias repair: extended applications and further experience with the onlay island flap urethroplasty. *J Urol* 143: 98, 1990

Humby G: A one-stage operation for hypospadias. *Br J Surg* 29: 84, 1941

Keating MA and Duckett JW: Failed hypospadias repair. In Cohen MS and Resnick M (Eds): **Reoperative Urology.** Boston, Little Brown and Co, 1995, p. 188

King LR: Hypospadias- a one-stage repair without skin graft based on a new principle: chordee is sometimes produced by the skin alone. *J Urol* 103: 660, 1970

Koff SA: Mobilization of the urethra in the surgical treatment of hypospadias. *J Urol* 125: 394, 1981

Kogan BA and Feustel PJ: What can we learn from pediatric urology certification logs? *Urology* 78: 147, 2011

Koyangi T, Matsuno T, Nonomura K and Sakibara N: Complete repair of severe penoscrotal hypospadias in 1 stage: experience with urethral mobilization, wing flap-flipping urethroplasty and "glanulomeatoplasty". *J Urol* 130: 1150, 1983

Long CJ, Chu DI, Tenny RW, Morris Ar, Weiss DA,Shukla AR, Srinivasan AK, Zderic SA, Kolon TF, Canning DA: Intermediate-term followup of proximal hypospadias repair reveals high complication rate. *J Urol* 197: 852, 2017

Mathieu P: Traitment en un temps de L'hypospadias balanique ou juxtabalanique. *Journal de Chirurgie* 39: 31, 1932

McNamara ER, Schaeffer AJ, Logvinenko T, Seager C, Rosokliga I, Nelson CP, Retik AB, Diamond DA, and Cendron M: Management of proximal hypospadias with 2-stage repair: 20-year experience. *J Urol* 194: 1080, 2015

Nesbit RM: Congenital curvature of the phallus: report of three cases with description of corrective operation. J Urol 93: 230, 1965

Nesbit RM: Operation for the correction of distal penile ventral curvature with or without hypospadias. *J Urol* 97: 729, 1967

Nicolle F: Improved repairs in 100 cases of penile hypospadias. *Br J Plast Surg* 29: 150, 1976

Nove-Josserand G: Resultats eloignes de l'urethroplastie par la tunnelisation et la greffe dermo-epidermique de l'hypospadias et la l'episadias. *J Urol Med Chir* 5: 393, 1914

Ombredanne L: Precis cliniqueet operatoire de chirurgicale infantile. *Libraires de L'Academie de Medecine* 654, 1923

Orkiszewski M: Urethral reconstruction in skin deficit. *Urologia Polska* 40: 12, 1987

Perlmutter AD and Vatz AD: Meatal advancement for distal hypospadias without chordee. *J Urol* 113: 850, 1975

Pfistermuller KL, McArdle J and Cuckow PM: Meta-analysis of complication rates of the tubularized incised plate (TIP) repair. *J Pediatr Urol* 11: 54, 2015

Pippi Salle JL, Sayed S, Salle A, Bagli D, Farhat W, Koyle M, Lorenzo AJ: Proximal hypospadias: a persistent challenge. Single institution outcome analysis of three surgical techniques over a 10-year period. *J Pediatr Urol* 12: 28e, 2016

Poulsen J and Kirkeby HJ: Treatment of penile curvature – a retrospective study of 175 patients operated with plication of the tunica albuginea or with the Nesbit procedure. *Br J Urol* 73: 370, 1995

Retik AB, Bauer SB, Mandell J, Peters CA, Colodny A and Atala A: Management of severe hypospadias with a 2-stage repair. *J Urol* 152: 749, 1994

Sarhan O, Saad M, Helmy T, and Hafez A: Effect of suturing technique and urethral plate characteristics on complication rate following hypospadias repair: a prospective randomized study. *J Urol* 182: 682, 2009

Smith CK: Correction of hypospadias. *J Urol* 40: 239, 1938

Snodgrass W: Tubularized incised plate urethroplasty for distal hypospadias. *J Urol* 151: 464, 1994

Snodgrass W and Bush NC: Staged tubularized autograft for primary proximal hypospadias repair with 30-degree or more curvature. *J Urol* 198: 680, 2017

Snodgrass W and Bush NC: Persistent or recurrent ventral curvature after failed proximal hypospadias repair. *J Pediatr Urol* 15: 344, 2019

Snodgrass W and Bush NC: Graft and skin complications in 342 primary proximal hypospadias repairs: STAG vs. STAC. Abstract presented to the ESPU, Naples, 2024

Stanasel I, Le HK, Bilgutay A, Roth DA, Gonzales ET, JR, Janzen N, Koh CJ, Gargollo P and Seth A: Complications following staged hypospadias repair using transposed prepucial skin flaps. *J Urol* 194: 512, 2015

Thompson A: Hypospadias: its effect and treatment. *Lancet* 2: 429, 1937

Van der Toorn F, De Mooij K, Nijman R, Van der Horst E, Callewaert P, Steffens M, Hoebeke P, Van der Heijkant M, Froeling F, Wildhagen M, Willemsem S, Bryan S, and de Gier R: The Dutch hypospadias study: complications and prognostic factors after distal- and mid- type hypospadias repair. Abstract presented to the ESPU, Prague, 2015

Van Hook W: A new operation for hypospadias. *Annals of Surgery* 23: 378, 1896

Van Horn AC and Kass EJ: Glanulosplasty and in situ tubularization of the urethral plate: a simple reliable technique for the majority of boys with hypospadias. *J Urol* 154: 1505, 1995

Zaontz MR: The GAP (glans approximation procedure) for glanular/coronal hypospadias. *J Urol* 141: 359, 1989

Ventral Curvature

Chapter 2

Straightening Ventral Curvature

Completely and durably straightening ventral curvature is the single most important step in hypospadias repair.

The foundation for a successful urethroplasty and future sexual function is a straight penis. Since it is often bent in patients with hypospadias, understanding what causes ventral penile curvature and knowing how it is most reliably straightened are essential for the surgeon who undertakes these repairs.

Many urethroplasty complications after distal repairs, and most that occur after proximal repairs, are due to persistent or recurrent ventral curvature exerting tension on the surgical field during natural erections postoperatively. These fistulas, glans and wound dehiscences, strictures and meatal stenoses often cannot be successfully corrected until the underlying curvature is straightened – a process that requires taking down the prior hypospadias repair for a staged reoperation beginning with ventral corporotomies.

Even if the urethroplasty heals without complications, residual curvature of only 20° increases the likelihood that the man will have difficulties during sexual intercourse, leading to anxiety and dissatisfaction with his penis (Menon et al, 2016).

Despite the critical importance of making the curved penis straight, much less attention has been paid to this aspect of hypospadias surgery compared to ways to make a neourethra. We will not make progress towards improving outcomes in hypospadias surgery without a better understanding of what makes the penis bent and how we should straighten it.

But we will never determine the best methods to straighten curvature until surgeons measure it objectively. Eyeballing the degree of curvature is accurate only at the extremes – we can see when the penis is straight or is bent 90°. But our estimates are not reliable for curvature between these, especially around 30° which appears to be the point at which dorsal plications become less reliably durable. We cannot determine with certainty if the change from dorsal plication to ventral corporotomies is best made at 25° or 30° or 35° or 40° if surgeons do not objectively measure it.

These issues are the subjects of this chapter.

Why the Penis is Bent

We explain to parents and older patients that the penis consists of 2 erection cylinders and the urethra enclosed by skin. When the penis is bent, the ventral skin, urethral tissues, and sheath enclosing the erection cylinders can all be short.

Physical examination of the hypospadias penis most often shows relative deficiency of the ventral prepuce and shaft skin, which often tilts the glans and bends the penis. These effects of short skin resolve spontaneously during degloving, and every hypospadias surgeon has observed how the ventral skin commonly retracts proximally when it is released.

This is not "hypospadias with chordee". It is more accurate for the surgeon, and clearer for the family, to simply refer to the "short ventral skin" that is usually part of hypospadias. In fact, the parents have already seen that there is less skin underneath than there is on the topside, and easily understand that the shorter skin can tether the penis.

Persistent bending after the skin is released potentially is due to a short urethral plate and/or short ventral corpora. The common observation that curvature is little changed by transecting the urethral plate and dissecting it free from the corpora proves that bending after degloving is most often due to short ventral corpora – what Duckett termed "corporal disproportion".

However, the term "corporal disproportion" could imply that erectile tissues are deficient. The cause of corporal bending is relative shortness of the ventral side of the tunica albuginea sheath which encloses the erectile tissues. Again, it is more accurate for the surgeon and clearer for the family to explain that curvature that persists after degloving is due to the ventral sheath enclosing the erectile tissues forming too short, similar to how the ventral skin formed too short.

Then it is easier to explain how straightening is accomplished either by making the longer side shorter by plication, or the shorter side longer by ventral lengthening.

It has been a surprise for us to read contemporary operative notes describing chordee excision for straightening. As discussed in Chapter 1, from the late 1800s until the early 1970s the near universal understanding of penile curvature was that "fibrous bands", later called "chordee", on the surface of the tunica albuginea restricted full expansion of the corpora. Meticulous removal of this tissue was supposed to correct the bending. But the advent of artificial erection proved that the penis usually remains bent despite complete excision of tissues off the surface of the corpora from the corona to the meatus. Continuing belief in chordee and chordee excision therefore leads to persisting ventral curvature, such as we found in nearly 85% of boys whose surgeons performed that to straighten the penis (Snodgrass & Bush, 2019).

In summary, most curvature associated with hypospadias is due to the shorter ventral skin. The curvature that persists after the skin is released is most often due to a short ventral corporal sheath.

Prevalence of Ventral Curvature with Hypospadias

In the first edition of this textbook, we wrote that VC less than 30° is found in 10% of hypospadias with a distal meatus and 33% with a proximal meatus. However, these observations were made in a time before we began objectively measuring curvature. Therefore, we underestimated the degree of bending. Furthermore, those boys with a distal meatus found to have VC estimated at more than 30° were considered proximal variants and were not tallied among others with distal hypospadias.

The prevalence of VC associated with a meatus on the distal shaft, corona, or glans has not been widely reported. Stojanovic et al (2011) said it occurred in 30% of these patients. We evaluated consecutive men with uncorrected distal hypospadias and found that 36% had penile curvature that averaged 30° (10° to 65°), of which three-fourths was ventral and the remainder lateral bending (Bush and Snodgrass, 2023).

We reported that VC occurs in 80% of patients with a proximal meatus (Snodgrass and Prieto, 2007), averaging 70° (30° to 120°) (Snodgrass & Bush, 2017).

However, the exact prevalence of VC in populations of boys is not the important issue. Rather, it is important for surgeons to know that *any* patient with hypospadias can have ventral curvature, regardless of the location of the meatus, and so artificial erection should be done in *every* patient.

This statement also applies to MIP hypospadias, which Duckett wrote was unique in having no VC. He based that statement on a series of only 14 boys (Duckett and Keating, 1989). However, the penis in patients with MIP hypospadias definitely can be bent (Figure 1), and so they, too, should all have artificial erection during repair.

Furthermore, a boy with a distal meatus can have curvature greater than 30°, while another with a proximal meatus can have a straight penis after degloving (Figure 2). For this reason, our algorithm for urethroplasty is based on the degree of curvature after releasing the shaft skin, and *not* the meatal location.

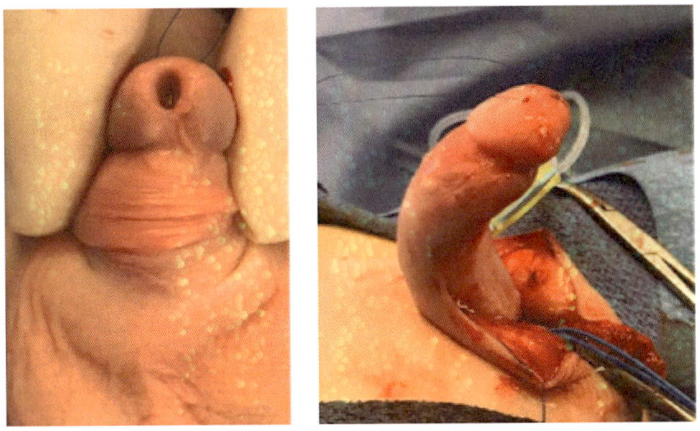

Figure 1. MIP hypospadias with ventral curvature. Boys with MIP hypospadias can have ventral curvature, as shown here which measured 60°. *All* patients with hypospadias should have artificial erection after degloving and before urethroplasty.

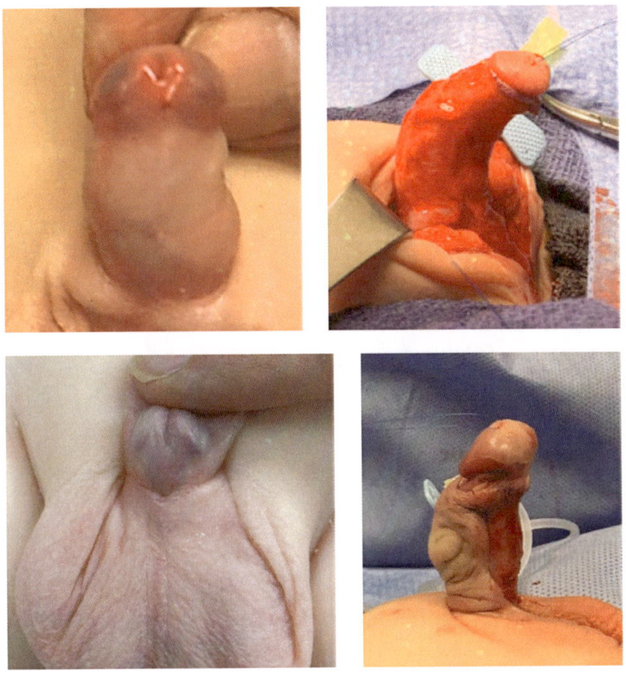

Figure 2. Meatal location does *not* predict the degree of ventral curvature.
A, coronal meatus in a penis found in B to have 45°ventral curvature. C, proximal-appearing meatus in a penis shown in D to be straight after degloving.

Artificial Erection

There are several options in performing artificial erection. A 25-, 23-, or 21-gauge butterfly needle can be used for injection. In teens and adults, an 18-gauge needle is used. The needle can be inserted into the corpora on one side, or through the glans. Injection can

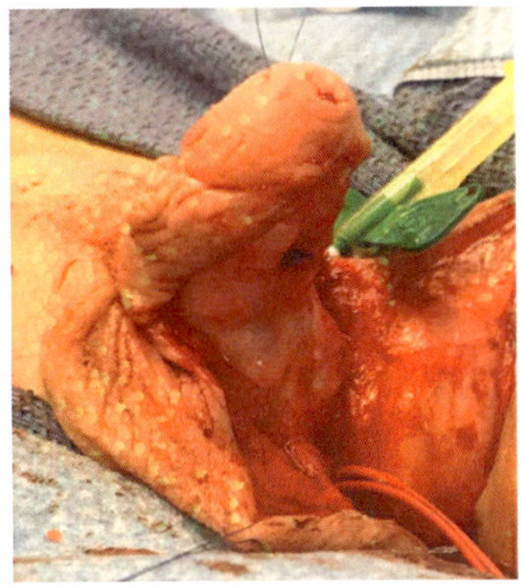

Figure 3. Ventral curvature at the penoscrotal junction. Most curvature occurs in the mid to distal shaft (at the purple mark), but it can be more proximal as in this example with bending at the penoscrotal junction indicated by the arrow. The original surgeon placed a tourniquet at the base before performing the artificial erection, which obscured the curvature. The patient subsequently had recurrent fistulas until the underlying cause was found and corrected. For this reason, we do the first artificial erection without a tourniquet to be certain any bending is located distal to where it will be placed.

be done without any compression on the penis base, while holding finger compression, or after applying a tourniquet. None of these details really matter, as long as the penis becomes completely firm and a low bend is not obscured by finger compression or a tourniquet.

For that reason, the first injection should be done without a tourniquet because curvature is sometimes found at, or just below, the penoscrotal junction. We have seen patients in whom VC was not diagnosed because of the tourniquet, who then developed recurrent urethroplasty complications (Figure 3).

Sometimes VC is not seen until near the end of the injection. Some people question if such curvature would occur naturally, believing artificial erection can "overfill" the corpora and induce a false curvature. However, natural erections fill the corpora completely and render them quite firm, and so curvature observed during saline injection is real and representative of what occurs during a spontaneous erection.

Artificial erection can also be induced by injecting vasoactive drugs intravenously, or directly into the corpora, although we have not routinely used either method.

Objectively Measuring Ventral Curvature

Optimal management of ventral curvature depends on its degree. In a 1999 survey of US pediatric urologists' preferences for straightening curvature, Bologna et al commented that such descriptions as "significant chordee" should be replaced by objective measurements obtained using a protractor as shown in Figure 4.

Nearly 20 years later we reviewed records from pediatric urologists across the US that proved little has changed. In a consecutive series of 73 patients originally operated elsewhere for proximal hypospadias, no operative records described measuring VC objectively. Only a third mentioned a numeric estimate of the degree, while the remainder categorized bending using such terms as "2+", "significant", "severe" or "extraordinary" (Snodgrass and Bush, 2019).

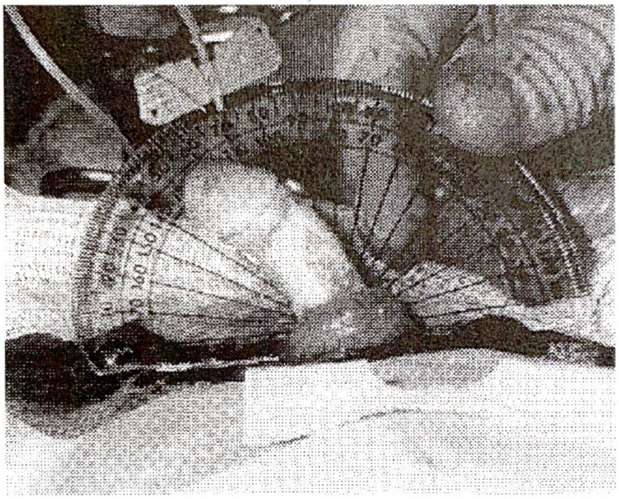

Figure 4. Measuring ventral curvature using a protractor.

We first used the goniometer to measure ventral curvature in late 2014 and soon realized that our visual estimates were not accurate, especially between 25° and 45°. The goniometer is an orthopedic instrument used to measure angles in fingers, and it needs a slight modification explained in Chapter 3 to adapt it to penis measurements in boys.

The goniometer should rest against the pubis and be aligned along the penile shaft, positioning the fulcrum at the point of maximum curvature (Figure 5). The mobile arm is then adjusted to the location on the glans where the neomeatus should be. We find this easiest to do with one surgeon taking the measurement while the other, or an assistant, keeps the artificial erection firm.

The accuracy of any measuring instrument depends upon using it correctly. The goniometer is a type of protractor which has been shown to accurately and reproducibly determine angles (Carter et al, 2009; Nussbaumer et al, 2010; Akizuki et al, 2016).

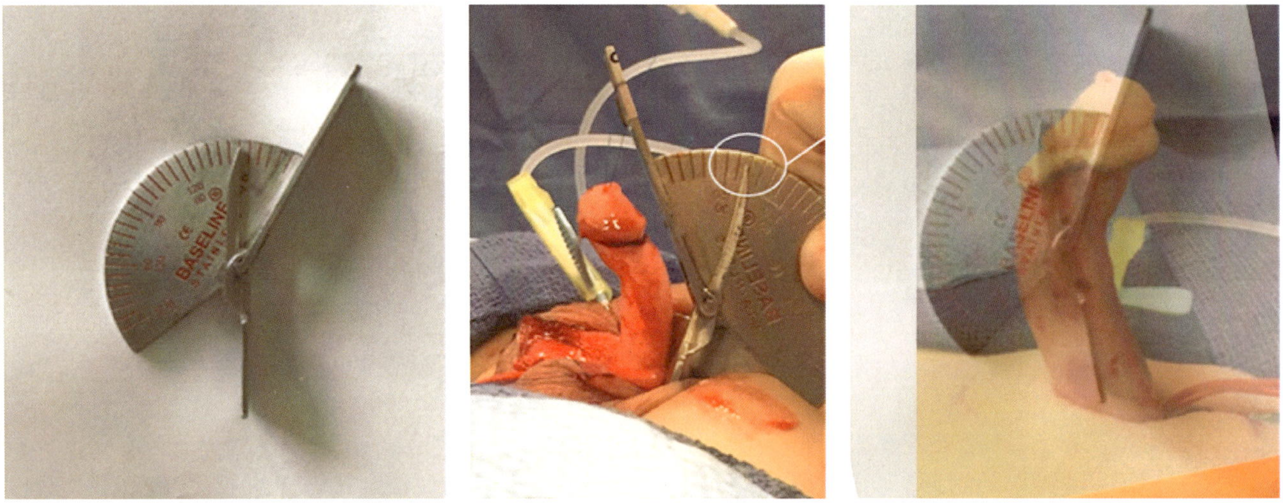

Figure 5. Measuring ventral curvature with a goniometer.
A, arrow indicates the arm which rests on the pubis for measurements, which has been shortened by 1cm. B, correct use of the goniometer, with one arm resting on the pubis and held parallel to the axis of the penile shaft. The other arm is adjusted to point towards where the meatus should be, as shown in C.

Some have suggested photo apps could measure curvature. We have not used those and suspect it might be difficult to take a representative lateral photograph in patients with severe hypospadias because the patient's thigh can obscure the penis. Furthermore, the direction the photograph is taken influences the appearance of the curvature, seeming to increase or decrease it. Regardless, surgeons should objectively measure VC, whether by using a goniometer, protractor, or, possibly, a photo app.

What Degree of Ventral Curvature Matters?

Persistent or recurrent VC potentially creates urethroplasty complications in the short-term, and sexual dysfunction in the long-term. The minimum curvature needed to pull open a fistula or cause a wound to dehisce is not definitely known, although the likelihood increases when it is 30° or more. A correlation between the degree of VC and various urethroplasty complications would require accurate measurement of the initial curvature, which is another reason surgeons should use an instrument to measure it.

In patients we evaluated after unsuccessful proximal repairs, 83% had persistent or recurrent VC. Of those, 100% had a urethroplasty complication in addition to the bending. Their recurrent VC was measured by goniometry during reoperations and averaged 50° (30°-90°) (Snodgrass and Bush, 2019). None had recurrent VC less than 30° which was, therefore, the threshold extent associated with urethroplasty complications in this series.

However, adults with even less VC may experience difficulties from it. One study specifically evaluated men reporting chordee without hypospadias, using drawings to represent varying degrees of bending (Figure 6). Men who indicated they had only 20° VC (Figure 6, no.3) described significantly more difficulties with sexual intercourse, greater dissatisfaction with their penis, and more unhealthy mental days than men who reported having a straight penis. When curvature reached 45° and 90° men were less likely to have had intercourse, or even to have kissed someone (Menon et al, 2016).

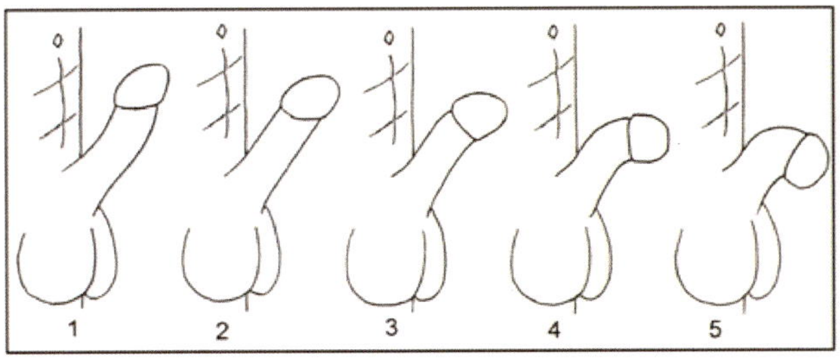

Figure 6. Drawings of penile curvature.
Drawings 3-5 represent 20°, 45° and 90°, respectively. Men with *any* degree of VC reported more difficulty with sexual intercourse, greater penile dissatisfaction, and more unhealthy mental days than men with a straight penis.

Our experience corroborates this report, as men with VC typically say the bending inhibited them from developing relationships which might lead to intimacy. Furthermore, a study of adults with congenital curvature which used a protractor to measure bending reported that 25° prompted men to request surgical straightening (Greenfield et al, 2006).

We suspect that many surgeons shown the sketches in Figure 6 might dismiss number 3 as not clinically significant, yet these reports show otherwise. The risk for urethroplasty complications, and future sexual dysfunction and the emotional issues related to that, together emphasize that the bent penis with hypospadias needs to be made straight.

Dorsal Plication VS Ventral Lengthening

VC due to a short ventral corporal sheath can be straightened by shortening the longer side with plication or lengthening the shorter side with corporotomies. It is far easier to do a plication, and repeat artificial erection intraoperatively usually shows the penis to be straight. However, plication does not correct the short ventral tunica albuginea sheath causing the curvature, but rather seeks to counteract the disproportionate forces that develop ventrally during erection in a bent penis to hold it straight. Viewed from this perspective, and knowing that it is not possible to bend an erect penis in any direction, it becomes obvious that there is a limit to the extent of curvature that plication can keep straight.

Intraoperative artificial erection described in 1974 made it possible for surgeons to better assess both the curvature and the immediate success of their methods to straighten it. Duckett was one of the first to realize from artificial erection that the most meticulous chordee excision that stripped away all the tissues down to and off the surface of the tunica albuginea did not make the penis straight. Like Nesbit before him, he faced the choice of shortening the longer side with plications or lengthening the shorter side. Plications were easier, and since removing the urethral plate did not straighten the penis, he saw additional benefit to plicating since it left the plate intact for urethroplasty.

Duckett described his evolving algorithm for straightening in 1990 (Hollowell et al). "Mild to moderate" curvature that persisted after degloving was corrected by dorsal TAP plication, leaving the urethral plate intact. When curvature was "more severe" he divided the urethral plate in addition to dorsal TAP. However, these descriptions were not precise, and eyeballing the bend often underestimates it. This was proven in Figure 1 of that article which showed VC that was nearly 90°, certainly more than "mild to moderate", yet Duckett straightened it using plications with the urethral plate intact. Then 4 years later, he further revised this algorithm to state that the urethral plate could be maintained and the penis straightened by plications in even the most severe hypospadias (Baskin et al, 1994). Duckett acknowledged ventral corporotomy with dermal grafting described by Devine and Horton, but said that he rarely found that necessary.

Duckett's influence was apparent in the 1999 survey of pediatric urologists mentioned above that found most used dorsal plication for VC of 30 - 40°, and half even for VC to 50°, the highest degree queried (Bologna et al, 1999). His influence continued after he died and a 2017 report on proximal hypospadias repair by his successors at CHOP stated nearly half the proximal hypospadias patients had plications with or without urethral plate division (Long et al). In a significant departure from Duckett, however, those authors said they no longer use plications for anything more than 15° of VC.

Others have also found ventral lengthening superior to plications. Braga et al (2008) reviewed 100 consecutive patients with proximal hypospadias repaired between 1996 and 2004 at Sick Kids in Toronto, reporting that 68% had dorsal plications. The others had single corporotomy with grafting, and those had significantly less recurrent curvature at a mean of 2 years later than did the patients who were plicated (9% vs 28%). We similarly published finding significantly less recurrent VC after ventral lengthening versus dorsal plication in proximal repairs (30% vs 70%) (Snodgrass & Bush, 2019). Finally, a recent meta-analysis of 17 articles with 582 patients confirmed the superiority of ventral lengthening over dorsal plications, which had *5 times* more recurrent curvature (Babu and Chandrasekharam, 2022).

All of these studies are limited by the fact that VC was not objectively measured, and so the question of when plications are effective and when ventral lengthening should be done could not be answered.

Why Should Vc < 30° be the Limit For Dorsal Plication?

The maximum extent of VC that can be reliably and durably corrected by dorsal plication is not known for 2 reasons. First, surgeons have not objectively measured curvature to accurately determine what they are straightening. Second, recurrent VC is often not recognized in prepubertal boys during postoperative examinations.

We base the decision to limit dorsal plications to VC less than 30° on several observations. Most patients with 30° or more curvature have proximal hypospadias, with penis length below average. Dorsal plication shortens the longer side of an already shorter penis, whereas ventral lengthening with 3 corporotomies increases penis length by an average of 30% (unpublished data). In addition, 50% of boys we evaluated whose original surgeons used dorsal plication for VC estimated between 30°- 45° developed recurrent VC (Snodgrass and Bush, 2019). Furthermore, we previously used dorsal plication in our own patients with objectively measured VC of 30°- 35° and encountered recurrent curvature postoperatively rarely seen after plications for less than 30°. Finally, we mimic plication using Adson forceps during artificial erection and observe that we can easily pull the penis straight

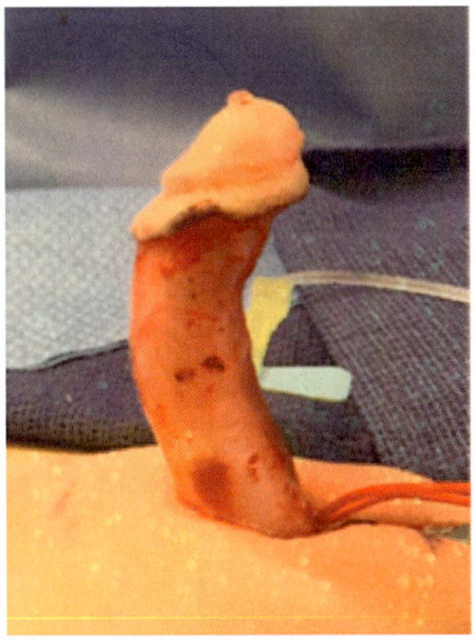

Figure 7. 30° ventral curvature.
Some surgeons might consider curvature with this appearance to be easily corrected with a dorsal plication. Certainly, that seems effective in the operating room, but plication for this degree of curvature does not reliably last. Using forceps to mimic a plication and pull a penis with 30° VC straight is difficult, and proves the tension which that degree of bending exerts during natural erections. This photograph also emphasizes again the need to objectively measure VC, rather than rely on eyeballing it.

when curvature is 25° or less, but it is nearly impossible to straighten when it is 30° or more.

Readers should also note the comment above that Duckett's successors no longer use plications when there is *15° or more curvature* (Long et al, 2017). They undoubtedly inherited patients from Duckett who grew into adulthood with bent penises from recurrent VC.

Nevertheless, some surgeons still wonder if 30° or 35° VC "needs" ventral lengthening and a staged urethroplasty, especially when the meatus is distal. In part, that is because 30° is not visually concerning (Figure 7). Perhaps feeling the force necessary to pull the erect penis straight with Adson forceps will be convincing.

The need to limit plications to lesser degrees of curvature is easily understood conceptually. Normally the penis is straight, and the internal forces generated during an erection are evenly distributed around the shaft. We ask parents to imagine bending an erect penis, and then to imagine pulling a bent erect penis straight. They immediately realize these are impossible, yet this is what surgeons are asking a plication stitch to reliably and durably accomplish.

A theme repeated throughout this book is getting it right the first time. When VC recurs, everything previously done usually has to be taken down and done over. The neourethra has to be transected and peeled off the corpora to expose the region that is bent. Corporotomies have to be made through the curvature to straighten the penis. Then the neourethra must be remade, which itself requires 2 stages. Therefore, reoperation for persistent or recurrent VC is often a 3-step process, as described in Chapter 17.

The penalty for a mistaken decision by the surgeon to straighten the penis by plication is high for the patient, which is another reason that plication should be limited to curvature < 30°, when it is most likely to work.

Straightening Ventral Curvature < 30°

We have heard surgeons dismiss curvature < 30° as clinically insignificant and not likely to bother the patient. However, reports mentioned above that men with only 20° of VC experience difficulties with sexual intercourse and the worries that come with that dysfunction, emphasize the need to straighten curvature that may appear "mild" to the surgeon.

As recounted in Chapter 1, dorsal plications began with Nesbit. In the first case, he simply plicated the tunica albuginea for a college student with lateral curvature. When the curvature recurred within a few months, Nesbit reoperated and excised horizontal ellipses of tunica albuginea which he closed with silk to shorten the longer side of the corpora. He subsequently corrected VC similarly, excising and then suturing closed horizontal ellipses in parallel rows on either side of the midline near the neurovascular bundles.

Rather than excise wedges of the tunic, Duckett made parallel horizontal incisions under the neurovascular bundles 4mm apart, and then sutured the incisions together while folding down the strip of tunic between them. Baskin worried that these transverse incisions made bilaterally near the neurovascular bundles might damage sensory nerves, and instead recommended plication be done in the midline without either excision or incision of the tunica albuginea.

Yachia also did midline plication but made an incision into the tunica albuginea that he closed in a Heineke-Mikulicz fashion. He explained that a healed incision would more likely maintain straightening than could a stitch alone (Yachia, 1990). This was later verified by a study that compared outcomes in adults with congenital curvature managed by either Nesbit (excisional) plication using 3-0 Vicryl to close the defect, or plication using 2-0 nylon without tunica incision or excision. Straightening was achieved in significantly more patients undergoing repair that involved tunica excision even though a smaller suture was used to close the defect (Poulsen and Kirkeby, 1995).

We similarly encountered recurrent VC in some patients with less than 30° bending that we initially corrected using Baskin plication. Consequently, we now do midline plications with tunica incision and Heineke-Mikulicz closure as described by Yachia.

Over the years we have gradually increased the size of the suture we use for plications, too. Before he started measuring VC, WS performed Baskin plications using a single 6-0 Prolene, thinking that if this did not straighten the penis, then ventral lengthening would be better. Now we measure curvature with the goniometer and also estimate the force needed for straightening using 2 forceps to mimic the plication. When VC measures < 30° and the forceps easily pull the fully erect penis straight, we use a 4-0 Prolene suture to better ensure the strength of the plication. Would larger sutures make plications durable for greater degrees of VC? The largest we have seen used is 2-0 nonabsorbable sutures in boys who nevertheless had recurrent curvature.

Regardless of the technique used we have observed recurrent VC after dorsal plications, meaning that even the most "aggressive" plication with incision or excision of the tunica albuginea for curvature ≥ 30° does not reliably withstand the tension exerted against it by spontaneous erections postoperatively. Rather, in some cases, plication moved the fulcrum of bending, resulting in an S-shaped penile deformity described below.

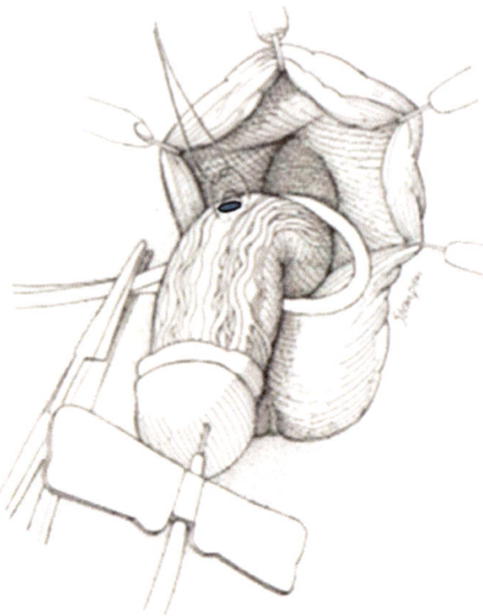

Figure 8. Heineke-Mikulicz (Yachia) midline plication. An 11-blade scalpel makes a 2mm long puncture through the tunica albuginea of the corpora in the midline opposite the point of maximum curvature. This incision is then closed using 4-0 Prolene, including 2mm of the tunic above and below it. The knot is buried into the incision, which is then covered by a small dartos flap to prevent penile skin from scarring to it.

Heineke-Mikulicz Plication (Yachia)

This method for dorsal plication is shown in Figure 8. A 2mm stab incision is made through the tunica albuginea in the midline opposite the point of bending. A 4-0 Prolene suture closes the puncture along with 2mm of tunic just above and just below it, burying the knot. To prevent overlying shaft skin from adhering to the suture, a small dartos flap then covers the Prolene. Repeat artificial erection is always done to confirm straightening.

Straightening Ventral Curvature ≥ 30°

We do not use any type of plication to straighten VC ≥ 30° confirmed by goniometry. Instead, corporotomies are done to lengthen the ventral side and relieve tension that develops there during erections.

Initially, WS made a single corporal incision through the bend from 3 to 9 o'clock and closed the defect with a dermal graft. However, when he transitioned from flap to graft urethroplasties he also had to change this method for straightening, since a urethroplasty graft cannot be placed at the same time onto a corporal graft. Rather than make a single corporotomy, he instead made 3 incisions across the arc of bending and allowed them to heal without grafting them. Straightening was achieved in all the boys in his first series (Snodgrass and Prieto, 2009).

Our recent experience with a large number of patients who had unsuccessful proximal hypospadias repairs makes clear that single corporotomy with corporal grafting does not give the same results as 3 corporotomies. We found that 33% of patients who had a single corporotomy with corporal grafting by other surgeons presented with recurrent VC measuring an average of 54° (30°-90°) (Snodgrass and Bush, 2019).

Boys with proximal shaft to perineal hypospadias have a mean of 70° VC (Snodgrass and Bush, 2017). Surgeons using a single incision corporotomy admit that one incision from 3 to 9 o'clock may not suffice for that extent of curvature. Instead, their incision is made from one dorsal neurovascular bundle across the ventral surface to the opposite neurovascular bundle when curvature exceeds 60° (Gong and Cheng, 2017). Typically, the edges of this incision are further undermined off the erectile tissues so that it will open more widely (Figure 9). Results were not reported, and so it is not known if this longer incision reliably straightens higher grades of bending, or if the integrity of the corpora is left intact.

Furthermore, all grafts have a potential to contract, which would cause recurrent VC in this situation. Similarly, biodegradable substances such as SIS that some use instead of dermis can also shrink the corporotomy incision.

In contrast, we reported that 3 corporotomies are successful in over 98% of cases having a mean of 70° VC and ranging to 120° (Snodgrass and Bush, 2017). Furthermore, we verify the penis is straight by artificial erection at each subsequent stage, and during all reoperations. We have not encountered difficult intra- or postoperative bleeding from not grafting the incisions, and the men we have straightened have not reported subsequent erectile dysfunction.

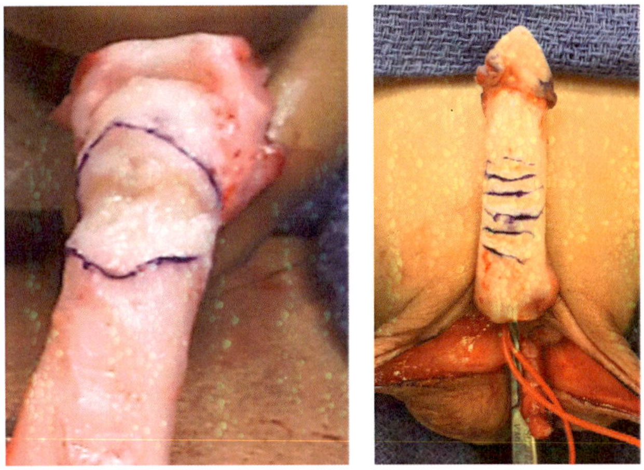

Figure 9. Corporal defects made by 1 versus 3 corporotomy incisions.
A, the large ventral defect created by a single incision extending from neurovascular to neurovascular bundle, vs B, lesser, yet more effective, defects after 3 incisions made from 3 to 9 o'clock.

3 Ventral Corporotomies

When artificial erection demonstrates 30° or more VC after degloving, the urethral plate is transected at the corona and dissected in continuity with the native urethra off the corpora proximally into the scrotum. Dartos and spongiosum attached to the urethral plate and urethra are preserved with them during this dissection. Then artificial erection is repeated, identifying and marking the point of maximum bending. Next, 3 lines are drawn horizontally from approximately 3 to 9 o'clock, the first across the point of maximum curvature and the other 2 approximately 4mm distal and proximal to it. With a tourniquet applied proximally, these 3 lines are incised through the tunica albuginea, exposing the erectile tissues (Figure 10).

It is important that these incisions be made *through* the tunica albuginea, as more shallow incisions done to facilitate a subsequent artificial erection risk making inadequate corporotomies to straighten the penis.

Buck's fascia enclosing the tunica albuginea is also shorter ventrally, and it too is incised transversely just lateral to the corporotomy incisions so that it lengthens and does not limit the widening of the corporotomies.

Next, the corporotomies are covered by a dartos flap raised from the adjacent shaft skin, which is sewn

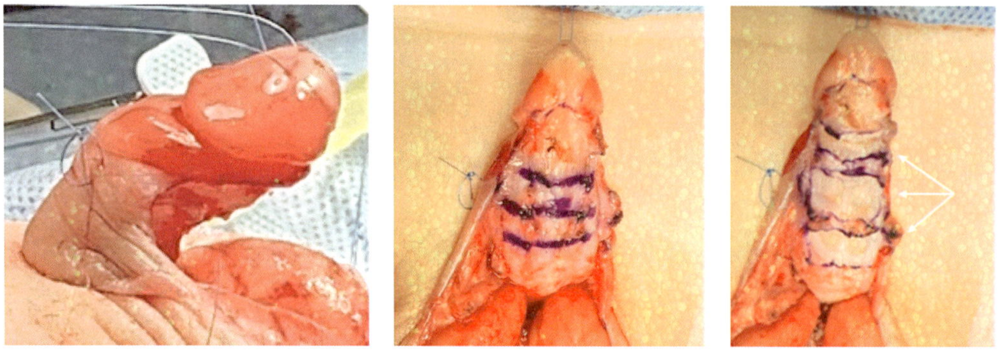

Figure 10. 3 corporotomies without corporal grafting.
A, 70° VC. B, lines drawn in the arc of curvature where the corporotomy incisions will be made. C, appearance after 3 corporotomy incisions (arrows).

around the perimeter of the incisions and to the isthmuses between them to contain any bleeding (Figure 11). Transverse 6-0 PDS mattress stitches are used to secure the dartos to the intact corpora to reduce gaps where blood could escape, circumferentially and at each isthmus. Then 1:1000 epinephrine is irrigated over the covered incisions, and the assistant holds pressure on them with a gauze as the tourniquet is removed.

We make 3 corporotomies in nearly every case with 30° or more curvature. The extent to which the incisions open varies according to the acuteness of the angle and degree of bending. The greatest increase in length is gained by the middle incision, while the distal incision usually achieves the least.

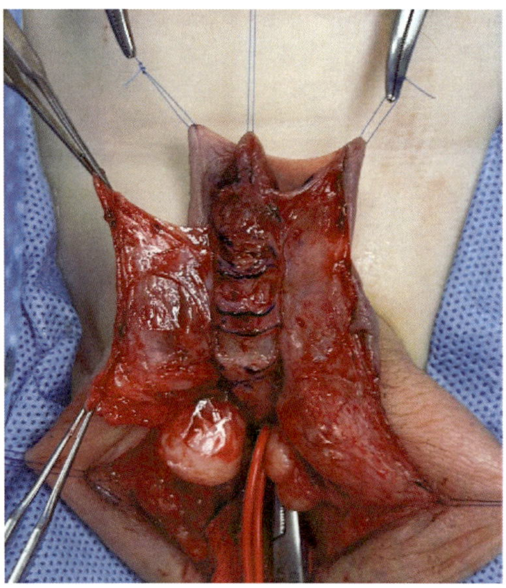

Figure 11. Dartos flap harvested in order to cover the 3 corporotomies.

Most often, the penis is curved in the midshaft, but sometimes the bending is more distal and a 3rd incision would be made at or even above the corona of the glans. In those situations, we rely on 2 incisions and never incise the corpora within the glans.

How to Determine the Penis is Straight

The penis will be straight if the surgeon makes the 3 corporotomies as we describe them. As mentioned, we confirm straightening at each subsequent stage of the repair.

But, since artificial erection is not reliable after making corporotomies, how does the surgeon learning this maneuver know that straightening has been accomplished? WS tried injecting saline through a 21-gauge butterfly to achieve a faster infusion of a larger volume, but that did not make the penis firm. Being unsure, he initially placed a single Baskin plication dorsally for insurance against a small degree of residual bending. However, shaft skin can fix to that suture, even when it is covered with dartos, so that it does not glide normally. Furthermore, plication likely will not prevent persistent curvature from inadequate corporotomies.

Wanting to avoid this dorsal "insurance" plication, NB had the insight to visualize the bent penis as a triangle. When the penis is straight, A+B should equal C. If it does not, then the incisions, especially the middle and most proximal, are extended ≤1mm further

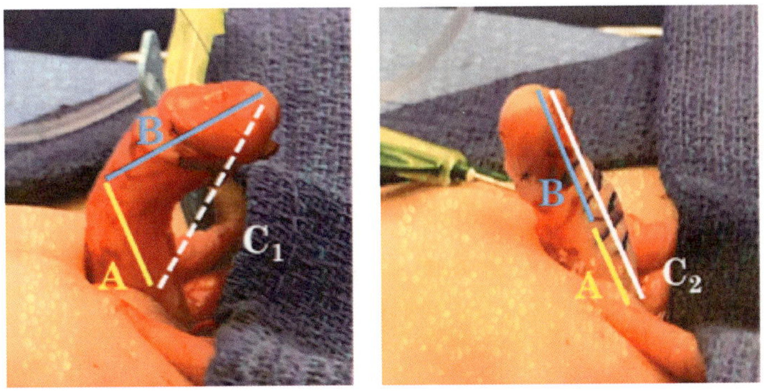

Figure 12. Bush's triangle to measure the penis is straight.
A, a suture is placed in the tunica albuginea where A and C_1 meet, while marks are made with a surgical pen on the dorsal midshaft where A and B meet opposite the bend, and at the meatus where B and C meet in this picture. Then lengths A and B are measured. B, after adequate incisions, A+B should equal, or slightly exceed, C_2, indicating the penis is now straight. This method works best when the penis is completely degloved.

---

laterally and the measurements repeated until A+B = C (Figure 12).

Triangular measurements are most easily made when the penis is completely degloved. After transitioning from STAG to STAC we no longer deglove dorsally in the first operation when bending is corrected, and so we no longer rely on these measurements to confirm the penis is straight. Again, our experience performing hundreds of 3 corporotomies and then confirming results with artificial erection at subsequent stages, proves this method nearly always straightens any extent of VC. However, surgeons first using 3 corporotomies should do the triangular measurements until they are certain they are making the penis straight.

Do The Corporotomies Bleed?

The 3 corporotomy incisions are made with a tourniquet in place. The dartos flap is then secured circumferentially. Then 1:1000 epinephrine is irrigated onto the incisions, the tourniquet is released, and the assistant holds pressure on a gauze over the corporotomies while the surgeon advances the urethra back distally to end in a urethrostomy.

Typically, there is minimal bleeding from under the dartos flap in boys, which can be controlled with additional stitches to better tack the flap to the corpora. If it remains bothersome, additional topical epinephrine and compression usually suffices to stop the bleeding. In rare instances the tourniquet is re-applied briefly. Regardless, at the conclusion of the operation a gentle compression bandage is applied which helps maintain hemostasis. Problematic postoperative bleeding should not occur.

Do Corporotomies Cause Erectile Dysfunction?

Surgeons who prefer plication worry that a single corporotomy with a corpora graft disturbs the integrity of the erectile cylinders and might impair future erections. Critics who prefer a single corporotomy with graft worry that 3 corporotomies without corporal grafting disturb the integrity of the erectile cylinders, possibly causing later erectile dysfunction.

However, we know of only 1 report describing temporary erectile dysfunction after a single corporotomy with grafting for lateral curvature in a 19-year-old (Badawy and Morsi, 2008), and in more than 20 years that we have used 3 corporotomies, including in numerous teens and adults, we have a single adult with postoperative erectile dysfunction currently undergoing further evaluation.

Artificial erection 6 months after 3 corporotomies is shown in Figure 13. Typically, the corporal surface is smooth, or has slight visible indentions where the incisions were made. The incisions appear to heal by ingrowth of tunica albuginea without visible scarring. At the graft surgery (STAC stage 2), VC ≤30° is present in 15% of patients, which is amenable to a single 4-0 Prolene Heineke-Mikulicz (Yacchia) dorsal plication. Recurrent VC thereafter has occurred in less than 1%, with management described in Chapter 4. Ballooning has only rarely occurred, always small, usually unilateral, and arising at the lateral edge of one incision, since the incisions are not grafted and heal maintaining the structural integrity of the corpora.

The same 3 corporotomies are used in postpubertal teens and adults (Figure 14). All are systematically queried about their postoperative erections and only a single patient has reported erectile dysfunction shortly after surgery with further evaluation underway. None have reported buckling during intercourse.

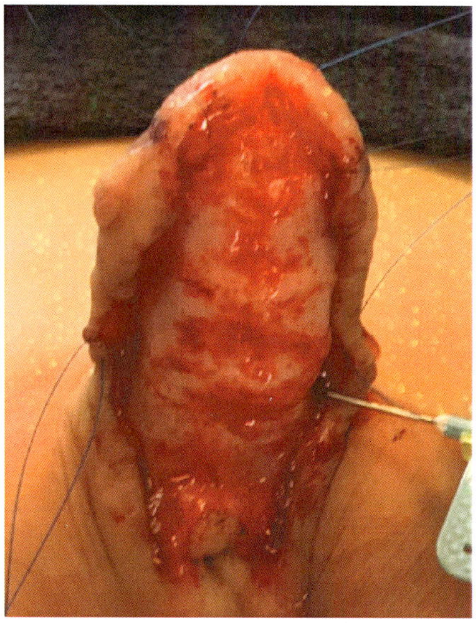

Figure 13. Artificial erection 6 months after 3 corporotomies for VC.
The penis is straight. Slight indentions are visible where the corporotomies were made, but there is no gross scarring and no ballooning from the healed incisions.

Critics of ventral lengthening cite a report by Husmann regarding ED in adult hypospadias cripples. 37% had ED, which was more likely in older men and associated with division of the urethral plate, ventral corporal grafting, and multiple DVIUs for strictures (Husmann, 2020). It is important to note that patients with ventral grafting comprised only 25% of all the men in that series with ED, and that multiple DVIUs was the greatest risk factor for this occurrence, occurring in nearly all of the patients with ED. No patient had straightening by 3 corporotomies.

Regardless, any potential for ED resulting from a single large ventral corporotomy with corporal grafting cannot be extrapolated to risk for 3 smaller corporotomies. We systematically query the patients if they have the ability to achieve and to maintain an erection before each step of a STAC repair. No older teen or adult has complained of ED after straightening by 3 corporotomies, with the exception of a recent postop patient in whom ED is present after a first stage STAC repair who is currently undergoing further evaluation. We have also tried using validated ED tools such as the IIEF to assess ED between stages, but most commonly these cannot be scored because

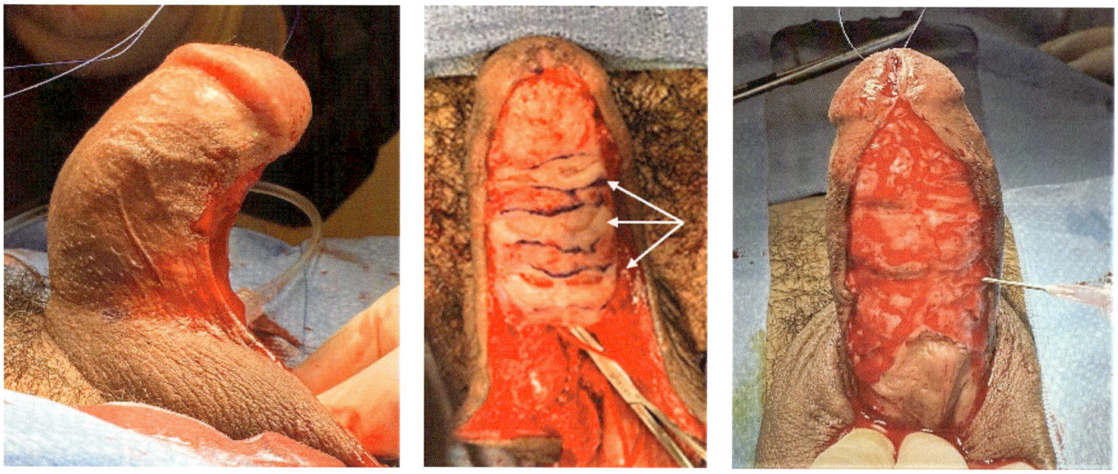

Figure 14. 3 corporotomies to straighten VC in an adult.
A, recurrent VC after childhood dorsal plication. B, 3 corporotomies have been made through the tunica albuginea indicated by the arrows. C, the patient reported straight erections, confirmed by artificial erection 6 months later. Slight indentions from the incisions are visible, but were not noticeable to the patient even before the urethral skin graft was placed.

many hypospadias patients are not sexually active when they have complications from childhood repair or when they are between stages, and therefore they leave most of the questions blank. Additional work to assess ED in patients in whom their hypospadias has affected their intimate relationships (or lack thereof) is therefore needed.

Results

We repeat artificial erection at each subsequent operation after straightening was done. Most often that demonstrates the penis is straight. Apparent persistent VC at the second operation is most often due to tethering by the urethrostomy and is relieved by releasing it off the corpora and dissecting it a centimeter or so proximally. Another common finding is thickened dartos on the surface of the corpora that needs to be excised anyway before urethroplasty grafting. Occasionally, bands of scar bridge across part of a corporotomy incision restrict expansion and are released by small transverse incisions. These measures straighten most 2nd stage bending, proven by another artificial erection.

We reviewed results in 224 consecutive patients undergoing 3 corporotomies during primary or reoperative STAC. VC averaged 66° (30-130). Of these patients, 23 were adults undergoing reoperations at a mean age of 25 years ranging to 40 years.

16% of these patients had residual curvature at stage 2, which averaged 23° and was successfully straightened with a HM dorsal plication. 99% had no persisting curvature at stage 3. No adult reported erectile dysfunction (Snodgrass & Bush, 2024).

Need to repeat corporotomies has been anecdotal, especially when we transitioned from STAG to STAC. Previously, contraction of the urethroplasty graft placed onto the 3 incisions during STAG occasionally also contracted the incisions so that 1 or more had to be made again.

Complications of Penile Straightening

Persistent or recurrent ventral curvature are the most common complications after penile straightening, and are found most often, in descending order, after chordee excision, dorsal plication, single corporotomy with corporal grafting, and 3 corporotomies without corporal grafting.

Surgeons should not assume a prior straightening procedure was effective, but rather must verify that the penis is straight by repeating artificial erection at each subsequent operation.

In addition, hypospadias surgeons must recognize the signs of persistent or recurrent ventral curvature in prepubertal boys, which are discussed and shown in Chapter 4.

Recurrent Ventral Curvature

Recurrent VC < 30° can usually be straightened by a Heineke-Mikulicz dorsal plication, assuming that an Adson test mimicking plication does not detect tension.

Recurrent VC ≥ 30° that persists after releasing the shaft skin most often indicates a short ventral corporal sheath. In a patient undergoing a 2nd stage repair who first had chordee excision or dorsal plication, the ventral corporal surface should be exposed and 3 corporotomies made across the bent area as part of a reoperative STAC procedure. The same is done when a patient previously had a single corporotomy with corporal grafting, with one of the 3 incisions usually going across the healed corporal graft.

If urethroplasty was completed management becomes more complex. Since the goal of hypospadias repair is to make normal anatomy, when the distal urethroplasty and glansplasty achieved that we first dissect the neourethra from the corpora down into the distal scrotum. Then repeat artificial erection is done to confirm curvature ≥ 30° persists and to accurately mark where the 3 corporotomy incisions should be made.

Typically, in a hypospadias reoperation, especially following a proximal repair, the neourethra has decreased elasticity and is best transected as part of the straightening process. When the neomeatus has a normal caliber and glans fusion the transection is made in approximately the midshaft, then 2 urethrostomies are created – one proximal and one distal urethrostomy, typically with the 3 corporotomy incisions made between them. A dartos flap covers the incisions and the shaft skin is closed, completing this first step of a Johansen-modified STAC (Figure 15).

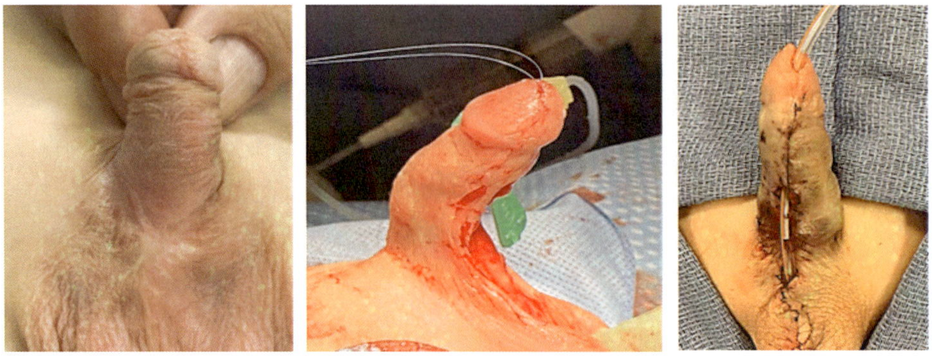

Figure 15. Johansen-modified STAC.
The patient had a TIP repair elsewhere and presented with a satisfactory glans and meatus but proximal shaft VC, as seen in A and B. The neourethra was divided in the midshaft region, 3 corporotomies were done for straightening and covered with a dartos flap, then the skin was closed between the proximal and distal openings in the urethra for a Johansen-modified STAC reoperation.

At the next operation artificial erection is repeated, and then the gap between urethrostomies is grafted using oral mucosa. This urethroplasty graft is tubularized to complete the neourethra at a 3rd stage.

Recurrent VC due to a short ventral corporal sheath is uncommon after 3 corporotomies made properly. When the bending measures 30° or less, an Adson test is done. We have found there is almost no resistance to this maneuver after prior corporotomies released ventral tension, and a Heineke-Mikulicz plication has successfully and durably straightened the recurrent bending.

If there is more than 30° recurrent ventral curvature after 3 corporotomies, or tension is found on the Adson test despite less curvature, one or more of the corporotomies are redone and STAC repair repeated. Urethroplasty grafting should be postponed until artificial erection demonstrates the penis is straight at the next operation.

"S" penile deformity

Dorsal plications can also distort the shape of the penile shaft, creating a "S"-shaped deformity. An example is seen in Figure 16.

Dorsal Curvature

Ventral lengthening by either single corporotomy with corporal grafting or 3 corporotomies can occasionally create dorsal curvature. There are several

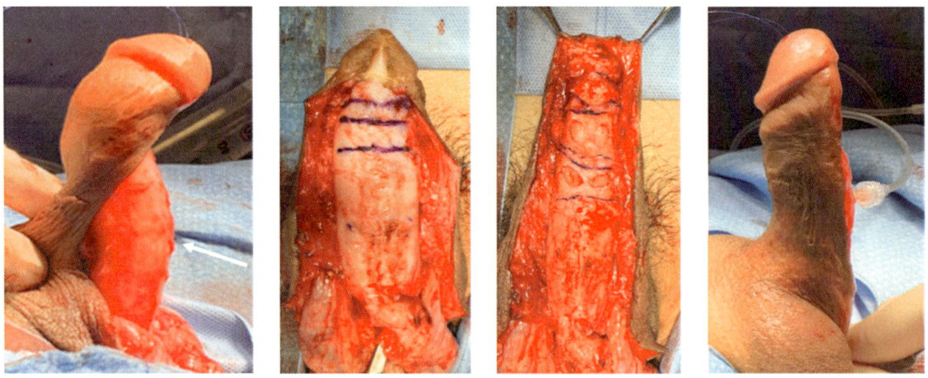

Figure 16. "S" deformity caused by dorsal plication.
A, "S" shape found during reoperation. B, C, 3 corporotomies done to straighten the distal curvature. The arrow in A indicates where ventral plication will also be needed to correct the dorsal bend from the plication. D, erection at the next stage proving the penis is now straight.

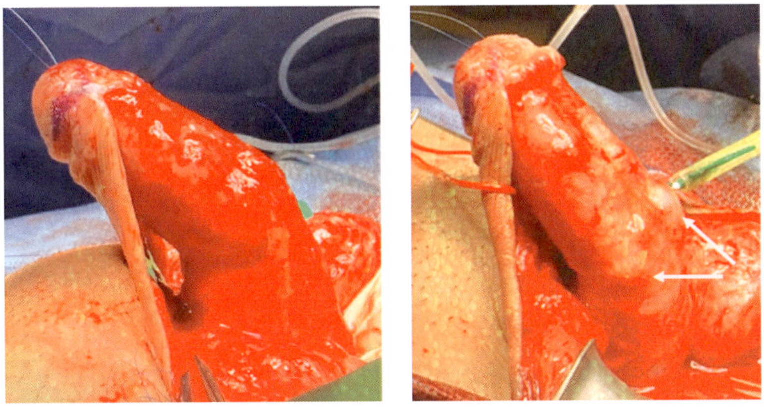

Figure 17. Dorsal curvature after a single corporotomy with corporal graft.
In this case dorsal curvature was caused by a diverticulum of the corporal graft, shown by the arrows in B. In this situation the diverticulum can be imbricated shorter or incised across its mid-region transversely and sutured as in an excisional Nesbit plication.

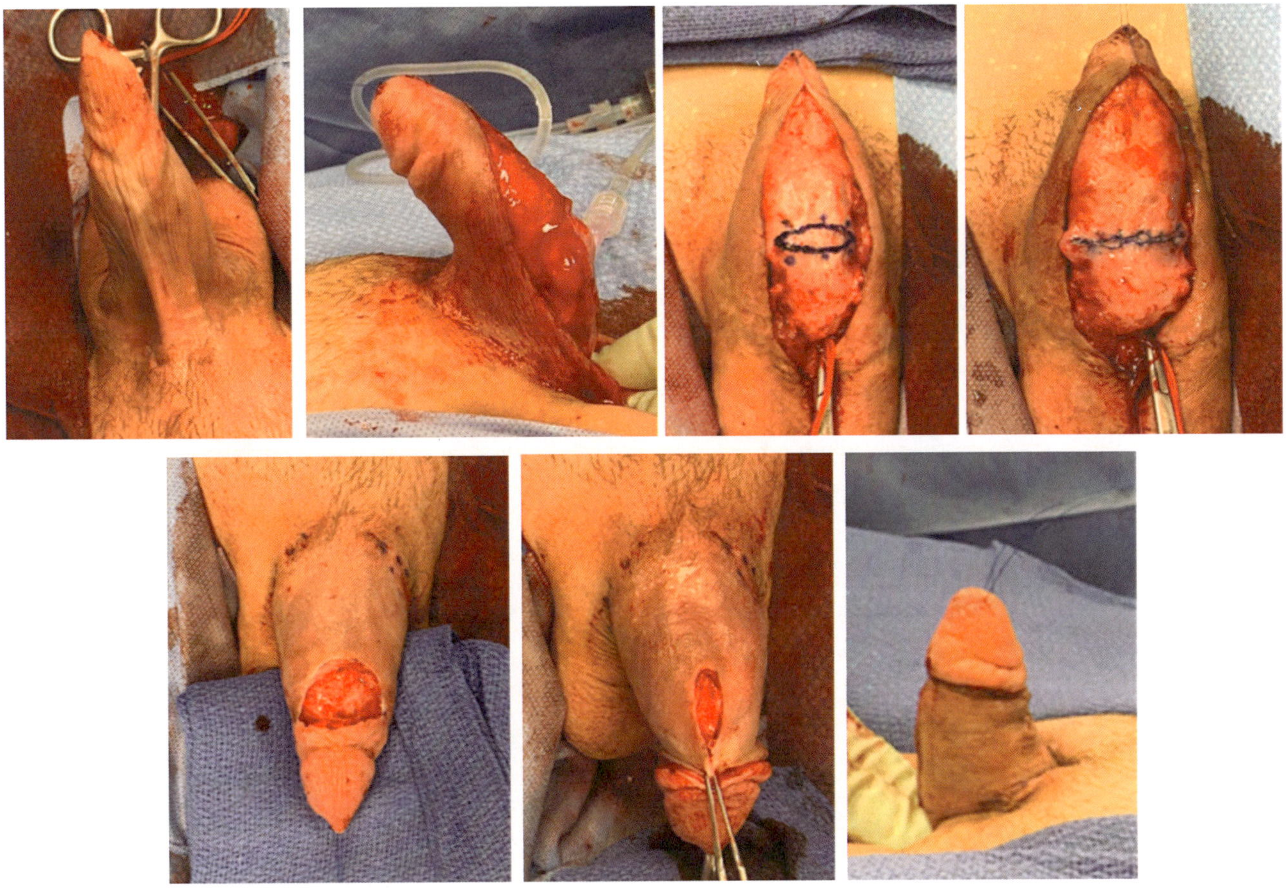

Figure 18. Correcting dorsal curvature and short dorsal skin.
A, stretching the penis shows tension bands which can pull on corporotomies during erections while they are healing, resulting in 45° dorsal curvature, seen in B. C, an ellipse was outlined over the healed corporotomy, which was then excised. D, the defect was sutured with interrupted subepithelial 2-0 Ethibond in this postpubertal patient, with a second epithelial layer of 5-0 Vicryl. The oral urethroplasty graft will next be placed over this. E, F, Heineke-Mikulicz lengthening of the dorsal short skin in the tension band can be made either near the glans as in this case, or at the penopubic junction. F, final result showing the penis is straight.

possible explanations. Either method can potentially overcorrect the bending, by making a single incision too large or by extending the 3 incisions past 3 and 9 o'clock. Sometimes a corporal graft does not provide sufficient tensile strength during postoperative spontaneous erections and a diverticulum develops (Figure 17). More often, short dorsal skin pulls the corporal graft longer, or the 3 corporal incisions wider, as they heal (Figure 18).

We approach dorsal curvature by first releasing the dorsal shaft skin from the corpora without degloving dorsally, which can reduce tension and allow skin scarred to the corpora to stretch. When it is obvious that short skin is still tethering the penis dorsally there are several options to consider: Dissection can continue under the skin above the pubis to further release it. Then the penopubic skin is advanced towards the penis and pexed to the base of the corpora to add length to the shaft skin. Another option is Heineke-Mikulicz lengthening of the short skin at either the corona or penopubic junction, shown in Figure 18. A third consideration is reversed Byars flaps to move ventral skin dorsally, assuming that the resulting ventral defect can still be closed. These skin management problems are discussed in Chapter 21.

Once any skin tethering is addressed, the dorsal bend is straightened. It hinges from a corporotomy, and is corrected by a Nesbit plication (Figure 18). When encountered at a second stage, the plication is done and the urethroplasty graft can then be placed over it. If dorsal curvature is first detected at the final stage, Heineke-Mikulicz plication is done ventrally on either side of the graft where the penis is most bent.

Dorsal penile curvature does not exert the same magnitude of tension on the hypospadias repair that ventral curvature does. In addition, mild dorsal curvature does not cause the same sexual dysfunction that ventral bending does. For these reasons dorsal bending that objectively measures < 30° may be acceptable.

Key Points

VC that persists after degloving most often is due to a short ventral corporal sheath – and not to "chordee". Bending less than 30° can be straightened by dorsal plication, making a midline tunica albuginea incision with a Heineke-Mikulicz closure. Bending greater than 30° is most reliably and durably corrected by making 3 transverse corporotomy incisions across the arc of the curvature.

We encourage surgeons to objectively measure curvature since visual estimates are not reliable to determine the degree of bending.

The penis needs to be straight for optimal sexual performance, with men reporting that VC as little as 20° interferes with intercourse and creates worry.

Persistent or recurrent curvature ≥ 30° is the underlying cause for many urethroplasty complications after distal repairs, and most complications following unsuccessful proximal repairs. Therefore, artificial erection should *always* be done during each stage of a repair, and in reoperations for any complication.

The risk for persistent or recurrent VC is greatest when initial straightening is done by chordee excision or dorsal plication. However, it can also occur in as many as 1 out of every 3 patients following single corporotomy with corporal grafting. Persistent or recurrent VC is least likely when straightening is done by 3 corporotomies.

The goal of getting it right the first time requires that ventral curvature be straightened using the most reliable and durable methods. Surgeons cannot be reluctant to do something that is new to them and continue doing what they are comfortable with when there is proof that it does not work good enough. The cost of persistent or recurrent VC is simply too high for the patient.

References

Akizuki K, Yamaguchi K, Morita Y and Ohashi Y. The effect of proficiency level on measurement error of range of motion. *J Phys Ther Sci* 28:2644, 2016

Babu R and Chandrasekharam VVS: A meta-analysis comparing dorsal plication and ventral lengthening for chordee correction during primary proximal hypospadias repair. *Pediatr Surg Int* published online, 2022

Badawy H and Morsi H: Long-term follow-up of dermal grafts for the repair of severe penile curvature. *J Urol* 180: 1842, 2008

Bologna RA, Noah TA, Nasrallah PF, and McMahon DR: Chordee: varied opinions and treatments as documented in a survey of the American Academy of Pediatrics, Section of Urology. *Urology* 53: 608, 1999

Carter TI, Pansy B, Wolff AL, Hillstrom HJ, Backus SI, Lenhoff M and Wolfe SW. Accuracy and reliability of three different techniques for manual goniometry for wrist motion: a cadaveric study. *J Hand Surg Am* 34:1422, 2009

Duckett JW and Keating MA: Technical challenge of the megameatus intact prepuce variant: the pyramid procedure. J Urol 141: 1407, 1989

Gong EM and Cheng EY: Current challenges with proximal hypospadias: we have a long way to go. *J Pediatri Urol* 13:457, 2017

Greenfield JM, Lucas S, and Levine LA: Factors affecting the loss of length associated with tunica albuginea plication for correction of penile curvature. *J Urol* 175: 238, 2006

Hollowell JG, Keating MA, Snyder HM, III and Duckett JW: Preservation of the urethral plate in hypospadias repair: extended applications and further experience with the onlay island flap urethroplasty. *J Urol* 143: 98, 1990

Husmann DA: Erectile dysfunction in patients undergoing multiple attempts at hypospadias repair: etiologies and concerns. *J Pediatr Urol* 17: 166e1, 2020

Long CJ, Chu DI, Tenny RW, Morris Ar, Weiss DA,Shukla AR, Srinivasan AK, Zderic SA, Kolon TF, Canning DA: Intermediate-term followup of proximal hypospadias repair reveals high complication rate. *J Urol* 197: 852, 2017

Menon V, Breyer B, Copp HL, Baskin L, Disandro M and Schlomer BJ: Do adult men with untreated ventral curvature have adverse outcomes? *J Pediatri Urol* 12: 31e, 2016

Nussbaumer S, Leunig M, Glatthorn JF, Stauffacher S, Gerber H and Maffiuletti NA: Validity and test-retest reliability of manual goniometers for measuring passive hip range of motion in femoroacetabular impingement patients. *BMC Musculoskeletal Dis* 11: 194, 2010

Poulsen J and Kirkeby HJ: Treatment of penile curvature – a retrospective study of 175 patients operated with plication of the tunica albuginea or with the Nesbit procedure. *Br J Urol* 75: 370, 1995

Snodgrass W and Bush NC: Staged tubularized autograft repair for primary proximal hypospadias with 30-degree or greater ventral curvature. *J Urol* 198: 680, 2017

Snodgrass W and Bush NC: Persistent or recurrent ventral curvature after failed proximal hypospadias repair. *J Pediatr Urol* 15: 344, 2019

Snodgrass W and Prieto J: Straightening ventral curvature while preserving the urethral plate in proximal hypospadias repair. *J Urol* 182: 1720, 2009

Stojanovic B, Bizic M, Majstorovic M, Kojovic V, and Djordjevic M: Penile curvature incidence in hypospadias: can it be determined? *Adv Urol,* 2011

Yachia D: Modified corporoplasty for the treatment of penile curvature. *J Urol* 143: 80, 1990

Chapter 3

Goniometry to Measure Ventral Curvature

How much curvature is too much to straighten by dorsal plication? Is it the same for a Baskin plication versus a Yachia Heinecke-Mikulicz plication versus a Duckett incisional TAP or a Nesbit excisional plication? How much persistent or recurrent curvature results in a postoperative fistula, wound dehiscence, or a neourethral stricture or meatal stenosis?

A study in which pediatric urologists were shown images of penis curvature and asked to estimate the degree of bending illustrates that point (Villaneuva, 2020). Participants answered with a wide range especially for curvature of 20° to 40°. This is the same extent of curvature that we found our own eyeball estimates were least reliable, yet this is where the boundary most likely lies between VC that can be successfully managed by plication and that which is better corrected using 3 ventral corporotomies. These results are shown in Figure 1.

Another study proved the need for surgeons to measure, rather than eyeball, penile curvature by asking pediatric urologists to simulate 30° VC with their index finger. Photographs of their responses were then assessed using both goniometry and a smartphone photo app. Only 33% of the participants accurately simulated 30°, even though that extent of curvature is commonly cited as important in decision-making. Another 44% simulated curvature that was greater than 30°, while the remaining 23% indicated curvature which was less than 30° (Mosa et al, 2022). These over- and under-estimates averaged a 10° difference, which would translate in nearly half of patients undergoing plication for what the surgeon considered to be no more than 30° VC, and nearly

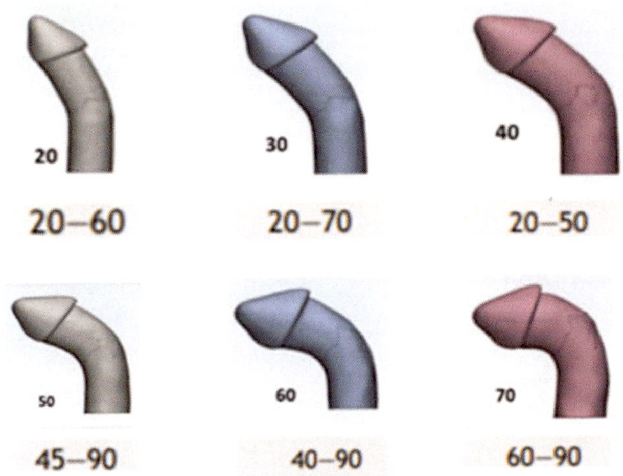

Figure 1. Visual estimates of ventral curvature by pediatric urologists.
The smaller numbers next to the diagram are the actual degree of curvature, while those in the grey boxes below are the range of eyeball estimates by study participants. If 30° is the point at which plication should not be done, these responses indicate there will be patients with less curvature who will have ventral corporotomies because their bending was overestimated, and patients with 30° or greater curvature who will have plications because their bending was underestimated.

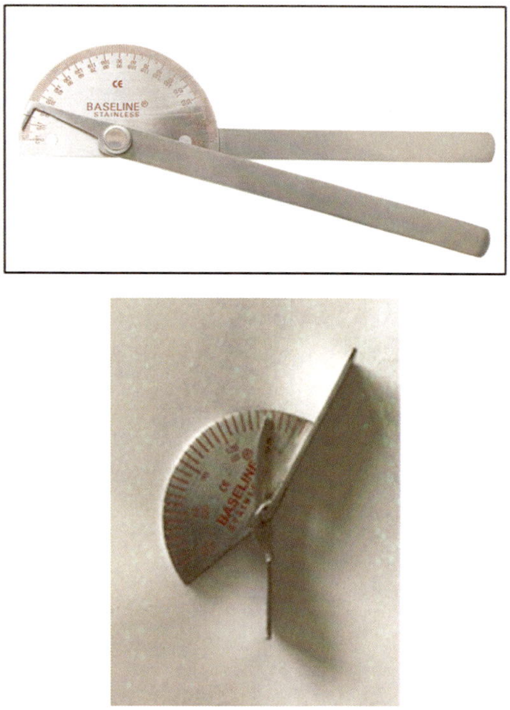

Figure 2. Different types of goniometers.
A, the goniometer used in the Villaneuva study vs B, the modified goniometer we use in patients.

25% having ventral lengthening for curvature that likely could be successfully managed by plication.

Nevertheless, some have questioned whether goniometry is actually more accurate than eyeball estimates. Villanueva created small-scale penis models with varying degrees of VC, and then asked pediatric urologists to visually estimate the bending before handing them a goniometer with brief instructions for its use to measure them. Those measurements also showed a wide range, and the author concluded that goniometry is no better than eyeballing.

However, other studies have shown that training and experience are necessary to properly use the goniometer, as is true of most instruments. The pediatric urologists Villanueva tested had no prior experience with the instrument, and were given the wrong goniometer to measure penile curvature, especially on models much smaller than actual penises (Figure 2). Despite experience using a goniometer, WS, who was a test subject, found the testing goniometer difficult and confusing to use. Nevertheless, the author concluded objective measurements using the goniometer risked over- diagnosis of curvature $> 30^\circ$. Others evaluating the accuracy of goniometry report that the range of error is only 5% with experience (Akizuki et al, 2016).

Furthermore, the greatest risk from inaccurate determination of the degree of VC is in *under-estimating* it. While it is preferable to complete a repair on a penis bent $< 30^\circ$ with a single TIP procedure, staged graft repairs also create a normal penis. In fact, Bracka strongly advocated 2-stage graft repairs for *all* hypospadias, even distal cases with a straight penis, because the available techniques before TIP did not make a normal glans and meatus (Bracka, 1995). Meanwhile, TIP repair with dorsal plication in a penis bent more than 30° is likely to result in recurrent curvature, urethroplasty complications, and ventral skin loss, all making reoperation to achieve a normal penis more difficult. Therefore, if an error is going to be made, it is better to over-estimate than to under-estimate VC.

Evidence reviewed in Chapter 2 indicates that dorsal plication should be limited to VC $< 30^\circ$, which both our clinical experience before using objective measurements and the studies by Villanueva and Mosa et al prove is not accurately identified by eyeball estimates.

Using the Goniometer Correctly

The stationary limb of the goniometer should rest on the pubis for stability and then align with the lateral midline of the penile shaft. The fulcrum of the instrument is placed at the point of maximum curvature and the moveable arm adjusted so that its end is in the same horizontal plane as the correct location for the neomeatus on the glans. It is best for the surgeon to manipulate the goniometer while an assistant maintains a firm artificial erection.

The correct alignment is shown in Figure 3.

When used properly, the goniometer has been found to have high inter- and intra-rater reliability (Carter et al, 2009). It also has been shown to have good test – retest reliability > 0.90 (Nussbaumer et al, 2010). Therefore, hypospadias surgeons can rely on these measurements and use them for intraoperative decision-making.

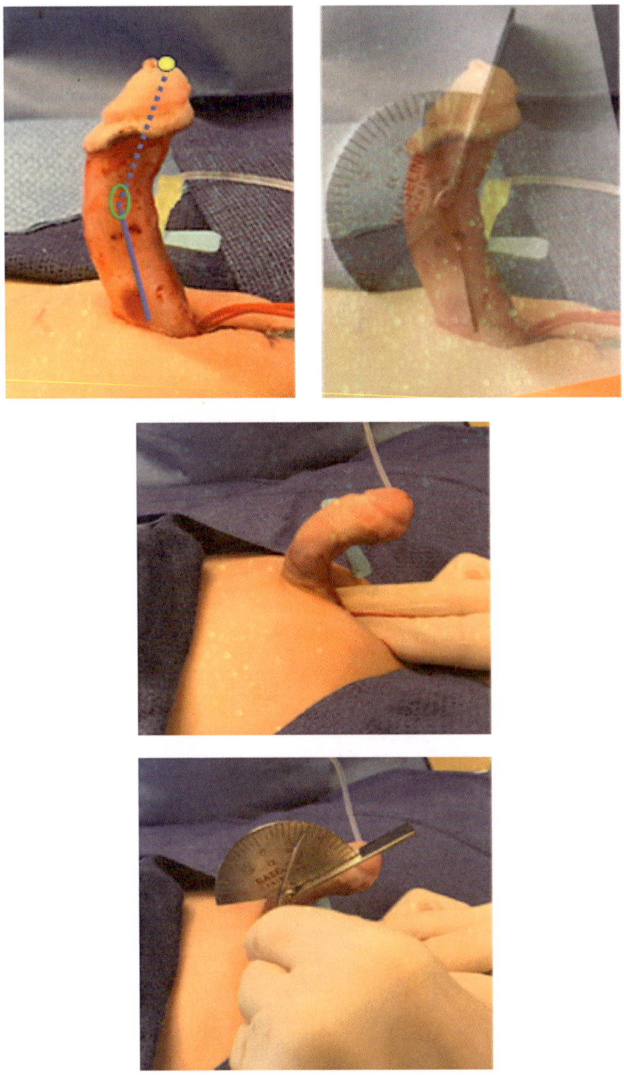

Figure 3. Using the goniometer correctly.
A, the green circle indicates the point of maximum curvature, with lines drawn along the shaft above and below. B, The fulcrum of the goniometer is placed at the point of curvature and the two arms aligned along the penile shaft as demonstrated. Note the moveable arm points to the location for the neomeatus. C, Another patient, with the goniometer properly aligned in D.

Modifying the Goniometer

The standard finger goniometer needs to be slightly modified before it is used to measure penile curvature. The stationary arm is too long, and so when it rests on the pubis the fulcrum is above the point of maximum curvature on the penis making it more difficult to accurately measure the angle.

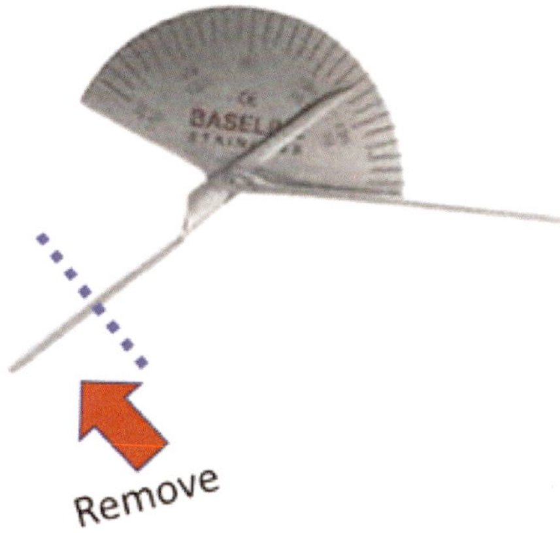

Figure 4. Modifying the goniometer.
The 2 arms of the goniometer are the same length. The stationary arm should be shortened by 1cm so that the instrument better fits a prepubertal penis.

To remedy that, 1 cm of the stationary arm is removed using a Dremel, as shown in a YouTube video on the Hypospadias Specialty Center channel. Alternatively, the persons who repair instruments and sharpen scissors often have the appropriate tools to cut the stationary arm to size. The correct location to shorten the arm is shown in Figure 4.

Alternatives to the Goniometer

The standard finger goniometer is readily available and inexpensive. But other alternatives do exist. One is the use of a standard protractor. These can be sterilized and used similar to a goniometer. Others have been investigating the use of photo apps to calculate the extent of penile curvature. This could also prove useful, but care must be taken as the degree of angulation changes based on the angle that the photograph is taken. Testing will need to be done to see if this is able to be standardized for the various users - assuming a circulating nurse in the operating room will be the one taking the photo and measuring the angle on the photo app. Additional work will need to be done to see if it is even possible to use a photo app on patients with severe hypospadias, where the lateral corpora and often the bend itself can be obscured by the thigh and therefore not able to be easily seen in a lateral photo.

Key Points

Given the critical role that straightening VC plays in successful hypospadias repair, and the inaccuracy of visual guestimates of the degree of curvature, surgeons should objectively measure the bending.

We prefer to use the goniometer, which, when slightly modified, is easy to use with reproducible results. A standard protractor can also be used.

For hypospadiology to progress, surgeons must begin systematically measuring penile curvature using instruments.

References

Akizuki K, Yamaguchi K, Morita Y and Ohashi Y. The effect of proficiency level on measurement error of range of motion. *J Phys Ther Sci* 28:2644, 2016

Bracka A: A versatile two-stage hypospadias repair. *Br J Plast Surg* 48:345, 1995

Carter TI, Pansy B, Wolff AL, Hillstrom HJ, Backus SI, Lenhoff M and Wolfe SW. Accuracy and reliability of three different techniques for manual goniometry for wrist motion: a cadaveric study. *J Hand Surg Am* 34:1422, 2009

Mosa H, Paul A, Solomon E, Garriboli M: How accurate is eyeball measurement of curvature? A tool for hypospadias surgery. *J Pediatr Urol* 20: published online ,2022

Nussbaumer S, Leunig M, Glatthorn JF, Stauffacher S, Gerber H and Maffiuletti NA: Validity and test-retest reliability of manual goniometers for measuring passive hip range of motion in femoroacetabular impingement patients. *BMC Musculoskeletal Dis* 11: 194, 2010

Villanueva CA: Ventral penile curvature estimation using an app. *J Pediatr Urol* 16: 437, 2020

Chapter 4

Recurrent Ventral Curvature

Persistent or recurrent VC is the most common complication, by far, after proximal hypospadias repair, and is often found after unsuccessful distal repairs, too. Tension generated by spontaneous erections when the penis is bent is the underlying cause of many urethroplasty complications.

This fact is not widely known; rather, it is commonly believed that straightening is reliable and durable, as seen by the fact that few surgeons repeat an artificial erection during second stages or reoperations. However, in the 1950s Culp wrote that the risk for persistent VC after chordee excision was sufficiently great to justify staging repairs to be certain the penis was straight before urethroplasty. Like us, Devine and Horton reported in the 1970s that persistent VC was the most common finding in unsuccessful hypospadias repairs. Jayanthi et al published a series of patients undergoing reoperations in the 1990s saying they all had recurrent hypospadias with varying degrees of VC.

Despite these warnings issued periodically over many decades, surgeons have not been taught this risk or how to recognize the signs of recurrent VC on physical examination in prepubertal boys. Furthermore, they may dismiss parental concerns that the penis is bent postoperatively because they believe the straightening maneuvers they use are durable.

The Scope of the Problem

Nearly 85% of patients we evaluated after primary proximal hypospadias repair done by other pediatric urologists had persistent, or recurrent, VC ≥ 30°, averaging 50°.

These boys presented for 2nd opinions having the usual complications of fistulas, glans or wound dehiscence, meatal stenosis and neourethral strictures. Nearly all parents self-referred, and 40% had no idea there was curvature in addition to the other complication(s) which prompted their consultation. Most said the first surgeon did not mention recurrent VC during postoperative evaluations. Others reported the surgeon reassured them their son's penis was straight when they expressed concern that it was not. Therefore, these patients with recurrent VC were not a selected or biased group for this complication, but rather are representative of patients undergoing proximal hypospadias reoperation today (Snodgrass and Bush, 2019).

The prevalence of persistent or recurrent VC varied by the method originally used for straightening:

Chordee Excision

Chordee excision was the 2nd most commonly used means for straightening, and the least successful procedure with 83% of patients having persistent VC. As discussed in Chapter 2, ventral curvature is *not* caused by chordee tissue on the surface of the corpora constricting their normal expansion during erection, and the most thorough dissection to excise all tissues from the tunica albuginea rarely straightens the penis. This fact was proven by artificial erection in the 1970s, and then emphasized by Duckett in the 1990s. Yet many surgeons still believe that ventral curvature is caused by chordee and straightened by chordee excision.

This misconception is not unique to specialists in the United States. Bracka taught that VC was straightened by chordee excision which included excising the urethral plate, supplemented by dorsal plication during the second stage if necessary. Following his example, a 2013 report from Europe said that meticulous excision of chordee tissue made it "unnecessary" to repeat an artificial erection. Nevertheless, the authors admitted that some patients undergoing staged repairs needed an intermediate operation to re-straighten curvature before urethroplasty, and, in their series that included only 9 patients with proximal hypospadias, 6 were diagnosed with a bent penis by puberty (Ekmark et al, 2013) This was almost certainly not new curvature that developed with penile growth as the authors suggested, but congenital curvature that was never properly straightened by chordee excision.

Dorsal Plication

The most used means to straighten ventral curvature in the patients we evaluated was dorsal plication, which remains the most popular method used worldwide. Plication was strongly encouraged by Duckett for nearly all curvature after he realized that chordee excision removing the urethral plate did not make the penis straight. Accordingly, he advocated preserving the plate for urethroplasty and straightening the bending with plication(s) (Baskin and Duckett, 1994).

However, the limits of curvature which can be reliably and durably made straight by plication are ill-defined. 70% of patients we evaluated after dorsal plications elsewhere had recurrent VC ≥ 30°, which Braga et al similarly found in 28% of boys who had plication mostly for curvature subjectively estimated to be <45°. Apparently Duckett's successors are encountering similar problems with recurrent VC, since they no longer perform plications when curvature is only 15° or more (Long et al, 2017).

Recurrent VC is especially likely when the urethral plate is preserved for urethroplasty, which both we and Braga et al reported. In fact, we stopped using TIP for proximal repairs when there is VC measuring ≥ 30° because of this risk (Snodgrass and Bush, 2021).

Only half of the patients we evaluated for complications after proximal repairs had another artificial erection done immediately after their plication to confirm success. When performed, repeat artificial erections most often show the penis is straight, meaning the plication was placed in the correct location. However, plication works by pulling the penis straight without relieving the ventral tension caused by erections when the sheath enclosing the erectile tissue is short ventrally. As a result, natural postoperative erections overcome the strength of the plication and the curvature returns. Our series found that happens after either Baskin or Nesbit plications using either absorbable or nonabsorbable sutures ranging in size to 3-0. Furthermore, we commonly encounter patients who had repeated dorsal plications when the first one failed, yet still present with VC ≥ 30°. An example is shown in Figure 1.

For these reasons we strongly discourage plication(s) to correct VC ≥ 30°.

Single Corporotomy with Corporal Graft

Ventral lengthening by a single corporotomy with grafting of the corporal defect is more successful than dorsal plication because it attempts to release the tension caused by a short ventral corporal sheath. Nevertheless, we found recurrent VC in 33% of patients

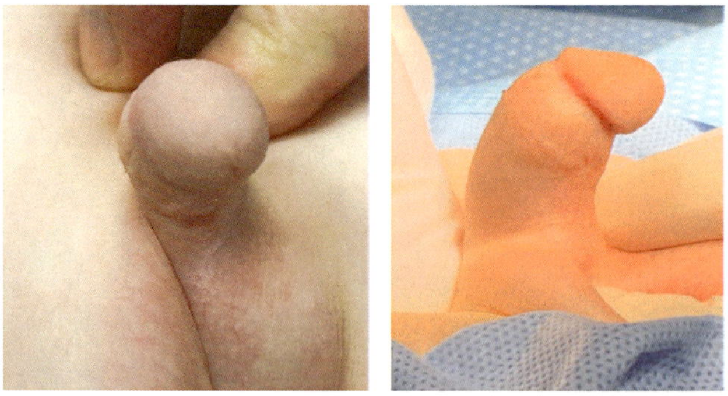

Figure 1. Recurrent ventral curvature after Baskin and then Nesbit plications.
VC recurred after a Baskin plication, and so a Nesbit plication was done. These pictures show recurrent VC that measured 60° after the 2nd plication.

who were straightened by that technique, which was possibly due to an inadequate corporotomy, curvature too great for a single incision to correct, and/or contraction of the corporal graft.

We reported that VC in proximal hypospadias averages 70° (Snodgrass and Bush, 2017), and this extent, or more, bending may be too much for a single corporotomy incision to straighten. In fact, Gong and Cheng (2017) wrote that the corporotomy incision must be made wider that the traditional 3 to 9 o'clock for curvature > 60°, and instead extend from neurovascular bundle to neurovascular bundle - meaning their incision travels from the dorsal side of the penis near 2 o'clock across the entire ventral surface and then back onto the dorsal side to 10 o'clock, leaving only a narrow bridge of intact corpora. Then they advise the opened tunica albuginea should be further mobilized from the erectile tissues to increase the width of the defect. The authors did not report either the success or complications of this maneuver.

A percentage of all grafts used for whatever purpose shrink, and so will at least some of those placed into the corporotomy defect, leading to recurrent VC. That problem is avoided by instead making 3 corporotomies without grafting the incisions.

3 Corporotomies without Corporal Grafting

The straightening maneuver with the least risk for persistent or recurrent VC is 3 corporotomies done without corporal grafting. Neither of the 2 patients in our series who had this method done elsewhere had recurrent curvature. Similarly, we reported recurrence in less than 1% of cases that we straightened with 3 corporotomies (Snodgrass and Prieto, 2009; Snodgrass and Bush, 2017, Snodgrass and Bush, 2024).

As with all techniques, the procedure has to be done correctly to work. As described in Chapter 2, the incisions we make extend *through* the tunica albuginea from approximately 3-9 o'clock to relieve tension in the corpora sheath. There is no need to further dissect the tunica albuginea from the erectile tissues to make the incision wider because these 3 incisions made across the area of greatest curvature reliably straighten the bend. Gong and Cheng wrote that they found the transverse incisions we make were "insufficient for curvature > 60°", but also said that they did not incise the tunica down to erectile tissues like we do. Failure to incise through the tunica albuginea sheath enclosing the erectile tissue will not reliably lengthen the ventral corpora and is a technical error.

Diagnosing Recurrent Ventral Curvature

VC is diagnosed postoperatively by the characteristic appearance and behavior of the penis. The penis is hunched over (Figure 2), and resists having the glans lifted cephalad, snapping back to its resting position when it is released. These findings are so reliable that surgery to confirm the diagnosis and straighten the curvature should be done whenever they are encountered, even if there are no other apparent complications.

Journal reviewers studying similar pictures that we submitted objected that the penises appeared to them to be straight or only minimally bent. In fact, some argued that they would be "quite satisfied" with those outcomes from a proximal repair. As we said above, the medical records of patients with recurrent VC rarely mention it, and few parents recalled the surgeon commenting that the penis was bent. Similarly, in nearly half the cases the parents also had not noticed the curvature. Skeptics replied that curvature not seen by surgeons or parents cannot be clinically significant, but we also did not previously recognize the signs of recurrent VC—in large part because we were not looking for it. Failing to recognize VC does not mean it is not there, or that the curvature does not pose a risk for future sexual dysfunction and dissatisfaction with the penis.

Spontaneous erections are also unreliable to detect recurrent VC, in part because they are not often observed in the outpatient clinic, and also because they can be misleading. We have encountered patients with low VC at or even below the penoscrotal junction whose penis looked straight during natural erection (Figure 3). This further emphasizes the need to *always* perform artificial erection during all stages after straightening, and at reoperations for complications even when curvature is not suspected.

Patients with the appearance shown in Figure 2, and all those with a postoperative complication, should be suspected of having recurrent VC. The fact that

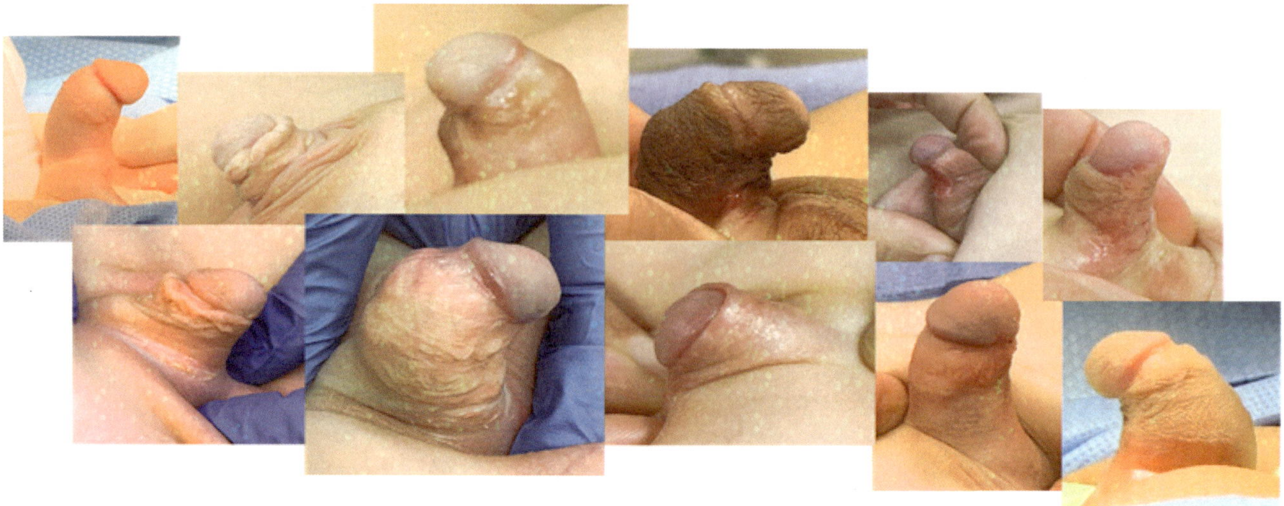

Figure 2. Typical appearance of recurrent ventral curvature.
These photographs show the usual appearance of recurrent VC, with the penis "hunched over". If the glans is lifted upwards resistance is felt which snaps the penis back to this position when it is released. Although this curvature might not seem significant, these boys all had bending ≥ 30°, averaging 50°.

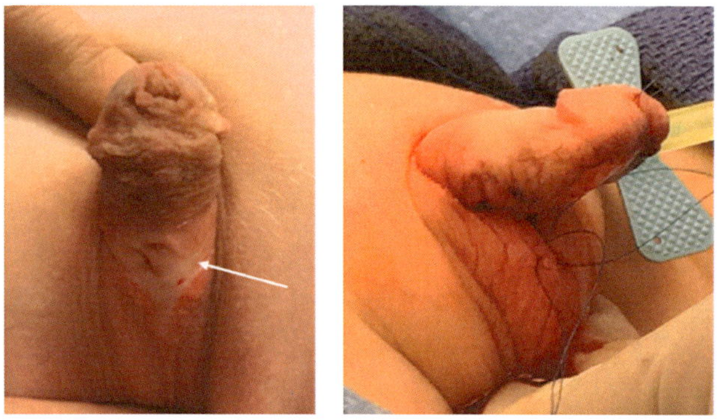

Figure 3. Recurrent ventral curvature at the penoscrotal junction.
Spontaneous erection appeared straight in this boy because the bend was just below the penoscrotal junction causing recurrent fistulas in the region indicated by the arrow. A senior pediatric urologist did not suspect or diagnose this curvature despite 2 failed fistula closures. A "normal" preoperative erection does not exclude recurrent VC, and so an artificial erection should always be done during hypospadias reoperations, especially for recurrent complications.

---

recurrent curvature is not often reported by other authors is explained by it being overlooked on examination and not systematically searched for by artificial erection during 2nd stages and reoperations. In the series reported by Texas Children's, Boston, and CHOP, initial straightening in boys with proximal hypospadias was done by degloving/chordee excision in over 50% in one (McNamara et al) which does not address the short ventral corporal sheath that most of them have. Dorsal plication was the main correction in from 50% to 70% in the other two (Long et al, Stanasel et al) which, as mentioned above, failed in nearly 3 of every 4 patients we evaluated with complications after proximal repairs. Nevertheless, one center did not mention recurrent VC, and the other two said it occurred in < 10% of patients. Yet, each described boys undergoing several reoperations for complications, which is almost pathognomonic for underlying persistent or recurrent VC. We have reoperated on multiple patients from each of these institutions and consistently found their penises still bent.

Our own experience shows how recurrent VC can be missed. WS relied on dorsal plication to straighten curvature in boys with proximal hypospadias so that he could do TIP urethroplasty. He rarely noticed recurrent VC, until we learned to recognize it better during examination and to search for it during 2nd stages and reoperations. Now we know that 1 of every 4 of those patients who had proximal TIP developed recurrent ventral curvature and suspect, in retrospect, that the prevalence was at least 1 of every 3. But we diagnosed half of these patients in just the past 5 years because we did not know to look for it sooner (Snodgrass and Bush, 2021).

It Doesn't Happen at Puberty!

Some speculate that "rapid" penile growth at puberty can cause the previously straight penis to bend. To our knowledge, the only published account asserting this was by Ekmark et al (2013), mentioned above, who reported new curvature during puberty in 6 (5%) of 114 patients followed to age 16 years. However, the authors stated that artificial erection was not routinely done during their childhood repairs, and that the curvature they recognized was corrected by chordee excision without repeat artificial erection to confirm successful straightening. Therefore, it is much more likely that the curvature they encountered at puberty was present long before then, and just not recognized.

We have yet to evaluate a man who stated his penis was straight until puberty and then started bending. Rather, we reported that all recurrent VC present in a consecutive series of teens and adults developed before puberty (Snodgrass & Bush, 2022).

It is likely that this idea of pubertal bending took hold because surgeons did not recognize recurrent VC in childhood until the penis grew larger and the curvature could no longer be overlooked!

Problems Associated with Recurrent Ventral Curvature

Not only did 85% of boys with urethroplasty complications after proximal hypospadias repair have persistent or recurrent VC, but 100% of those who were bent also had a urethroplasty complication. These included fistulas, glans dehiscence, meatal stenosis and neourethral stricture, many of which were recurrent (Figure 4). These complications were typically found in the region of maximum tension created by erections, which was believed to be the main, or at least a contributing, factor to their occurrence.

Recurrent VC after chordee excision or dorsal plication has also been identified in patients with complications after distal repairs (Figure 5).

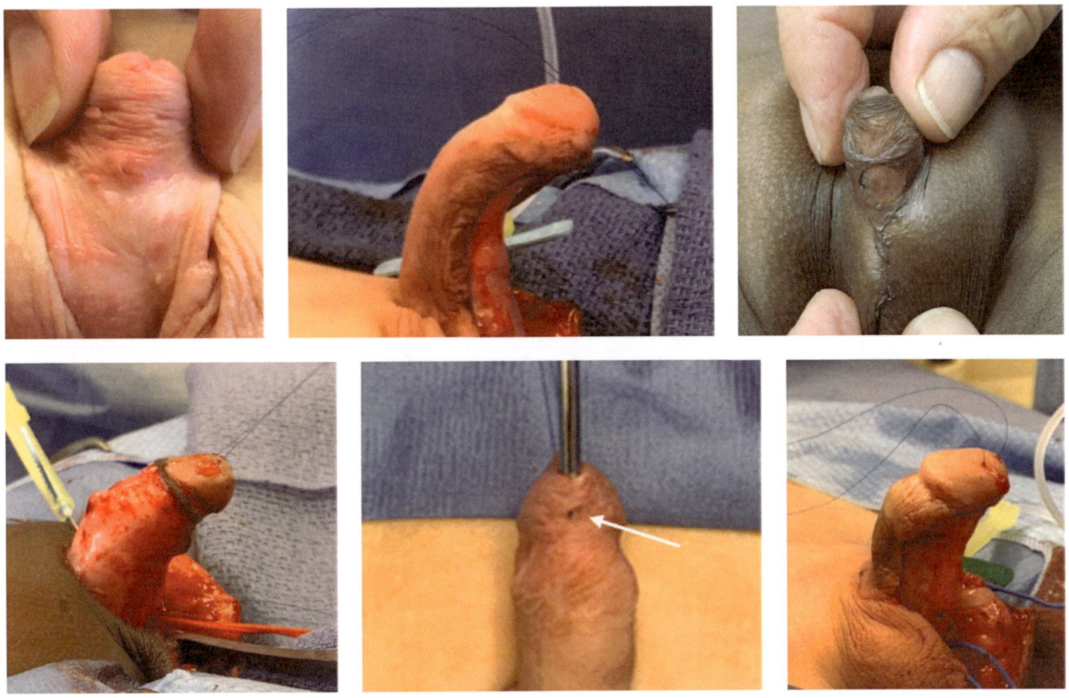

Figure 4. Urethroplasty complications with recurrent ventral curvature.
A,B, recurrent fistulas are visible in the midshaft of the penis in a boy with 60° VC. C,D, wound dehiscence in the region of bending in a patient with recurrent VC measuring 55°. E,F, coronal fistula and a neourethra stricture in the region shown by the arrow in a patient with 35° recurrent VC. VC can recur within weeks of surgery and exert tension on the healing wounds to pull open fistulas or entire wounds. Most urethroplasty complications after proximal repairs are associated with recurrent VC, as are many following distal repairs.

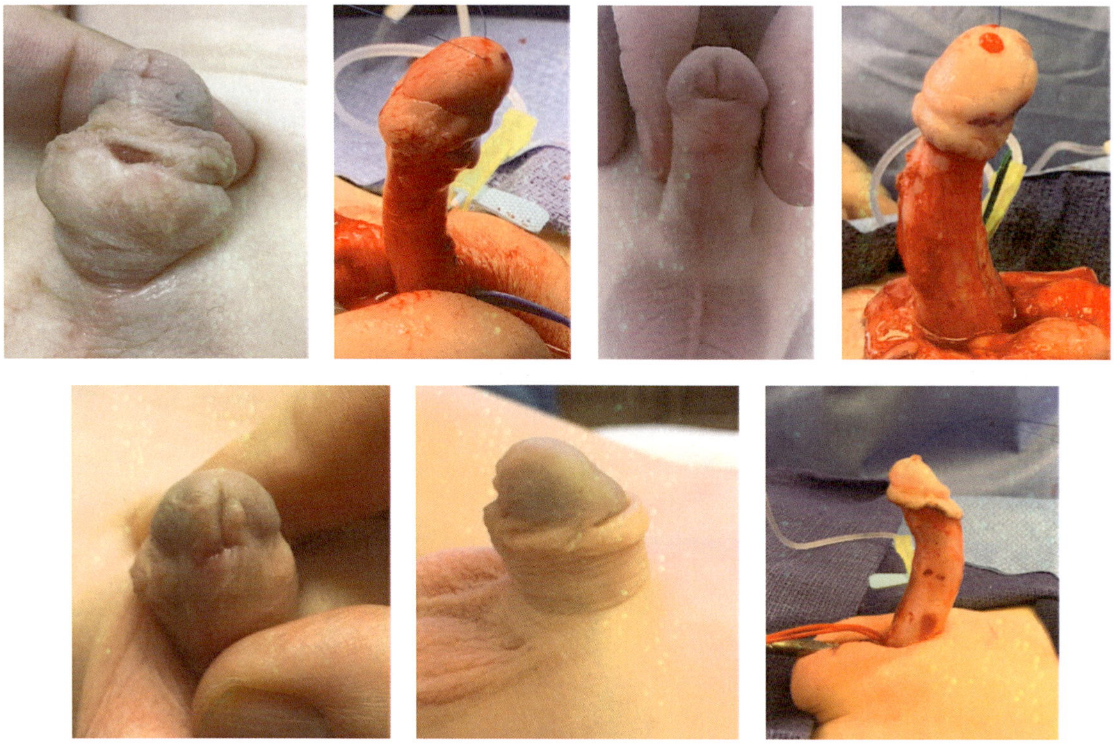

Figure 5. Recurrent ventral curvature and urethroplasty complications after distal repairs.
A,B, fistula in the region of maximum VC which measured 30° following chordee excision at the first operation. C,D, glans dehiscence in another patient with recurrent VC measuring 35° after dorsal plication. E,F,G, recurrent glans dehiscence in a straight-appearing penis found to have 30° of VC despite prior dorsal plication.

As we wrote in the preceding section, all complications should prompt another artificial erection during reoperation, and recurrent complications nearly always indicate there is recurrent VC. These reoperations often continue to fail until the underlying curvature is corrected.

But even if the urethroplasty heals without complications despite persistent or recurrent VC, the repair cannot be considered a success knowing that bending as little as 20° (Figure 6) causes sexual dysfunction and associated worry in adults (Menon et al, 2016).

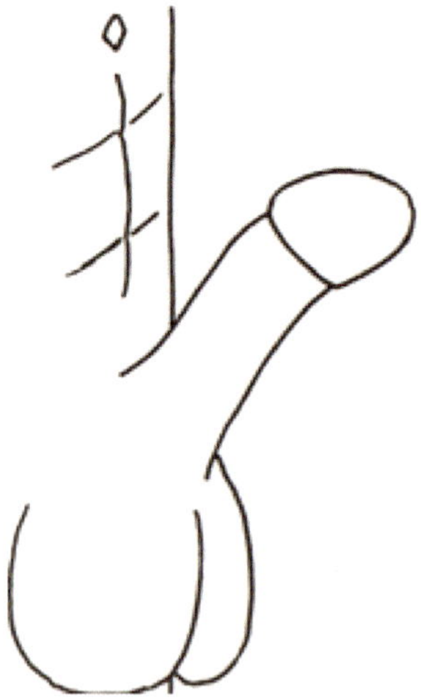

Figure 6. Men with 20° ventral curvature reported sexual dysfunction and worry.
It cannot be over-emphasized that what might appear trivial to surgeons can cause significant sexual dysfunction and related worry to men, according to those who self-reported their penis looked like this (Menon et al).

Managing Recurrent Ventral Curvature

Curvature measuring 30° or more after chordee excision or dorsal plication should be managed with 3 ventral corporotomies. We have seen countless patients similar to the boy shown in Figure 1 who had recurrent VC after dorsal plication and then had

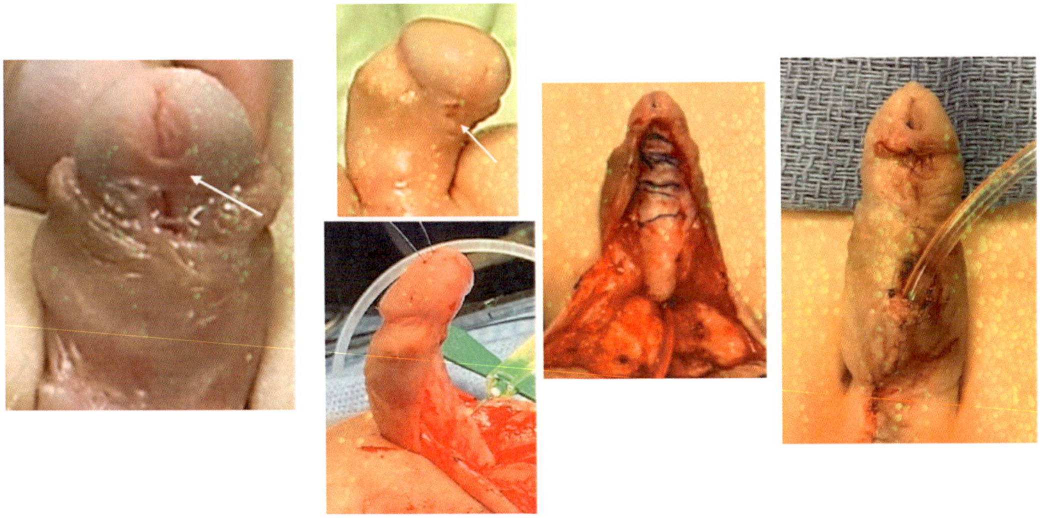

Figure 7. Straightening recurrent VC.
A, this patient presented with partial glans dehiscence leaving a 2mm band across the wings, and a pseudomeatus with open neourethra continuing proximally below the corona (arrow). B, in addition, there was distal ventral curvature that created tension on the repair (arrow) and pulled it apart. C, after ventral degloving the curvature measured 50°. D, 3 corporotomies have been made across the arc of bending. Note that all 3 are on the distal shaft, with the most distal just below the corona. The glans was not disturbed, but will be laid open at the STAC 2 grafting to place a lip graft all the way from the urethrostomy to the tip of the glans. E, a urethrostomy is completed and the penile shaft skin closed to complete STAC 1 repair. Note how low the meatus is along the shaft after correction of the curvature. After the corporotomies heal and the skin stretches during spontaneous erections, STAC 2 and 3 will complete a lip graft urethroplasty.

another, or even a third, plication, often using a different technique - yet remained bent.

In most cases the neomeatus is also abnormal. Consequently, the neourethra is transected distally at the corona and then peeled off the corpora to access the curved area. Three corporotomy incisions are made to straighten the penis, which usually exacerbate the ventral skin deficiency that most of these patients also have (Figure 7). Therefore, the most reliable reoperation in these situations is STAC repair, to first make the penis straight with symmetric circumferential penile shaft skin, and then to complete the graft urethroplasty ending in a normally-positioned neomeatus. Reoperative STAC is discussed in more detail in Chapter 17.

Occasionally, prior surgery has created a normal distal neourethra and meatus. In those cases, access to the bent corporal sheath is gained by transecting the urethra in the midshaft region to perform the 3 corporotomy incisions for straightening. Both the distal and proximal cut ends of the urethra are brought to the skin as temporary urethrostomies, and the penile skin is closed between them, in a Johansen variation on STAC repair (Figure 8).

When recurrent VC in the range of 20° to 30° is found in a patient who had a ventral corporotomy (ies), we perform an Adson forceps test with the penis erect to determine the tension a plication would have to withstand. We have observed that previous corporotomies release most the ventral tension so that the erect penis is quite easily pulled straight - meaning a Heineke-Mikulicz plication will likely be durable.

If the Adson test is uncertain, or clearly demonstrates there is too much tension for a plication to pull and keep the penis straight, then 3 corporotomies need to be made, or remade, across the area of greatest curvature. That also requires transecting the neourethra and peeling it away from the corpora to expose the bent area for a STAC reoperation.

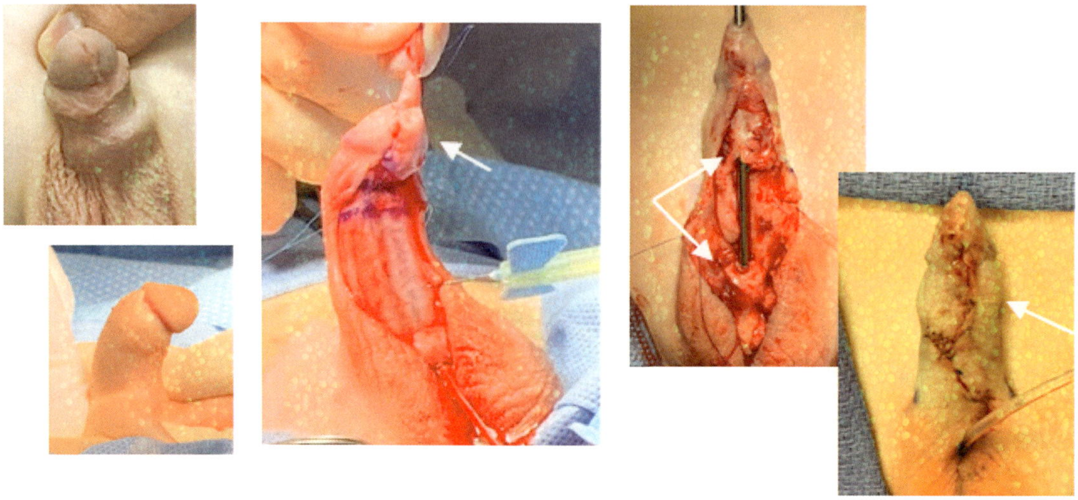

Figure 8. Johansen variation of STAC.
A, normal neomeatus after TIP repair. B, distal ventral curvature which, after degloving, measured 65°. C, urethra has been transected to gain access to the corpora. Arrow indicates the distal urethra lifted up to mark the corporotomy incisions. D, after the corporotomies are made, the distal urethra is laid back down over them and both a distal and proximal urethrostomy are made as indicated by the arrows. E, straightening the penis also creates ventral shaft skin deficiency and so reoperative STAC repair is done to allow the skin to heal and stretch during natural erections. STAC 2 and 3 will then complete a lip graft urethroplasty between the urethrostomies. This Johansen-modified STAC repair retains the normal distal neourethra and glansplasty from the initial operation.

The fact that ventral lengthening with staged urethroplasty is most often needed for persistent or recurrent VC measuring 30° or more emphasizes again that the first operation needs to be done in the best way. That means straightening ventral curvature using 3 corporotomies when it is ≥ 30°.

Key Points

Recurrent VC is the most common complication after proximal and many distal repairs, especially when straightening was done by chordee excision or dorsal plication. VC ≥ 30° should be straightened using 3 ventral corporotomies during the initial repair.

Persistent or recurrent VC is widely underreported, in large part because surgeons have been taught that chordee excision, dorsal plication, and single corporotomy with corporal grafting are all successful. Consequently, they do not recognize recurrent VC, and do not repeat artificial erections during subsequent stages or at reoperations for complications.

Traditional hypospadiology focuses mostly on urethroplasty. However, making the penis straight is the greater challenge, and failure to achieve that most often means the urethroplasty will also be unsuccessful.

Hypospadias repair can be compared to building a house. No matter the skill of the builder, a house resting on a poor foundation will develop problems—just as a urethroplasty constructed in a bent penis nearly always has complications. The foundation of successful hypospadias repair is a straight penis.

References

Baskin LS and Duckett JW: Dorsal tunica albuginea plication for hypospadias curvature. *J Urol* 151: 1668, 1994

Braga LHP, Lorenzo AJ, Bagli DJ, Dave S, Eeg K, Farhat WA, Pippi Salle JL and Khoury AE: Ventral penile lengthening versus dorsal plication for severe ventral curvature in children with proximal hypospadias. *J Urol* 180:1743, 2008

Culp OS: Surgical correction of hypospadias. *J Urol* 79: 279-92, 1958

Devine CJ Jr, Franz JP, Horton CE: Evaluation and treatment of patients with failed hypospadias repair. *J Urol* 119: 223-6, 1978

Ekmark AN, Svensson H, Arnbjornsson E, and Hannsson E: Postpubertal examination after hypospadias repair is necessary to evaluate the success of primary reconstruction. *Eur J Pediatr Surg* 23: 304, 2013

Gong EM and Cheng EY: Current challenges with proximal hypospadias: we have a long way to go. *J Pediatr Urol* 13: 457, 2017

Jayanthi VR, McLorie GA, Khoury AE and Churchill BM: Can previously relocated penile skin be successfully used for salvage hypospadias repair? *J Urol* 152: 740-3, 1994

Long CJ, Chu DI, Tenny RW, Morris Ar, Weiss DA, Shukla AR, Srinivasan AK, Zderic SA, Kolon TF, Canning DA: Intermediate-term followup of proximal hypospadias repair reveals high complication rate. *J Urol* 197: 852, 2017

McNamara ER, Schaeffer AJ, Logvinenko T, Seager C, Rosokliga I, Nelson CP, Retik AB, Diamond DA, and Cendron M: Management of proximal hypospadias with 2-stage repair: 20-year experience. *J Urol* 194: 1080, 2015

Menon V, Breyer B, Copp HL, Baskin L, Disandro M, Schlomer BJ: Do adult men with untreated ventral penile curvature have adverse outcomes? *J Pediatr Urol* 12: 31, 2016

Snodgrass W and Bush NC: Staged tubularized autograft for primary proximal hypospadias repair with 30-degree or more curvature. *J Urol* 198: 680, 2017

Snodgrass W and Bush NC: Persistent or recurrent ventral curvature after failed proximal hypospadias repair. *J Pediatr Urol* 15: 344, 2019

Snodgrass W and Bush NC: Recurrent ventral curvature after proximal TIP hypospadias repair. *J Pediatr Urol,* 17: e pub, 2021

Snodgrass W and Bush NC: Do new complications develop during puberty after childhood hypospadias repair? *J Urol,* 208: 696, 2022

Snodgrass W and Bush NC: Three Corporotomies to Straighten Ventral Curvature in Proximal Hypospadias. Abstract Presentation, Pediatric Urology Fall Meeting, Kentucky, 2024

Snodgrass W and Prieto J: Straightening ventral curvature while preserving the urethral plate in proximal hypospadias repair. *J Urol* 182: 1720, 2009

Stanasel I, Le HK, Bilgutay A, Roth DA, Gonzales ET, JR, Janzen N, Koh CJ, Gargollo P and Seth A: Complications following staged hypospadias repair using transposed preputial skin flaps. *J Urol* 194: 512, 2015

Repair When Ventral Curvature Is Less Than 30°

Chapter 5

Distal Hypospadias: Which Need Surgery, and Which Do Not?

There are 3 potential reasons for distal hypospadias repair arising from the disordered anatomy: abnormal urination, sexual dysfunction, and body image concerns. However, different surgeons evaluating the same patient may not agree that the anatomy is sufficiently abnormal to affect function, and some will advise parents that a repair in their son would be primarily "cosmetic".

Parents hearing that word may worry that the possibility of complications outweighs any benefit for changing the appearance of an organ that is usually concealed. Activists argue that "cosmetic" surgery should not be done in children before they are able to give their own consent.

It is also distressing for parents when one pediatric urologist recommends surgery and another tells them it is not necessary.

These varying opinions arise because objective criteria have not been used to decide who needs surgery and who does not. Proceeding from the premise that abnormal anatomy increases the risk for abnormal function, those criteria can be defined.

Normal Versus Abnormal Anatomy

The goal of surgery is to change the abnormal anatomy of hypospadias into normal penile anatomy. The normal anatomy of the glans and meatus was defined by Hutton and Babu (2007) in prepubertal boys, who reported that the meatus is enclosed by the glans with a distance from the ventral lip to the corona which exceeds 2.5mm, averaging 4.5mm. Therefore, hypospadias with > 2.5mm glans fusion already has normal glanular anatomy and, therefore, little risk for urine spraying (Figure 1).

However, hypospadias with < 2.5mm glans fusion has abnormal anatomy with an increased likelihood for a spraying or deviated urine stream (Figure 2).

In addition to glans fusion enclosing the meatus, the normal penis is also straight. Although all hypospadias surgeons know that some patients with distal hypospadias have ventral or lateral penile curvature, the prevalence and severity of those, and their impact on sexual function, have not been well-defined.

This chapter addresses the question does abnormal glans fusion and/or penile curvature cause functional problems that warrant distal hypospadias repair?

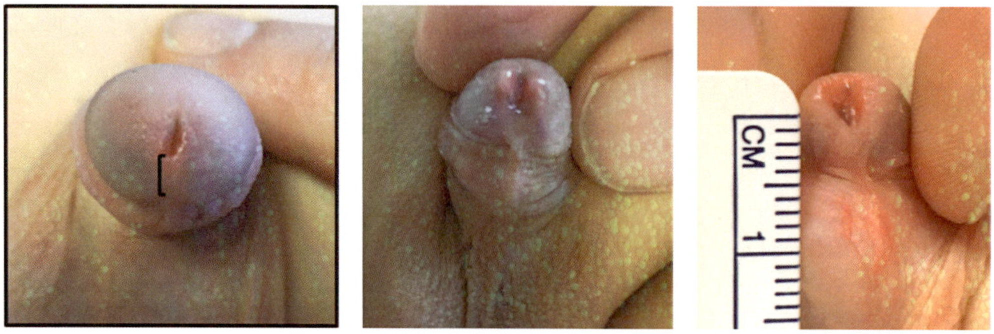

Figure 1. Normal glans fusion.
A, normal penis with normal glans fusion between the meatus and the corona shown by the bar. The glans fusion in this example measured 4mm, within the normal range that is > 2.5mm and averages 4.5mm. B, hypospadias with 3mm glans fusion, and therefore normal glans anatomy. C, MIP hypospadias also with 3mm glans fusion. Because both these boys in B and C have normal glans fusion, neither is likely to have urine spraying.

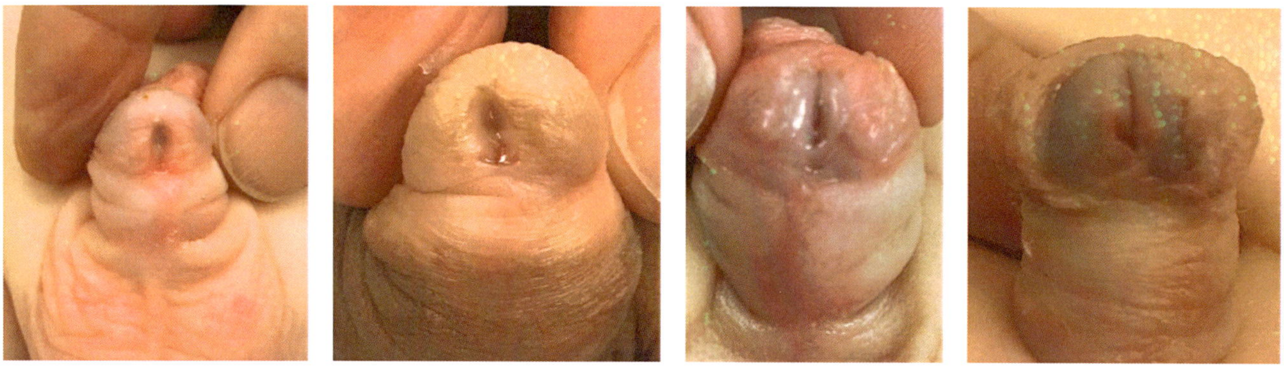

Figure 2. Hypospadias with no, or < 2.5mm, glans fusion.
Each of these cases has abnormal glans fusion, ranging from 0 to 1mm. Consequently, they all are likely to have problems from a deviated or spraying urine stream.

Abnormal Function From Abnormal Anatomy

Urine Spraying

Abnormal glans fusion increases the risk for urine spraying. Although some parents of infants with hypospadias and abnormal glans fusion report the stream appears compact and straight to them, with time the stream usually becomes less reliably compact. Other parents already notice that their infant's steam is deflected downwards. If the hypospadias is not corrected, deviation and spraying seem to become apparent around 8 years of age, possibly as boys reach a height where their penis is no longer within the bowl of the toilet when they urinate.

Men with uncorrected, or unsuccessfully repaired, distal hypospadias offer insights regarding the impact of their abnormal anatomy. We reviewed the complaints of consecutive men presenting with uncorrected distal hypospadias. None of them had normal glans fusion, as shown in representative photographs in Figure 3, and 80% reported urine spraying (Bush & Snodgrass, 2023). Similarly, Ching et al (2010) noted that 86% of men they evaluated with uncorrected hypospadias reported abnormal urination, including spraying. Of men we reviewed who had abnormal glans fusion due to subterminal correction or glans dehiscence of their childhood hypospadias repair, 92% had urine spraying (Snodgrass & Bush, 2022).

Although most of these men voided standing at least part of the time, they described significant bother urinating. Typically, they explained the stream was compact initially when it was most forceful, but sprayed and splattered near the end of urination when pressures decreased, or when they voided with a less full

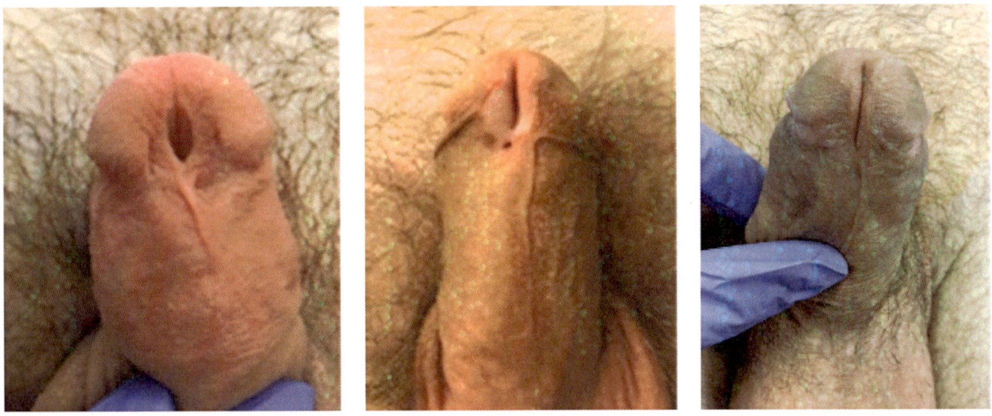

Figure 3. Men with uncorrected hypospadias and urine spraying.
None of these men have normal glans fusion enclosing the meatus, and all of them complained of urine spraying.

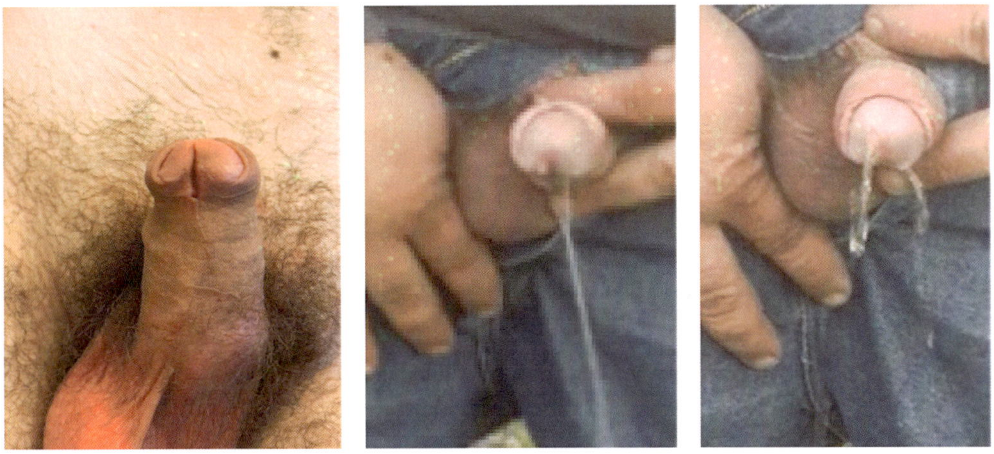

Figure 4. Urine spraying in a man with uncorrected distal hypospadias.
A, there is no glans fusion. B, the urine stream is initially deflected downwards and sprays. C, splattering of his stream near the end of urination.

bladder. Several provided videos showing their abnormal stream, and pictures taken from one of those are seen in Figure 4. Furthermore, the variable nature of the stream added worry, since many could not reliably anticipate when it would spray and so they always had to take precautions to avoid splattering on themselves or others standing nearby. Some described first checking if a public toilet was empty before standing at a urinal and using a stall when it was occupied. Others said they pressed close to urinals to keep the stream inside them. One man with unsuccessful surgery voided into his hand so that he could urinate standing in public. Another reported holding his "foreskin handle" as the only means to urinate standing up as seen in Figure 5. These discussions made clear that standing to void is not the same as voiding normally, and the simple question if a man urinates standing may not capture the real nature of his voiding.

These data give a different perspective than conclusions reached by 2 earlier studies of men with uncorrected hypospadias. Fichtner et al (1995) reported that the meatus was located below the tip of the glans in half of men they evaluated who were thought to be normal. They, and another 16 who had coronal or subcoronal hypospadias, were reportedly all able to urinate standing with a straight steam. Dodds et al (2008) found that a third of men with uncorrected or unsuccessfully corrected distal hypospadias had urine spraying or deflection and that a few preferentially sat to void, yet they were not interested in surgery. The

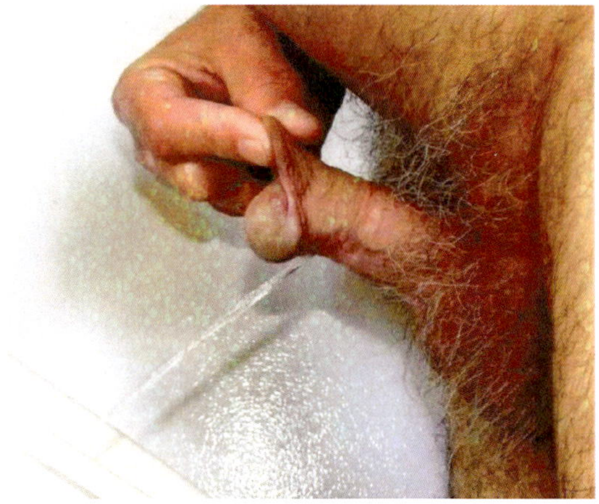

Figure 5. The "foreskin handle" used by a man with uncorrected distal hypospadias to help direct his urine stream. He reported he made this photo in order to show his "urination process" to his urologist.

average age of men in their study was 53 years and the authors concluded they had adapted to their condition. However, the men with uncorrected hypospadias in our study had an average age of 44 years and wanted their condition corrected. Furthermore, many said they were initially discouraged from undergoing surgery by the adult urologists they first consulted, which could be another explanation why the men in the study by Dodds et al did not request repair. Finally, the impact of intact foreskin, or even partial foreskin that can be held as a "handle" while voiding, vs. the impact of circumcision on urinary function in adults with uncorrected hypospadias has not been evaluated to our knowledge. One patient with MIP form of hypospadias, who typically voided without retracting his foreskin, reported having normal urinary function until he underwent a circumcision in adulthood, at which point his urinary spraying became untenable and so he sought repair of his hypospadias.

Penile Curvature and Sexual Dysfunction

As mentioned above, the prevalence of penile curvature in distal hypospadias is not well-defined. We previously published that ventral and lateral curvature occurred in 11% and 2%, respectively, and that all ventral bending was < 30° (Snodgrass & Bush, 2010). However, that underestimated the actual prevalence and severity, since patients found to have > 30° were considered proximal hypospadias variants and not included in the study sample, and the actual degree of curvature was visually estimated rather than objectively measured. A recent study reported ventral curvature in 31% of distal hypospadias, although the degree of that bending was not stated (Stojanovic et al, 2011).

36% of the adults with uncorrected distal hypospadias in our series had ventral penile curvature which measured an average of 30° (15-65). Another 10% had lateral bending. Nearly half of these men reported difficult penetration and/or discomfort for themselves or their sexual partner.

Of all the men in our study, 32% described painful sexual activity. In some that related to their penile curvature, but there were others with a straight penis who complained of irritation in the exposed urethral tissues during intercourse, while 1 man said his scrotal web irritated his wife's introitus.

Many of these men reported inhibitions as teens and young adults from worries about what a new lover might think of their penis. Therefore, they refrained from developing relationships which might lead to intimacy, causing them regret that their hypospadias was not repaired earlier.

Supporting our observations, men responding to an online survey who self-identified as having distal hypospadias also reported more penile curvature, more difficulties with sexual intercourse, and worse SHIM scores compared to men self-identified as being normal (Schlomer et al, 2014).

Body Image Concerns

Although it was not the chief complaint in any of our patients, 60% of the men in our series with uncorrected distal hypospadias also mentioned dissatisfaction with the appearance of their penis. Several of these were newly single and wanted repair before they started dating again. One man was embarrassed that the last words his wife said as she left him were, "I don't want a man with a broken dick."

The online survey of men by Schlomer et al similarly found that those self-identified with uncorrected distal hypospadias reported more dissatisfaction with their glans and meatus and their penile shaft axis than did men identifying as having a normal penis.

"Cosmetic" Versus "Reconstructive" Surgery

Surgeons commonly say "cosmetic" when they mean the "appearance" of the penis, and often tell parents that a distal hypospadias repair in their son would be "mostly cosmetic" when they believe there will be no functional improvements. However, parents hearing this often equate "cosmetic surgery" to something unnecessary and not worth the risk of complications, however small.

Plastic surgery societies have defined "cosmetic" and "reconstructive" operations. For example, the American Society of Plastic Surgeons describes cosmetic surgery as procedures done to "enhance and reshape *normal* body structures to improve appearance and confidence". In contrast, reconstructive procedures "treat body structures affected aesthetically or functionally by *congenital defects*".

> **By this standard, hypospadias repair is always "reconstructive", even if it is done primarily for appearances.**

Therefore, it is not medically correct to describe a repair as "mainly cosmetic", or even to refer to the "cosmetic outcomes" of hypospadias surgery. This caveat also applies to hypospadias publications, in which nearly all authors refer to the "cosmetic results" of surgery, rather than the "aesthetic outcomes".

WS wrote of the "superior cosmetic results" of TIP compared to meatal-based and onlay flap repairs in the first article describing the new operation (Snodgrass, 1994). For many years he used "cosmetic result" and "appearance" interchangeably in his publications, unaware of the negative connotations that the term "cosmetic" has for some parents.

Only in the past few years did he realize the confusion caused by these descriptions when he gave second opinions to parents told by the first pediatric urologist that their son did not "need" surgery for his distal hypospadias and that a repair would be "cosmetic". Their common response was that the penis would not be seen by others like a cleft lip will be, that they could not bear the guilt if their son developed any complications from a cosmetic operation, and that they were uncertain if they had the right to make this decision for their son when it was all about how his penis looked. It is interesting that parents of children with cleft lip rarely question the need for reconstructive surgery, even though cleft lip (unlike cleft palate) rarely causes functional issues and is primarily performed for "cosmetic" reasons.

Decision-Making For or Against Distal Hypospadias Repair

The surgeon evaluating an infant with hypospadias should measure the glans fusion and also determine if the penile shaft is straight or bent. Patients with abnormal anatomy are at risk for abnormal function, specifically urine spraying and /or sexual dysfunction, and the emotional impact both of those cause. Consequently, it is reasonable for surgeons to recommend repair to make the anatomy normal. As discussed in Chapter 23, distal hypospadias repair evokes more anxiety and causes more pain in teens and adults than it does in infants and children, and older patients typically are angry that surgery was not done when they were young. We have yet to encounter the teen or adult with uncorrected hypospadias who said, "I'm happy my parents waited so that I could make this decision."

Conversely, since the goal of hypospadias repair is to make normal penile anatomy, patients who already have a straight penis with normal glans fusion do not need urethroplasty and glansplasty, although the partial foreskin usually is managed by either circumcision or prepucioplasty.

Prevalence of These Functional Symptoms

Some might ask if the men with uncorrected hypospadias that we and Ching et al evaluated with uncorrected distal hypospadias are representative, or outliers from a larger group of asymptomatic unoperated adults. That question cannot be answered definitively as either yes or no. To our knowledge, neither the total number of boys born each year with distal hypospadias, nor the total number of primary repairs performed in them has been reported.

We can only extrapolate estimates of these. If this birth defect occurs in 1 of every 200 males (CDC Birth Defects), then approximately 10,000 newborns are diagnosed each year in the US, of which at least 70%, or 7000, have distal hypospadias (Duckett and Baskin, 1996). From case logs submitted to the Board of Urology by urologists seeking pediatric urology certification reviewed by Kogan and Feustel (2011), we can calculate the number of distal repairs by pediatric urologists to range from at least 5000 to approximately 6750, plus repairs done by general urologists and pediatric surgeons in the US. That suggests that few boys born with hypospadias reach adulthood without repair and that the pool from which our patients came is small - meaning they were more likely representative than outliers.

Regardless, informed consent requires surgeons to inform parents of newborns with hypospadias who have subnormal glans fusion and/or penile curvature that at least some will grow into men with functional voiding problems, sexual dysfunction, and dissatisfaction with their penis if it is not corrected. Furthermore, the finding that a third of our patients and those of Stojanovic et al, as well as a significant number of those reported by Schlomer et al, had penile curvature means that pediatric urologists evaluating infants with hypospadias cannot only look at the meatus to decide if surgery is needed; they must also determine if the penis is straight before recommending against reconstructive surgery.

Key Points

Data show that abnormal anatomy increases the likelihood for abnormal urinary and sexual function. Surgeons assessing infants with hypospadias should measure glans fusion and evaluate for penile curvature when making a recommendation for or against repair. Using objective criteria will reduce variation in the advice different pediatric urologists give parents.

Although the penis with hypospadias also looks abnormal, and surgery is done, in part, to impart a normal appearance, hypospadias repair is never "cosmetic". Realizing the confusion that term causes parents, surgeons should simply refer to penile "appearance" rather than its "cosmetic appearance".

References

State of the urology workforce and practice in the US, 2018. AUA, 2019

Ching CB, Wood HM, Ross JH, Gao T, and Angermeier KW: The Cleveland Clinic experience with adult hypospadias patients undergoing repair: their presentation and a new classification system. *BJU Int* 107: 1142, 2010

Dodds PR, Batter SJ, Shield DE, Serels SR, Garafola FA, Maloney PK: Adaptation of adults to uncorrected hypospadias. *Urology* 71: 682, 2008

Duckett JW and Baskin LS: Hypospadias. In Gillenwater JY (Ed) **Adult and Pediatric Urology**, 3rd Ed, 1996, pp 2549-2589

Facts about hypospadias. CDC Birth Defects.

Fichtner J, Filipas D, Mottrie AM, Voges GE, and Hohenfellner R: Analysis of meatal location in 500 men: wide variation questions need for meatal advancement in all pediatric anterior hypospadias cases. *J Urol* 154: 833, 1995

Hutton KAR and Babu R: Normal anatomy of the external urethral meatus in boys: implications for hypospadias repair. *BJU Int* 100: 161,2007

Kogan BA and Feustel PJ: What can we learn from pediatric urology certification logs? Urology 78: 147, 2011

Schlomer B, Breyer B, Copp H, Baskin L, DiSandro M: Do adult men with untreated hypospadias have adverse outcomes? A pilot study using a social media advertised survey. *J Pediatr Urol* 10: 672, 2014

Snodgrass W: Tubularized incised plate urethroplasty for distal hypospadias. *J Urol* 151: 464, 1994

Snodgrass W, Bush N and Cost N: Tubularized incised plate hypospadias repair for distal hypospadias. *J Pediatr Urol* 6: 408, 2010

Snodgrass W and Bush NC: Lessons from adults with uncorrected hypospadias: functional and aesthetic concerns. Abstract presented to SPU, Las Vegas, 2021

Stojanovic B, Bizic M, Majstorovic M, Kojovic V, and Djordjevic M: Penile curvature incidence in hypospadias: can it be determined? *Adv Urol*, 2011

Chapter 6

Urethroplasty When Ventral Curvature Is Less than 30°

We emphasize throughout this textbook that decision-making in hypospadias repair is based on the degree of VC. This chapter describes urethroplasty when the penis is straight, or has less than 30° VC measured objectively. That determination is made after degloving and before beginning the urethroplasty. As shown in the algorithm for primary repairs, these patients undergo TIP regardless of their meatal location.

Another theme in this textbook is that urethroplasty is best done using TIP or staged graft repairs. Together these 2 techniques manage all hypospadias and share many common steps. Consequently, surgeons can master those steps and more rapidly gain expertise to repair the spectrum of phenotypes comprising this condition. Gone are the days when a surgeon had to so carefully evaluate each patient and then choose from several techniques based on how he or she subjectively characterized the anatomic findings - a "wide" glans groove, a "healthy" urethral plate, "good" spongiosum, or "dysplastic" ventral tissues.

Throughout this book we also emphasize the importance of getting the repair right the first time. Complications are more often due to technical errors made in key steps of the right operation than they are from surgeons choosing the wrong operation for the patient. Therefore, complications can be reduced by doing each step in the best way. This chapter describes those for TIP.

The Goal of Hypospadias Repair

The goal of every hypospadias repair is to make the abnormal anatomy into a normal penis. That means the penis is made straight. The meatus is a vertical slit at the tip of the glans with normal glans fusion below it to the corona. The penile shaft is covered symmetrically by penis skin. There are no lingering complications, and no scars outside of the circumcision and/or median raphe lines.

Distal TIP Repair

TIP repair tubularizes the urethral plate into the neourethra. To make the neourethra a normal caliber, a midline incision is *always* made through the epithelium extending down to the underlying corpora. The final depth of that incision varies according to how deeply grooved the urethral plate is naturally - but whether it is essentially flat or deeply grooved to near the corpora, we always make a midline incision from within the hypospadiac meatus to the tip of the plate and down to the tunica albuginea of the corpora to ensure there will be a normal-sized neourethra.

From the beginning some have worried that this incision might scar, resulting in meatal stenosis or neourethral stricture. Consequently, they hesitate to incise the entire length of the urethral plate, or to extend the TIP incision deeply to the surface of the underlying corpora. But failure to incise the urethral

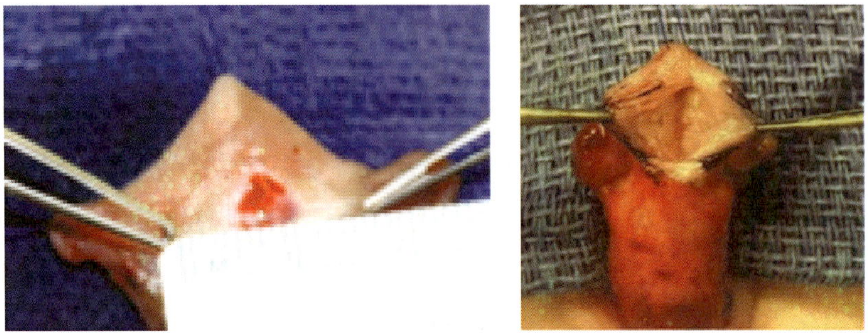

Figure 1. Incorrect versus correct TIP incision.
A, this minimal incision into the urethral plate made by Sarhan et al will not widen it sufficiently to create a normal caliber neourethra. B, correct TIP incision by Bush and Snodgrass opens the urethral plate much wider and will create a normal caliber neourethra.

plate correctly is the most common technical error surgeons make doing the procedure, which, ironically, *increases* the risk for the meatal stenosis or neourethral stricture they were trying to avoid.

We reported doing *no other operation* besides TIP in 426 consecutive patients with distal hypospadias, and none of them developed meatal stenosis or a stricture (Snodgrass and Bush et al, 2010). A subsequent meta-analysis of 3621 distal TIP repairs found 3.6% meatal stenosis and 1.3% urethral strictures (Pfistermuller et al, 2015). That should be proof enough that the TIP incision nearly always re-epithelializes without creating obstruction.

Later, some worried that a urethral plate which measured <8mm wide before TIP incision increased risk for complications (Holland and Smith, 2000; Sarhan et al, 2009). In response, we measured plate width before incision in 224 consecutive patients with distal hypospadias and found that 85% were <8mm. The pre-incision width averaged 6.1mm (2-11), compared to a post-incision width of 12mm (10-16), an increase of 116% (Bush and Snodgrass, 2017).

It is apparent that Sarhan et al did not incise the urethral plate correctly, since they reported only a 57% increase in width - half what we observed. This is clearly seen in representative photos from their versus our article (Figure 1).

This is another example of complications being the result of technical errors, rather than the fault of the anatomy or the operative method. Grahame Smith, who was the first to publish that pre-incision urethral plate <8mm might be a contraindication to TIP, later admitted he did not make the incision as deeply as did Snodgrass after watching him in a live-surgery workshop (Snodgrass and Bush, 2016).

More recently, Pippi-Salle has wondered if a subset of patients he describes as having an "unfavorable" plate that is "narrow" with "poor spongiosum" might be better repaired by G-TIP (Abbas and Pippi Salle, 2018). However, in a prior study rating urethral plate appearance for TIP, he reported poor agreement between pediatric urologists (El-Hout et al, 2010), which means different surgeons would judge "narrow" and "poor spongiosum" differently. In addition, no study has reported significantly decreased complications after G-TIP versus TIP. On the other hand, grafting the urethral plate incision may encourage some surgeons to incise it more deeply, i.e., to do TIP right. This topic is discussed below.

A colleague once told WS, "If there are 30 surgeons, there are 30 different ways to do a TIP." That is the heart of the problem when surgeons have complications in more than 10% of their distal TIP repairs. For many years we have emphasized the most common errors we read in the operative notes of other surgeons after a failed distal TIP: not incising the entire urethral plate from meatus to its distal tip deeply down to the corpora, tubularizing the plate too far distally, not covering the neourethra with a dartos flap.

To those we will add another: doing a dorsal plication and TIP repair when there is ventral curvature $\geq 30^\circ$ - regardless of meatal location. In other words,

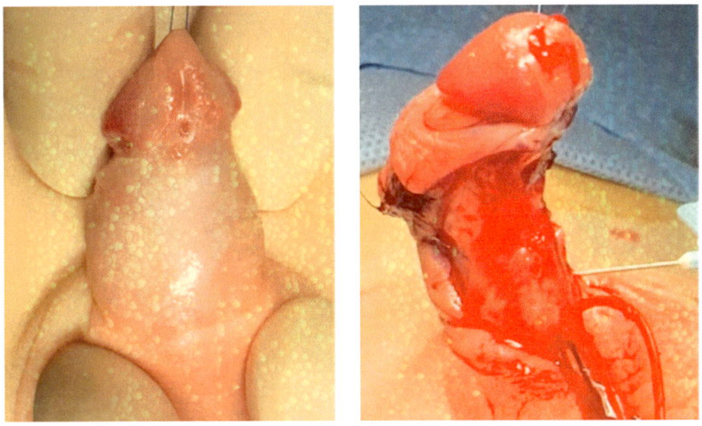

Figure 2. Ventral curvature > 30° despite a coronal meatus.
Regardless of meatal location, a patient with ventral curvature ≥ 30° should *not* have TIP repair. We inform *all* parents before a distal repair that it will be a staged operation if we encounter ventral curvature ≥ 30°.

a boy with a distal meatus whose penis is bent 30° or more should have either a STAC-TIP or STAC repair depending on the elasticity of the penile urethra as discussed in Chapter 10 (Figure 2).

Surgical Technique

Degloving

A holding stitch of 5-0 Prolene on an RB1 needle is placed horizontally in the glans. This size suture is sufficient both for maneuvering the penis and securing the urethral stent, and the monofilament does not scar the glans. "Snake-eyes" are rarely encountered postoperatively using this suture.

Then an 8Fr sound is passed into the distal urethra to detect a "thin" appearing area. This finding indicates a deficiency of dartos and spongiosum covering the urethra. When encountered, the initial skin incision is deviated proximally below this area to avoid inadvertent entry into the urethra.

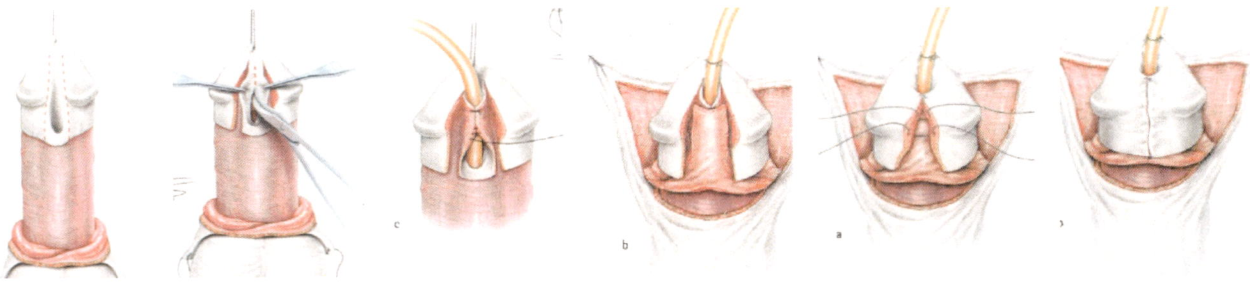

Figure 3. Distal TIP repair.
A, mirror image incisions are outlined along the visible edges of the glans wings where they join the urethral plate. The glans wings are then dissected laterally to 3 and 9 o'clock along the surface of the corpora, with additional dissection superiorly as needed to release downward tension on them. B, midline urethral plate incision is made to the underlying corpora from within the meatus to the tip of the plate. C, tubularizing the urethral plate starts distally at approximately the mid glans, at least 3-4mm from the end of the plate. The neourethra is sewn in 2 subepithelial layers with a continuous 7-0 Vicryl. The opening should be oval, and not round. D, a dartos flap is dissected ventrally and sutured over the neourethra. E, the neomeatus is created by approximating the glans wings over the neourethra using 3 interrupted, subepithelial 6-0 Vicryl sutures placed from the mid glans to the corona. The second stitch includes a bite of the dartos flap to hold it in place. The glans is *not* sutured to the urethra. *No* sutures are placed through the glans epithelium. F, after glansplasty, the inner prepucial collar is sutured together using subepithelial 7-0 Vicryl and an epithelial 9-0 Vicryl at the corona

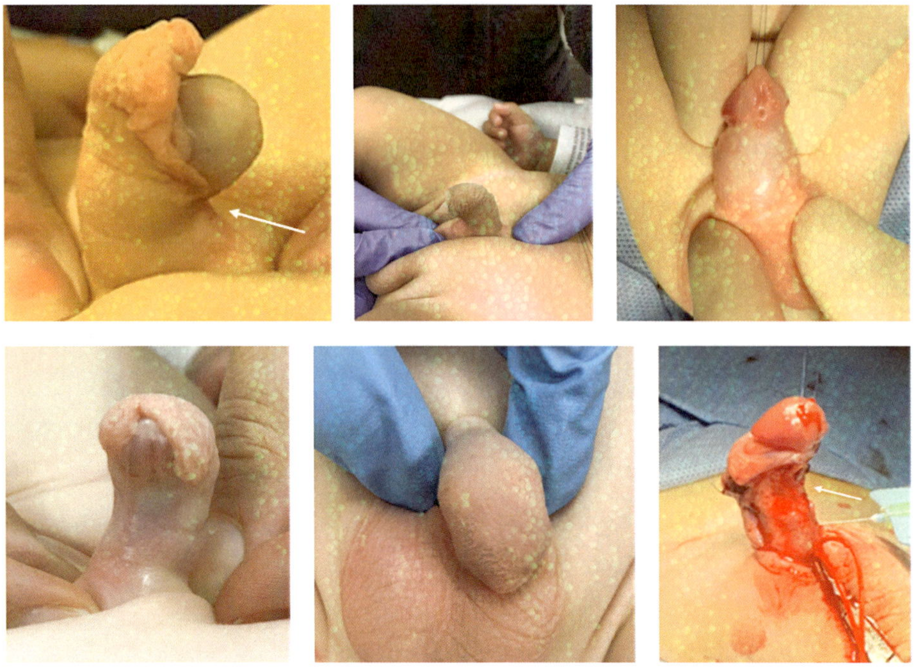

Figure 4. Warning signs of ventral curvature 30° or greater.
A, obviously deficient ventral shaft skin (arrow) may indicate VC ≥ 30° from short ventral corpora. B, a skin hump near the midshaft (arrow) is another sign of possible VC. C, different patient with a coronal meatus noted on exam to have apparent ventral curvature in D, with a dorsal midshaft skin hump opposite the bend as seen in E. He was found during artificial erection to have 35° of VC in the midshaft as indicated by the arrow in F. Note that he was degloved ventrally until artificial erection was done and the extent and location of the bending was identified.

For many years we made a traditional circumferential degloving incision in all boys with distal hypospadias whose parents wanted the end result to be a circumcised penis. That was based on the presumption that most of these patients had either a straight penis, or VC < 30° that could be straightened by dorsal plication (Snodgrass & Bush, 2011). However, as mentioned in Chapter 2, we now know that 1 of every 3 patients with a distal meatus has VC, which in half of those is ≥ 30°. These 15% should be considered to have a proximal variant and managed by STAC-TIP or STAC repair as mentioned above.

Often there are signs predicting VC ≥ 30° in a patient with a distal meatus. These include markedly deficient ventral shaft skin and dorsal skin humps located on the midshaft, as shown in Figure 4.

However, we have encountered patients in whom there were no signs of curvature until artificial erection was done. For that reason, today we begin all primary hypospadias repairs using a ventral incision as shown in Figure 5. There is no downside to beginning the operation in this manner, and, in fact, various abnormalities of the penoscrotal junction often seen in boys with distal hypospadias, including scrotal webs extending up the penile shaft and penile torsion, are more readily corrected via a midline raphe incision.

Other advantages of ventral degloving are that it facilitates urethral mobilization down to within the scrotum during STAC-TIP and maintains the foreskin for urethroplasty grafting should that be necessary when VC ≥ 30° is encountered. It is also the correct skin incision for those who desire foreskin reconstruction for the final aesthetic result.

Since this VC can be found unexpectantly, we inform all caregivers of the possibility repair will require more than 1 operation.

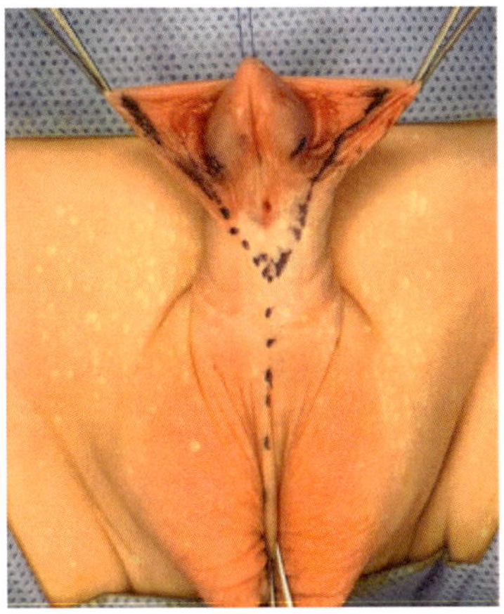

Figure 5. Ventral degloving incision for distal hypospadias repair.
Incision lines are marked along the ventral edge of the prepuce taking care to preserve 4mm of inner mucosal collar away from the corona, which is also marked. Those lines extend alongside the urethral plate and then meet in the median raphe and continue down to the scrotum. The initial dissection is done close to the skin on one side, preserving its underlying dartos along the corpora to make a coverage layer for the neourethra if TIP is done. Dissection on the other side releases dartos from the surface of the corpora to preserve with the skin in order to create a dartos flap to cover corporotomy incisions if STAC-TIP is done. Once the skin is released and artificial erection is performed, degloving can be completed dorsally when the penis is straight or has VC < 30°. When there is VC ≥ 30° the 1st stage of STAC-TIP is done, keeping the foreskin hood in place.

Whether the initial incision is ventral or circumferential, it preserves 4mm of the inner prepuce along the glans ventrally, which will later become part of the "mucosal collar". This collar should be symmetric around the glans to mimic the appearance of a normal, circumcised penis when that end result is desired.

In the past we made these collars approximately 1cm in width since that is a typical size created by Gomco and plastibell circumcisions. However, the inner prepuce will sometimes swell disproportionately and remain enlarged and unsightly when healing is complete. It is interesting that European surgeons usually leave no collar, but instead sew the shaft skin just under the corona. We have chosen a middle ground of a 4mm wide collar.

That decision takes into account that the inner prepucial collar has an importance beyond aesthetics. It also protects the urethroplasty and glansplasty from tension if the ventral shaft skin is sized too short or contracts somewhat postoperatively. Otherwise, that tension can result in a coronal fistula or glans dehiscence.

We use the Beaver 69 blade to make the skin incision. It is important to cut the ventral part of the incision near the midline just through the skin, avoiding injury to the distal urethra. We do not inject epinephrine before incising the skin in distal repairs, and we also do not insert a catheter into the urethra during degloving. A catheter elevates the ventral wall of the urethra towards the degloving dissection, whereas dissecting right under the ventral skin avoids the urethra as it drops away.

Previously we dissected ventrally just under the skin, preserving the underlying dartos to make a coverage flap for the neourethra. Today knowing that some boys will be found to have VC resulting in a STAC-TIP, we dissect immediately under the skin on one side, but deeper on the surface of the corpora on the other in case a dartos flap is needed to cover corporotomies.

We do not dissect with either a cautery or a tourniquet since there is little bleeding from surgery within the correct planes.

Artificial Erection

Next, artificial erection is done *in every case*. We do not apply a tourniquet initially since it can conceal low bending near the penoscrotal junction. If artificial erection suggests curvature low on the shaft, the ventral skin is further divided down the median raphe into the scrotum to better expose that region. Then the erection is repeated.

Any apparent curvature is next measured. We prefer the goniometer as discussed in Chapter 3, but a protractor or other method to objectively determine its extent can also be used.

VC measuring < 30° is straightened using a dorsal Heineke-Mikulicz plication described in Chapter 2. VC ≥ 30° results in a staged STAC-TIP with straightening by 3 corporotomies, and is described in Chapter 10.

We emphasize that the penis should *always* be evaluated for VC by artificial erection, and that curvature found should *always* be straightened before urethroplasty. We have encountered VC during reoperations when the prior surgeon reported spontaneous erection or an erection induced by finger compression at the penile base appeared straight, and presume the penis was not fully erect. As mentioned in Chapter 2, artificial erection does not overfill the corpora to create false curvature.

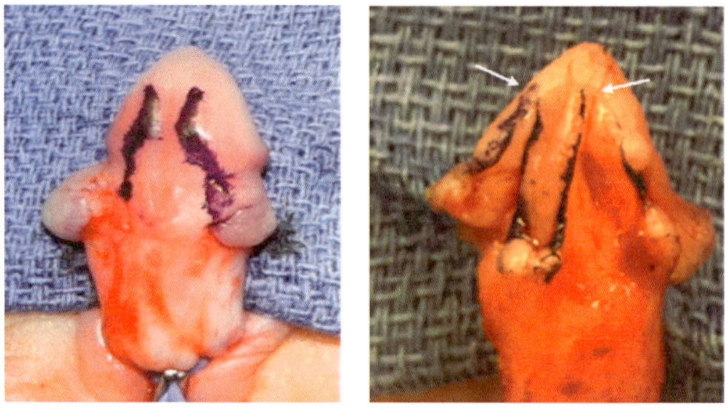

Figure 6. Incision lines to create glans wings.
A, incision lines to separate the urethral plate from the glans wings are marked along their visible junction as shown. Next 1:100,000 epinephrine will be injected. Note there is also a tourniquet in place. It is important to minimize bleeding so that the surgeon can clearly see the correct plane for dissecting the glans wings. B, the glans wings incisions extend to the distal end of the urethral plate as shown by the arrows.

Making Glans Wings

If a tourniquet has not been applied already, it is placed now before glans incisions are made. The lines for those incisions are marked along the visual junction of the urethral plate to the glans on each side (Figure 6). We do not measure the width of the plate to decide where these incisions will be made, nor do we make the incisions wider into the glans if the urethral plate appears to be narrow. We simply mark from the end of the plate down along its margin and across the inner prepuce.

1:100,000 epinephrine is then injected along these lines. This makes it easier to find the correct plane for dissection than when a tourniquet is used alone. Similarly, epinephrine injection alone does not provide the same bloodless field for dissection that the combination of injection plus a tourniquet provides. It is important that the surgeon sees this plane clearly. Some surgeons are reluctant to inject epinephrine while others avoid tourniquets, but we always use both and can attribute no complications to that longstanding practice.

We incise just though the glans epithelium with the Beaver knife, and then continue glans dissection using scissors. The plane between the urethral plate and glans is identified, taking care to avoid making a hole in the side of the plate or leaving the glans wing thin and more difficult to suture later. Each wing is mobilized from the corpora laterally to approximately 3 and 9 o'clock (Figure 7). Additional dissection is done as needed along the surface of the corpora superiorly to release any downward tension on the wings, which can cause the glans to dehisce.

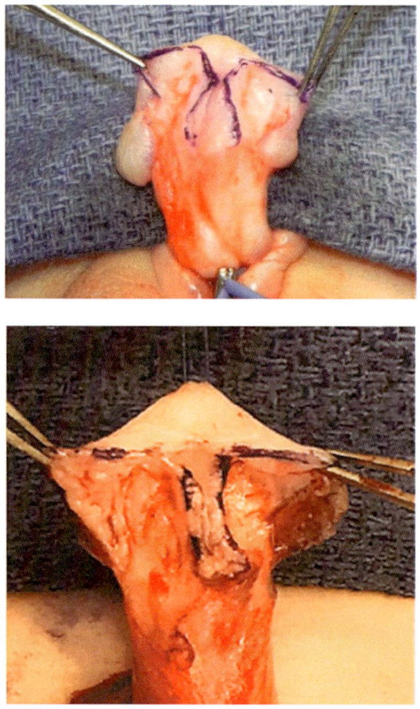

Figure 7. Mobilization of the glans wings.
A, the glans wings should be mobilized at least to 3 and 9 o'clock, as shown here. However, we have learned that additional dissection distally at 3 and 9 o'clock releases downward tension and decreases the likelihood for glans dehiscence. Consequently, today our completed dissection more often resembles the appearance shown in B. Note the thickness of the glans wings after dissection in the correct plane, which makes suturing during glansplasty more secure.

Occasionally a hole is made in the side of the urethral plate as the glans wings are created. We close the defect using interrupted 9-0 Vicryl, knowing it will later

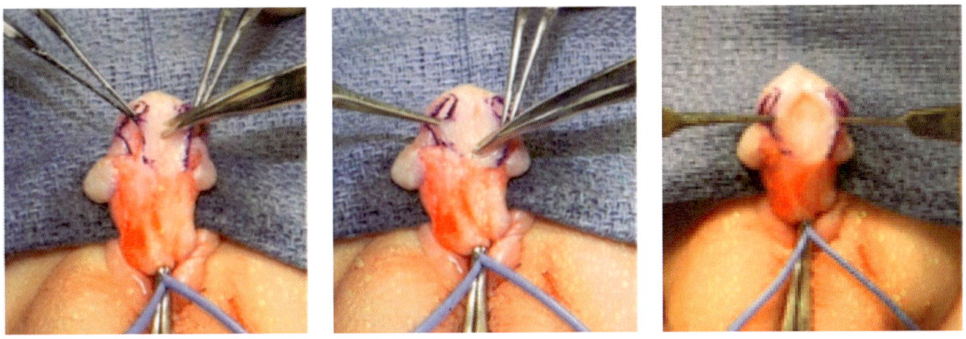

Figure 8. Urethral plate incision.
A, with counter-traction by the surgeon and assistant delineating the midline, the plate is initially incised at its midpoint using tenotomy scissors. B, incision continues down to within the meatus as shown, and then distally to the end of the plate, recognized by the junction of shiny plate to more granular glans tissues. C, dorsal plate incision is completed. Note it extends from within the meatus to (but not into) the visible glans distally, and deeply to the corpora. Tubularization will create a neourethra with normal caliber. The "raw area" left by the TIP incision re-epithelializes during healing without scarring into meatal stenosis or a stricture. The surgeon does not have to worry about the relative widths of the skin strips on either side versus the incised area.

be covered by both the dartos flap over the neourethra and the ipsilateral glans wing during glansplasty.

TIP Incision

Next, the urethral plate is held by the surgeon and the assistant on either side with 0.5mm Castro-Viejo forceps, gently stretching it laterally to delineate the midline. Tenotomy scissors incise the plate beginning in the middle and then extending proximally to within the meatus and distally to its tip. This incision is carried from the epithelial surface down to near the tunic of the corporal bodies underneath (Figure 8). We *always* make this TIP relaxing incision through the entire length of the plate down to the corpora. Not only does it widen the urethral plate, but it also releases longitudinal tension within the plate which can be observed while the tissues are being cut.

We state again that the most common technical error during TIP repair is failure to incise the urethral plate throughout its length and down all the way to the corpora. Visitors who have problems with meatal stenosis routinely comment after watching us that they thought they were making a deep TIP incision until they saw ours! Surgeons who worry about the size of the "raw area" that must re-epithelialize and are concerned the incision will scar and stenose hesitate to make it deep throughout the plate, preferring to do just what seems enough to roll the neourethra. This reasoning ignores results from centers worldwide showing that meatal stenosis and urethral stricture following TIP are uncommon. Ironically, it is the failure to incise deep that makes these complications more likely.

WS has made the TIP incision from within the meatus to the end of the plate and deep to the corpora for over 20 years, yet our incidence of either meatal stenosis or neourethral strictures is less than 1%. Similarly, meta-analysis of distal TIP results found meatal stenosis in only 3.6% and strictures in 1.3% of over 3600 repairs (Pfistermuller et al, 2015).

Tubularizing the Urethral Plate

A 6Fr stent (5Fr when the glans width is < 14mm) is passed into the bladder and tied to the glans holding suture. This stent is only used to provide urinary drainage. It is *not* a template for sizing the caliber of the neourethra, which will be greater than 8Fr, and usually more than 10Fr, when the TIP incision is done right. Nor is it necessary to tubularize the neourethra over a larger stent to ensure it will have a normal caliber and then exchange that stent for a smaller one.

Urethral plate tubularization begins distally at the mid glans, always more than 3mm from the tip of the plate (Figure 9). The first stitch is through epithelium, and then the remainder of the closure is subepithelial. In coronal and subcoronal repairs we run the

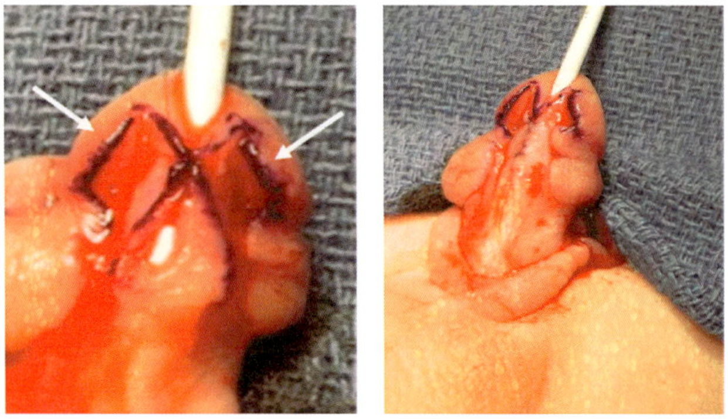

Figure 9. Urethral plate tubularization.
A, the first stitch is placed in the urethral plate adjacent to the midpoint of the glans (arrows), no closer than 3mm from the end of the urethral plate. The opening should be oval, not rounded. B, tubularization is completed in 2 subepithelial layers. Note again that the opening distally is wide, which helps prevent meatal stenosis.

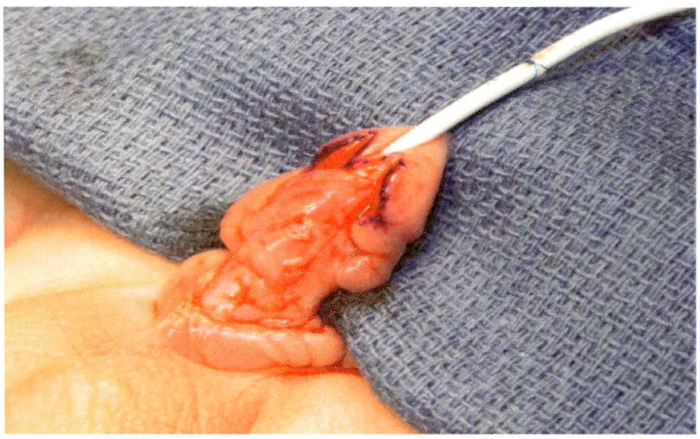

Figure 10. Ventral dartos covering over the neourethra.
A dartos barrier flap *always* covers the neourethra to decrease likelihood for a fistula.

suture proximally, tie a knot, and then run the second layer back distally using the same stitch. When the meatus is lower on the distal shaft we interrupt the first layer and then run the second.

We use 7-0 Vicryl on a TG 140-8 needle because we prefer that small, precise needle to the larger ones on monofilament sutures.

Dartos Flap Coverage Over the Neourethra

Next a ventral dartos flap is mobilized proximally to distally to cover over the neourethra. The distal edges are sutured lateral to the meatus with 9-0 Vicryl (Figure 10).

When degloving is done in the correct plane just under the ventral skin there is sufficient ventral dartos to create a barrier flap. If not, a dorsal dartos flap can be harvested from the shaft skin, button-holed, and transposed ventrally.

Occasionally we read an operative report stating there was not enough room between the glans wings and neourethra to place the dartos flap. We never encounter this situation, regardless of glans size, which most likely means the glans wings were not adequately mobilized.

We also read reports in patients presenting with fistulas that "adjacent tissues" were used to cover the neourethra, rather than an actual dartos flap. There is no reason not to make a dartos flap for the barrier layer between the neourethral sutures and those in the overlying skin and glans closures.

Glansplasty

The glans wings are stretched again to test for tension, and additional dissection along the corpora is done when needed to relieve any residual tension. Glansplasty sutures the glans wings directly to each other beginning distally where the ventral lip of the meatus should be.

We first place a 9-0 Vicryl stitch though the epithelium at approximately the midpoint of the glans wings to properly align them. The distance from that stitch to the corona should be 3-5mm to create normal glans fusion.

Then a 6-0 Vicryl on an S29 needle is placed subepithelially under the 9-0 suture. Next, 2 more interrupted 6-0 Vicryl stitches are placed subepithelially. The 2nd includes a small bite of the dartos flap to hold it in place, and the 3rd approximates the coronal margin (Figure 11). Blue marks delineating the corona on each side (not shown in the figure) help guide suture placement and correct alignment of the glans wings. This total of 3 glansplasty stitches reliably creates normal glans fusion, averaging 4mm.

We *never* do a second layer closure through the epithelium, because it is unnecessary and to ensure that the glans surface remains smooth as it is normally.

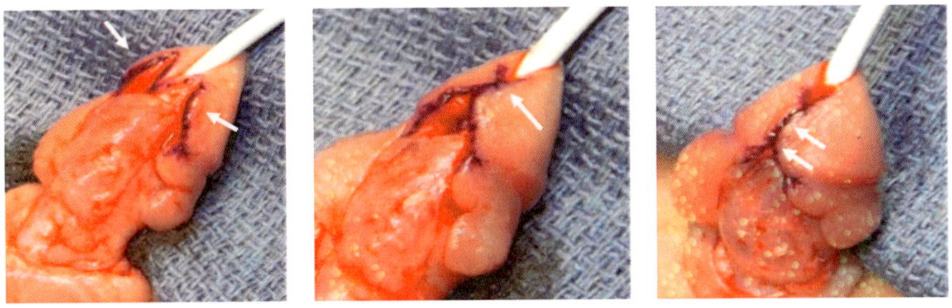

Figure 11. Glansplasty.
A,B, the first stitch is placed at the mid glans, indicated by the arrows, to create the glanular meatus in its normal location. The glans wings are *not* sutured to the tubularized urethral plate beneath. C, an additional 2 interrupted subepithelial stitches complete glansplasty from the neomeatus to the corona as shown by the arrows. The 2nd stitch includes a bite of the dartos flap to help hold it in place distally. An epithelial layer is *not* needed in the glansplasty and can leave visible marks in the skin. Mattress stitches that include the skin of the glans should *never* be done.

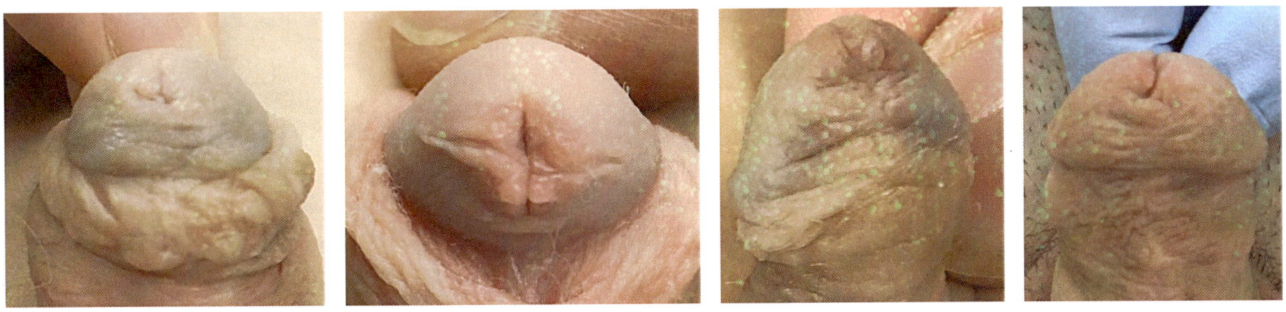

Figure 12. Avoidable scars created by suture closure of the glans epithelium.
A,B,C show typical transverse scars from closing the glans epithelium. These do not happen with subepithelial glans wings approximation. D, these scars persist into adulthood.

Suturing through the glans epithelium for a second layer closure can create transverse scars (Figure 12), which do not occur when sutures are placed subepithelially. These scars last a lifetime, reminding the boy grown into a man that he was born with a defect of his penis, and worrying him that a lover will ask why the head of his penis has scars.

Although WS was taught to approximate the glans with mattress sutures which included the epithelium, terrible scars can result from these (Chapter 16, Figure 8), especially if the surgeon is trying to overcome tension on the glans wings or ties the sutures too tightly. When tension is felt on the glans wings further dissection should be done to relieve it, rather than placing mattress sutures to overcome it.

In flap repairs the neourethra is sewn to the glans wings. However, in TIP and graft repairs the glans should *not* be sewn to the neourethra (Figures 11,13). Typically, the first stitch of the glansplasty is placed a

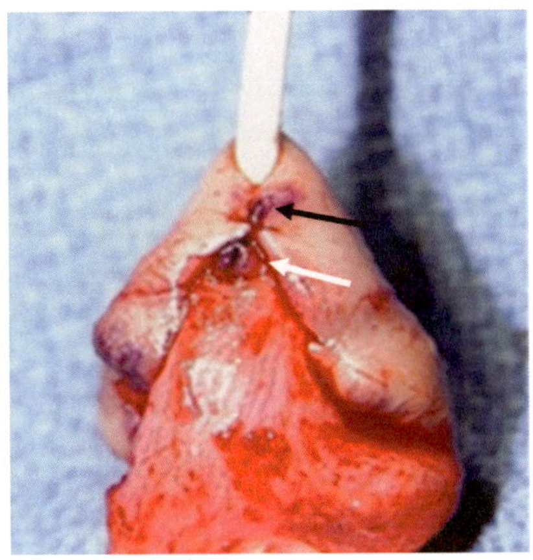

Figure 13. Glansplasty over the neourethra.
The glans wings are approximated *over* the tubularized neourethra - *not sewn to it*. The black arrow shows the first glansplasty stitch, beyond the end of the neourethra indicated by the white arrow. This gap heals spontaneously and without complications, in part because the remaining glansplasty covers over that space.

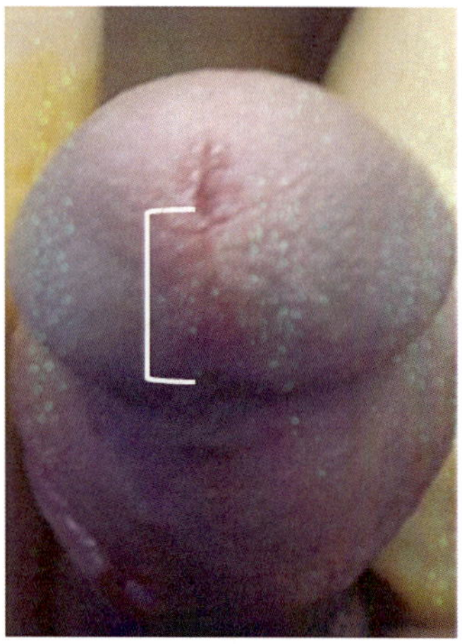

Figure 14. Normal glans wings approximation.
The glans wings approximation (white line) from meatus to corona should be more than 2.5mm long, and averages 4mm after TIP glansplasty.

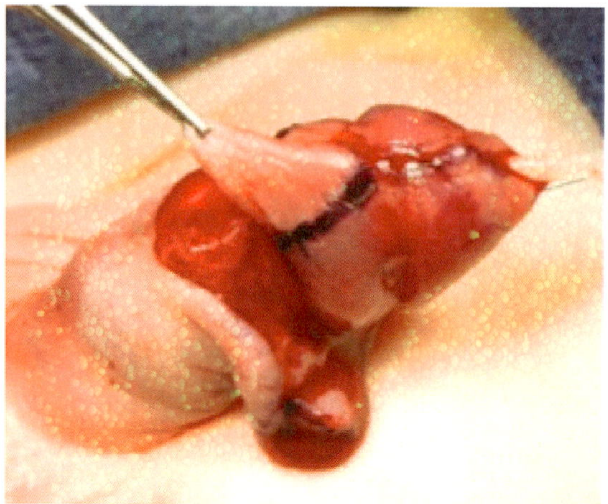

Figure 15. Shaft skin is excised from the mucosal collar.
Shaft skin which originally connected to the hypospadias meatus is excised so that the inner prepuce can be approximated to itself. There should be no tension on the closure of the mucosal collar.

short distance beyond the opening in the tubularized neourethra (Figure 13). The gap between glans and the tubularized urethral or graft plate heals spontaneously without stricture or fistula. In fact, the 2nd and 3rd stitches of the glansplasty approximate the glans wings over and proximal to the end of the neourethra. A surgeon determined to sew glans wings to the underlying neourethra may tubularize the plate too far distally to achieve that - thereby creating iatrogenic meatal stenosis.

The length of the glans closure, from the ventral lip of the meatus to the corona, should be more than 2.5mm, which is the lower limit of normal in boys without hypospadias (Hutton and Babu, 2007). The usual length after TIP repair is 4mm (Figure 14). Normal glans closure is necessary for both normal aesthetics and urinary function, specifically to avoid urine spraying.

Uniting the Mucosal Collar

The next step after glansplasty is to bring the inner prepuce together in the ventral midline to create the mucosal collar. First, remnant shaft skin from near the original meatus is cut off as shown in Figure 15, taking care to not remove so much that the subsequent closure will be tight. Next, we use 9-0 Vicryl to approximate the collar just below the corona, placing it through the epithelium since it is often too thin here for subepithelial suturing. Then the remainder of the collar is sewn using interrupted subepithelial 7-0 Vicryl. The width of the mucosal collar should be uniform circumferentially. We usually create an approximately 4mm collar, but previously we created one that was 8-10mm.

There should be no tension on this mucosal collar approximation, which is the site where most fistulas occur. Tension from a tight closure can also promote glans dehiscence. On the other hand, failure to make a collar can also contribute to these complications by exposing this critical area to tension from the shaft skin.

Shaft Skin Closure

There is a variable extent of ventral shaft skin deficiency to reconcile during closure, ranging from a short gap from the skin to the mucosal collar, to finding the skin is absent between the penoscrotal junction and the mucosal collar. The goal is to provide symmetric penile skin coverage around the penis as is found in a boy with a normal penis. The dorsal foreskin hood and any skin humps serve as tissue repositories to provide the needed skin ventrally.

Boys and men typically have a ventral median raphe, and skin closure during hypospadias repair should provide this aesthetic, concealing the wound in a natural skin line. Figure 16 shows the steps involved,

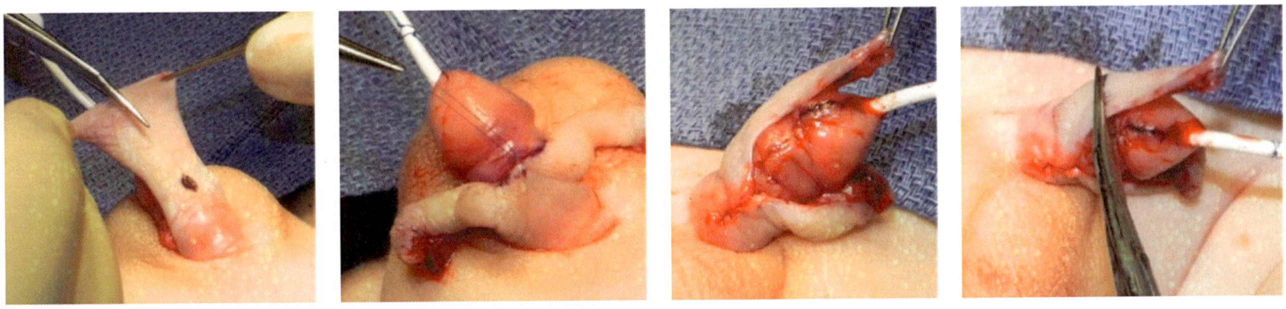

Figure 16. Shaft skin closure.
A, the foreskin hood is incised down its midline to the mark denoting the level of the corona. B, the dorsal shaft skin is sutured to the mucosal collar at 12 o'clock using a subepithelial 7-0 Vicryl. C, then the ventral skin is closed up the midline from proximally to distally with interrupted subepithelial 7-0 Vicryl to create a median raphe. D, excess skin is excised to finish the circumcision.

including a relaxing incision down the foreskin hood to the corona so that skin can be rotated ventrally.

It is important to keep the penoscrotal junction from riding up the shaft as the skin flaps are being sized, as that will result in the surgeon cutting the ventral skin too short. A suture placed at the penoscrotal junction and then held with a hemostat while the ventral skin is sized and closed helps to prevent this. We usually place 5-0 PDS sutures at the 3 and 9 o'clock positions subepithelialy along the penoscrotal junction as well to hold the skin in place, particularly for those with a large suprapubic fat pad. It is also important to keep the penis on maximum stretch during closure so that the skin will be cut to the length needed during erections.

Some surgeons prefer to close the ventral shaft skin up the median raphe first and then make the dorsal relaxing incision and excise the excess skin. The end result is the same: symmetric skin coverage circumferentially around the penile shaft, closed without tension.

When tension is felt despite careful sizing of the skin flaps, additional length can be gained by making short oblique cuts through or near the tight region ventrally. Excision or incision into the underlying dartos along the skin edges will often additionally release tension.

When there is penile torsion or lateral curvature in addition to distal hypospadias, skin closure is more difficult, as discussed in Chapter 21. In these circumstances, leaving a longer mucosal collar can help with the left skin deficiency.

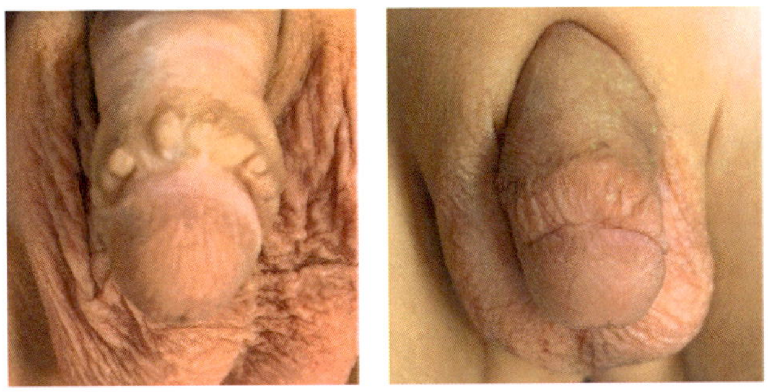

Figure 17. Ugly skin closure from 'baseball' stitching. A, ruffled scars from a running epithelial skin closure. These scars remain indefinitely unless skin revision is done. B, subepithelial closure heals in a smooth line that resembles the scar after a newborn clamp circumcision.

We *strongly encourage* subepithelial skin closure, no matter which suture is used, to reduce likelihood for suture tunnels. Those fill with keratin, becoming more unsightly and malodorous, and remain indefinitely unless they are cut open.

We also *strongly discourage* "baseball" stitching, which might save a few minutes of the surgeon's time at the cost of a ruffled, unsightly circumcision line as seen in Figure 17. As mentioned above regarding glansplasty, these abnormal scars disturb teens and adults, reminding them, and their lovers, that they were born with a penis defect. The healed closure should resemble a newborn clamp circumcision, with smooth incision lines.

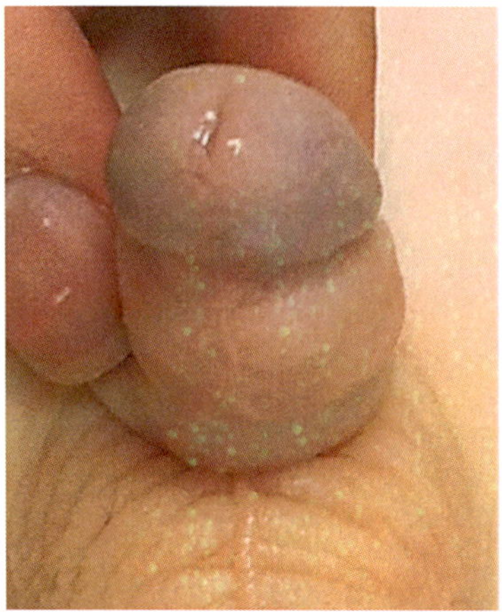

Figure 18. Normal anatomy after distal TIP repair. Distal hypospadias repair should create a normal penis: straight, with a slit meatus and normal glans fusion, and no visible scars outside of the circumcision line and median raphe. No other technique so reliably achieves this as does TIP repair.

Surgeons must also be able and willing to reconstruct the foreskin during distal hypospadias repair for parents who prefer that to circumcision. Those who feel differently should not discourage those parents with warnings that prepucioplasty increases complications, since published evidence proves otherwise, but rather simply refer the patient to another surgeon who will reconstruct the foreskin. Prepucioplasty is described in Chapter 8.

The goal of hypospadias repair is to make abnormal anatomy normal. In addition to a straight penis with a vertical meatus and normal glans fusion, that includes having no unsightly ruffles or divots, or scars outside the circumcision line and ventral median raphe.

TIP is the most reliable repair to achieve these goals for distal hypospadias when the penis is straight or has less than 30° ventral curvature. A typical postoperative result is shown in Figure 18.

Postoperative Care

Urinary Diversion

We use a 5Fr or 6Fr stent for urinary diversion in all prepubertal boys for 1 week after distal TIP repair, the size varying according to glans width less than or greater than 14mm. We emphasize that the neourethra is *not* sized around the stent; rather, deep TIP incision creates a neourethra with a normal caliber which is always greater than 8Fr and usually more than 10Fr. A larger stent is not needed for urine drainage, even in older boys approaching puberty, and potentially exerts pressure on the repair early after surgery when tissues are edematous.

The stent drains urine during this period of early postoperative edema. However, if it falls out prematurely we do not replace it unless urinary retention or extravasation develop, which are both rare. In fact, for a period of time we did not use postoperative stents after distal TIPs and confirmed that urethroplasty complications are the same with versus without urine diversion. However, we found more skin complications, especially edema causing secondary phimosis, that we surmised occurred because the bandage leaving the meatus clear for voiding provided less compression to the penis immediately after surgery. Therefore, we resumed postoperative diversion so that we could place a better bandage.

We also stress that suprapubic drainage is *never* needed after hypospadias repair, whether distal or proximal. Furthermore, we never use a balloon catheter after urethroplasty in a child, in part from superstition that active boys might forcibly dislodge it and disrupt the urethroplasty. Furthermore, a 6Fr stent provides adequate urine drainage but a balloon catheter the same size has a much smaller lumen for urine to pass since the channel to inflate the balloon takes some of the internal space.

Bandage

A medium Tegaderm™ is wrapped around the penis. Then gauzes are placed on the ventral side of the penis to provide gentle compression against the abdomen. These are held in place by a larger Tegaderm (Figure 19). This bandage falls off spontaneously and is not changed or replaced. There is no medical reason to use more complex bandages, especially something that requires sedation to remove.

Nerve Blocks and Medications

We do not give a preoperative antibiotic for primary hypospadias repair in prepubertal boys. All patients have a caudal nerve block before surgery begins, or a penile nerve block for those too old or with a spinal

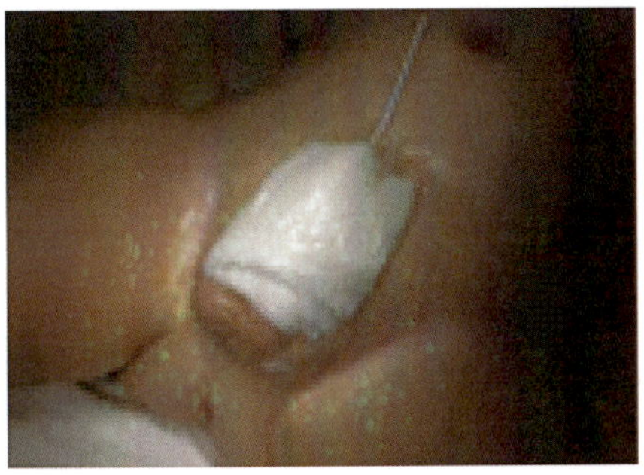

Figure 19. Postoperative bandage.
This bandage includes a medium Tegaderm™ wrapped around the penis, and a larger Tegaderm™ placed over gauze to hold the penis against the abdomen with gentle compression.

anomaly which precludes a caudal. Penile blocks comprise injections in the dorsal penopubic region to both sides of midline, and additional injection in the scrotal median raphe near the perineum. A disadvantage of penile blocks is that the dorsal injections can track inferiorly under the shaft skin and distort it. For that reason we prefer caudals.

In addition, all patients receive intraoperative ketorolac.

Following surgery, boys less than 1-year old receive alternating acetaminophen and ibuprofen every 3 hours, except when asleep, for 48 hours. This regimen begins with the first dose of acetaminophen given 3 hours after surgery, when intraoperative ketorolac and the caudal nerve block are wearing off.

Boys over 1 year of age are provided hydrocodone with acetaminophen as a substitute for acetaminophen alone to use as needed, although few require a narcotic before age 18 months.

We do not routinely prescribe oxybutynin for bladder spasms in infants less than 1 year of age. Boys 1 to 3 years of age are given 2mg/kg twice daily, while boys older than 3 are dosed three times daily with liquid, or the extended release oxybutynin once daily when they can swallow a small pill.

For many years we prescribed sulfamethoxazole/trimethoprim once daily during urinary diversion, despite knowing there were few data supporting this antibiotic prophylaxis. Both wound and urinary infections are uncommon, and a study confirming these occur in less than 5% of patients with no benefit from postoperative antibiotic prophylaxis (Doersch et al, 2022) convinced us to stop using it after distal TIP.

On the day of catheter removal, boys old enough to swallow a small pill can benefit from starting pyridium 4mg/kg for 2 days as an analgesic when voiding.

Hospitalization

There is no medical reason to admit otherwise healthy patients to the hospital after hypospadias repair. Ambulatory surgery has been the standard in the US since the mid-1980s, and there are no data suggesting complications are increased by that practice. We realize that some health care systems incentivize hospitalization, in which case every effort should be made to reduce bother and worry to the patient and parents, especially since there is no medical necessity for him to be in hospital.

Some surgeons respond that their parents demand hospitalization, fearing they will be unable to properly manage their son at home. We reassure such parents that there is no special care given in hospital that they will have to provide at home.

Dilations

We do not do, and WS has never done, therapeutic meatal dilations following TIP repair. The neourethra swells internally after surgery, similar to the penile skin externally. Accordingly, the meatus may appear small and the stream thin, observations that sometimes concern the parents. However, if the patient voids without straining and does not have UTIs, we reassure that these are normal, temporary findings. The stream becomes more full with time as the edema subsides.

This course of events has been documented by uroflowmetry showing a significant increase in Qmax between studies obtained at 2 months versus repeat studies 12 months after distal TIP repair (Holmdahl et al, 2006).

The improvement that some attribute to early dilations almost certainly is the result of resolving edema and would have happened without those treatments. Patients we have evaluated for 2nd opinions because of a "small-appearing" meatus and/or "fine" stream who do not have symptoms (straining) or signs of

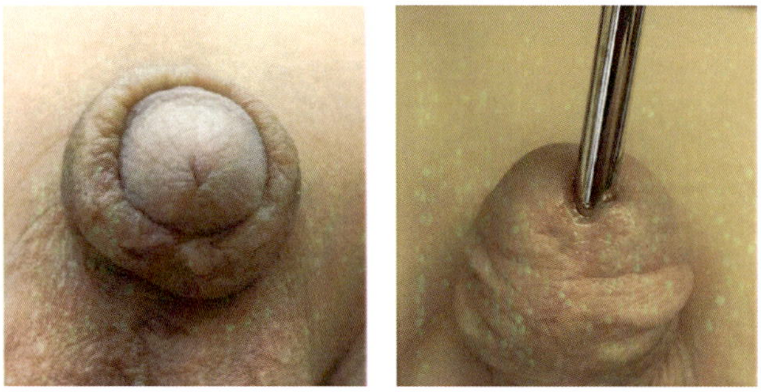

Figure 20. Small-appearing but normal-sized neomeatus.
A, small- appearing meatus after distal TIP repair in a patient without stranguria, UTI, or retention. B, the same patient, showing that a 12Fr sound passes easily. Therefore, this small- appearing meatus is normal-sized.

obstruction (UTI, retention) calibrate a normal size (≥ 8Fr). An example is shown in Figure 20.

Results After Distal Tip Repair

No other distal hypospadias repair has been scrutinized more closely than TIP. Similar results reported by multiple institutions worldwide indicate the deep TIP incision heals without creating meatal stenosis or urethral stricture. They also show the operation makes normal anatomy regardless of a wide or narrow, or flat versus deep urethral plate. These data, reviewed below, should be convincing to surgeons who fear that deep incision, or some anatomic feature such as a narrow or flat plate, increases risks for complications.

Rather than unfavorable anatomy, the main cause of urethroplasty complications after distal TIP, or any method of hypospadias repair, is technical errors made by the surgeon.

Common Technical Errors

Here are some errors that surgeons made, gleaned from the operative reports of patients with complications. They straightened "moderate chordee" with a dorsal plication and the VC recurred along with a fistula or glans dehiscence. The TIP incision was not cut deeply, or only included a portion of the urethral plate, in patients with meatal stenosis or a strictured neourethra. The plate was tubularized proximally to distally continuing too far so that it could be stitched to the glans wings and created meatal stenosis. A single-layer tubularization was done, or the neourethra was not covered with a dartos flap, contributing to a fistula. The glans wings were approximated with a single stitch at the corona and dehisced. Or they were closed with mattress sutures that gouged into the glans, or with epithelial stitches that made visible scars.

All of these can be avoided. There may be other ways to do the various steps than we describe that *give the same result.* However, we have carefully monitored our outcomes for nearly 30 years and know that TIP repair done as explained above should achieve the same urethroplasty and aesthetic results as ours.

Therefore, it is important that surgeons who do TIP differently review their results to confirm they have less than 10% urethroplasty complications. Those who believe they perform TIP repair as we describe but find they have more than 10% complications should watch our surgical videos on YouTube and/or visit our center to observe us and learn what steps they are doing differently.

Urethroplasty Results

We have not used a different operation than TIP for distal hypospadias with less than 30° VC in more than 30 years. We published results in 426 consecutive boys with follow up, finding urethroplasty complications in 4% that were equally divided between fistulas and glans dehiscence. There were no strictures and the 1 patient with meatal stenosis developed it secondarily 6 years later from BXO (Snodgrass and Bush et al, 2010).

Similarly, a meta-analysis reviewed 3621 patient outcomes following primary distal TIP reported in 49 publications from 1994 to 2012. At a mean of 16 months postoperatively 4.5% (3-7.5) of patients had reoperations. Fistulas occurred in 5.7% (4.0-8.2), meatal stenosis in 3.6% (1.7-7.4), and strictures in 1.3% (0.8-2.2) (Pfistermuller et al, 2015).

These data show that surgeons performing distal TIP repair should have less than 10% complications.

However, the complication rate of most surgeons is not known, in part because those with more usually do not publish them. Many parents tell us their

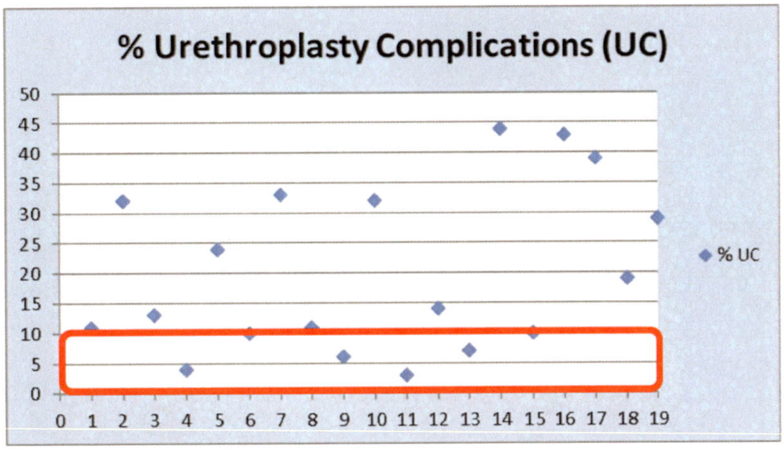

Figure 21. Complication rates after distal hypospadias repair.
The red box indicates surgeons in the Dutch Hypospadias Study whose documented complication rates were ≤ 10%.

surgeon quoted 95% success for distal repairs. But a report from the Dutch Hypospadias Study is sobering (Figure 21). They systematically collected and analyzed pre-determined outcomes from surgeons repairing distal hypospadias using mostly TIP at major centers around the Netherlands and found the average rate of complications in 814 boys was 19%, ranging as high as 44%. Only 16% of surgeons had 95% success, and only a third had complications in 10% or fewer of their patients (Van der Toorn et al, 2015).

The Dutch are certainly not uniquely poor surgeons. Instead, it is likely that a similar study done in other countries, including the US, would find similar results. In most cases this is not from surgeons choosing to do the wrong operation for the anatomy, but rather from surgeons not doing TIP in the best way.

Influence of Urethral Plate Characteristics

Some blame their complications on "unfavorable" anatomy of the patient. There is historic precedence for this conclusion. For example, Duckett wrote the MAGPI could be used for all cases on the distal shaft to the glans. However, Gibbons and Gonzales (1983) defined "meatal variants" that were not suitable for the procedure. Subsequently, the belief grew that most complications occurred because the surgeon chose the wrong operation for the specific anatomy of the patient (Duckett and Keating, 1995).

If that is true, then it is important that different surgeons evaluating the same patient reach the same conclusion regarding the type of anatomy he has. But a study that showed photographs to pediatric urologists and asked them to assess urethral plate suitability for TIP reported poor inter-rater agreement (El-Hout et al, 2010).

WS trained during the time when Gibbons and Gonzales were studying indications and contraindications for MAGPI and recalls their frequent uncertainty if the anatomy of a given patient was amenable for that repair. This became such a common problem among surgeons that Duckett organized a postgraduate hypospadias course at the AUA in which photos of different patients were shown for invited "experts" to comment on which repair was best for the anatomy. Their disagreements provided entertainment, but not much clarity, for the audience of urologists wanting to know which operation to do.

Depth of the Urethral Plate Groove

The first TIP article mentioned that all 16 patients had a urethral plate that could be described as "flat" or with a "cleft", yet there were no complications in that series (Snodgrass, 1994). We subsequently reported that there was no difference in outcomes in 426 consecutive distal TIP repairs based on the urethral plate groove being "deep", "cleft" or "flat" (Snodgrass and Bush et al, 2010).

Two other studies have also found these characterizations of the urethral plate did *not* predict urethroplasty complications (Holland and Smith, 2000;

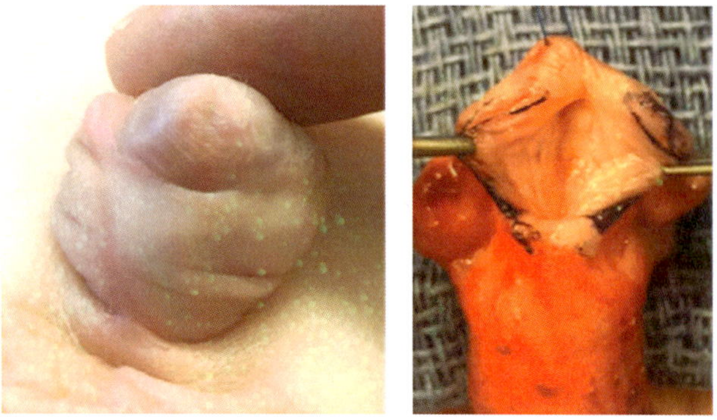

Figure 22. TIP for a flat urethral plate.
There is no groove in the urethral plate, yet TIP incision increased its width and depth to create a normal neourethra.

Sarhan et al, 2009). Therefore, TIP can be used in patients with a "flat" urethral plate (Figure 22), and all other variations of the natural groove in the plate.

Pre-Tip Incision Width < 8mm

Holland and Smith reported that a urethral plate < 8mm wide before TIP incision was associated with significantly more fistulas than when the plate was > 8mm wide.

Sarhan et al also said that pre-incision plate width < 8mm, which they found in half their patients, was a significant risk factor for complications. They concluded that a wider urethral plate was "essential" for successful TIP repair.

This is not our experience (Figure 23). Rather, these results indicate the authors made the technical error of not incising the plate down to the underlying corpora. Several years later Smith watched one of our live-surgery webinars and emailed that our theory was correct - that he thought he was making a deep incision like we did until he saw us actually making that incision. Inadequate TIP incision, whether by mistake or intention fearing a stricture, increases complications. Photographs from the article by Sarhan et al show they also made inadequate TIP incisions (Figure 23).

We subsequently measured pre-incision urethral plate width at its widest point in 224 consecutive patients with primary, mostly distal, hypospadias who all had TIP repair. 86% of these boys had pre-incision width < 8mm; if the recommendation of Sarhan et al

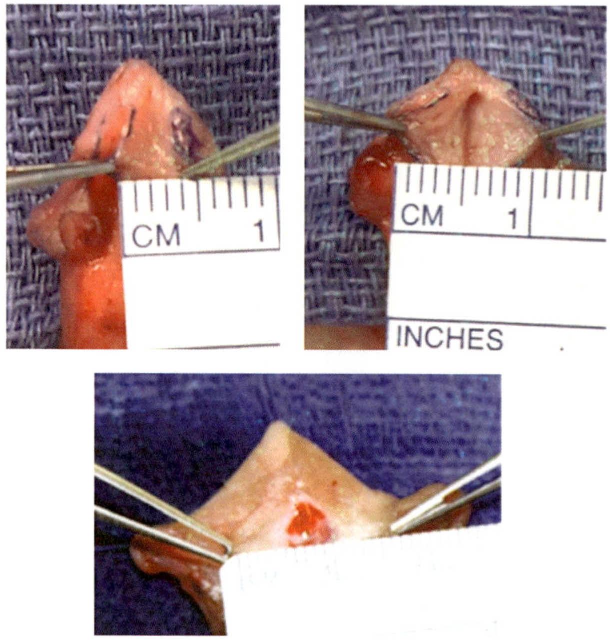

Figure 23. Proper vs inadequate TIP incision for UP width <8mm.
A, pre-incision urethral plate width measures 4mm. B, after correct, deep TIP incision the width measures 11mm (11Fr) straight across, and approximately 12mm when the depth to the corpora is taken into account. C, shallow incision made by Sarhan et al did not adequately widen the urethral plate.

was followed, few could have had a TIP repair. Proper TIP incision increased the width by an average of 116% in our series, versus the 57% increased width reported by Sarhan et al. Complications developed in 6%, with no difference when the plate was < 8mm versus > 8mm (Bush and Snodgrass, 2017). Sarhan et al found complications in 14%, *more than twice our rate*, with more fistulas and meatal stenosis caused by their shallow urethral plate incision. These observations should put this matter to rest, especially when one visibly compares the TIP incision done by Sarhan et at to ours, shown in Figure 23.

Urethral Plate "Quality"

The fact that at least 5% of distal TIP repairs develop complications despite each step apparently being done correctly has caused some to wonder if these cases indicate a urethral plate that is somehow not suitable for the repair. Since neither the depth of the urethral plate groove, nor the pre-incision width of the plate, relate to complications, Pippi Salle asked if there is some other factor of urethral plate "quality" yet to be defined.

He described an "unfavorable" plate as "narrow with poor spongiosum" but admitted that different urologists do not agree if a plate is "favorable" or "unfavorable" after examination. Consequently, he recommended G-TIP when urethral plate epithelium would comprise less than half the circumference of the neourethra but reported no supporting data for either this theory or practice (Abbas and Pippi Salle, 2018).

Subsequently, Abbas et al (2024) stated a "POST" score derived from measurements of the urethral plate to distinguish "favorable" from "unfavorable" plates correlated with distal TIP urethroplasty complications. However, there were several methodologic concerns that questioned their conclusions including that fistulas, the most common hypospadias complication, were not included in their definition of complications, 25% of their patients had midshaft hypospadias which has higher complications, and only 13% of their distal cases had a coronal / subcoronal meatus in contrast to the 80% we reported in our series of 551 consecutive distal repairs (Snodgrass and Bush et al, 2010).

In summary, we have used TIP for distal repairs in consecutive patients and not found an "unfavorable" urethral plate configuration to preclude its use. The findings by others described above can be explained by selection bias. Again, this is an important point: modern surgeons do not have to return to the 1980s when choosing the appropriate distal hypospadias repair depending upon analysis of the urethral plate anatomy. TIP can be used unless there is VC ≥ 30°.

Should the TIP incision be grafted (i.e. G-TIP)?

There are several reasons proponents give for doing a G-TIP repair. One is that the TIP incision will scar and cause neourethral stricture or meatal stenosis if left to re-epithelialize. Another is to make a shallow urethral plate more suitable for tubularization, while a third is to better position the neomeatus at the glans tip, especially when the plate appears to end lower.

Concern that TIP incision would heal with scarring was expressed at the beginning when surgeons compared it to internal visual urethrotomy for a stricture, which usually heals with recurrent scarring. It is ironic that deep TIP incision does *not* lead to meatal stenosis or urethral stricture, but hesitance to make the incision deep can secondary to tension on tissues.

As discussed above, we reported no strictures or meatal stenoses in a large series of boys after distal TIP (Snodgrass and Bush et al, 2010). The meta-analysis done by Pfistermuller et al similarly found a low incidence of these complications. Clearly, there is little inherent risk for obstruction after TIP repair when the procedure is done correctly. Without doubt, G-TIP encourages some worried surgeons to make the TIP incision deeper than they might do otherwise.

This same explanation applies to the argument that grafting is needed after incising and tubularizing a "flat" or "shallow" plate. Obviously, a deeper incision is needed when the plate is relatively flat, because its surface is further from the underlying corpora than when it is more deeply grooved. Surgeons worried the "large de-epithelialized" defect will scar may incise deeper knowing they will graft it.

Other surgeons are less concerned with creating obstruction than leaving the neomeatus below the normal location. They extend the TIP incision beyond the end of the plate and into the glans, and then graft to prevent the glans from scarring back together. However, we measure the glans fusion achieved by TIP repair without incision beyond the plate into the glans and find that it is always normal - averaging 4mm, which means the meatus is properly positioned.

Only two small studies directly compared distal G-TIP to TIP repair. In one, 70% of the patients had midshaft to perineal hypospadias (Shimotakahara et al, 2011) and results for those with distal hypospadias were not reported separately. The second also included patients with proximal hypospadias, but outcomes of those with distal repairs could be determined separately with no difference in G-TIP vs TIP (Mouvaras et al, 2014).

Furthermore, it is inevitable that a few grafts will contract and others may protrude out the meatus (Figure 24). We have seen both these complications after G-TIP done elsewhere. G-TIP also adds time and complexity, and makes prepucioplasty difficult for patients who prefer that option.

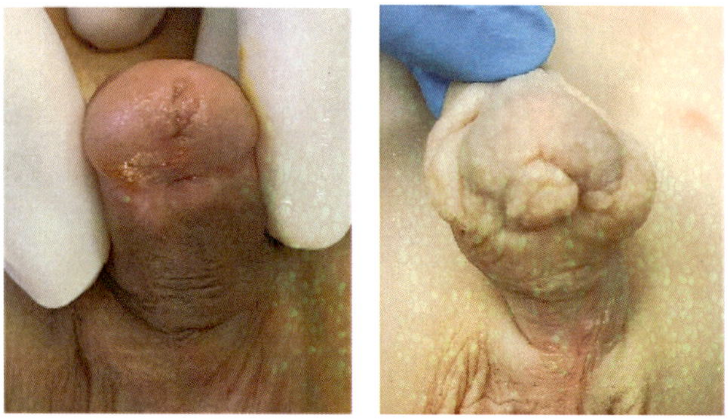

Figure 24. Graft protrusion after G-TIP.
A, foreskin protrudes outside an intact meatus, deflecting the urine stream. B, glans dehiscence with unsightly exposed graft.

The main benefit of G-TIP appears to be encouraging surgeons to incise the urethral plate deeply.

Functional Urethral Obstruction

One surgeon reported that 50% of patients he evaluated after unsuccessful TIP repair had "obstructive voiding", characterized by dysuria or recurrent fistulas, despite 8Fr calibration of the neourethra. The author opened the neourethra and observed a scar from prior TIP incision. He concluded that a sound could push past the scar but the urethra was functionally narrow. Urethrography was said to objectively diagnose this complication but was not done in 90% of the patients. The author concluded Mathieu repair was preferred for distal repairs (Hadidi, 2013). Whether or not the author evaluated for penile curvature in these patients was also not reported.

Patients with obstruction from any cause after any method of hypospadias repair present with straining, retention and UTIs, none of which were described in these patients. As stated above, both meatal stenosis and neourethra strictures are uncommon complications after distal TIP reported by surgeons worldwide. In our experience, recurrent fistulas after hypospadias repair nearly always indicate underlying ventral curvature and not distal obstruction.

Certainly, we have not seen patients with any evidence of obstruction in whom an 8Fr sound passes easily without resistance, and there is no other similar published report of patients with presumed "functional" obstruction. Furthermore, if obstruction commonly

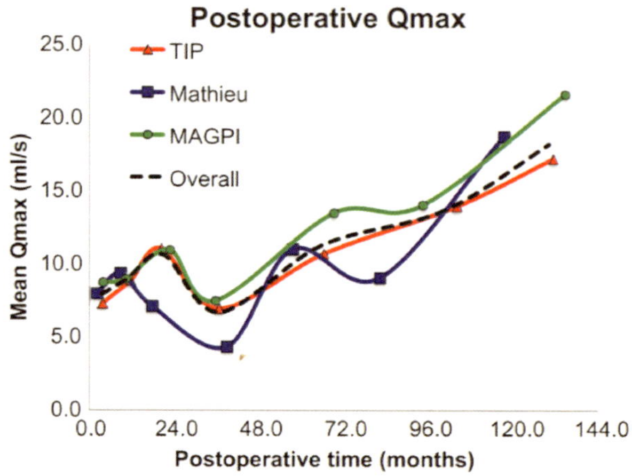

Figure 25. Uroflowometry 10 years after TIP, Mathieu, and MAGPI distal hypospadias repairs.
This chart shows increasing Qmax over time following TIP, Mathieu and MAGPI repairs, with no difference between them. Certainly, if TIP created either an anatomic or functional obstruction one would not expect long-term Qmax to *increase*.

occurs after distal TIP, one would expect long-term uroflowmetry studies to demonstrate a decreasing Qmax. However, as discussed in the next section, the 10-year uroflowmetry study reported by Hueber et al found that Qmax *increased* over time after distal TIP, and that it was the *same* as observed after MAGPI or Mathieu repairs (Figure 25).

Since TIP is the most commonly used repair for distal hypospadias, it is not surprising that surgeons who frequently manage patients with complications will see many who had TIP done. If 5% of patients develop a complication and many of those subsequently are managed by one surgeon in a referral center, that tertiary surgeon's practice will have a much higher percentage of patients with that complication.

As stated throughout this book, the most common reason for complications is technical error by the surgeon, and not an inherent problem with the operation.

TIP versus Mathieu

We have already established that TIP can be used to correct any distal hypospadias when there is less than 30° ventral curvature. And that there is value in surgeons worrying less about what operation to do than how to do the best operation in the best way.

Nevertheless, some surgeons continue to do Mathieu repairs either routinely, or in cases they believe have an "inadequate" plate or "too small a glans" for TIP. As emphasized above we have not encountered a case of distal hypospadias in over 30 years that had either an inadequate plate or too small a glans for TIP repair.

Some who do Mathieus say that TIP has not been followed adequately to know its early results stand up over time. However, a systematic literature review of published articles between 1990 and 2009 compared results for 1872 distal TIP and 1496 Mathieu repairs. Both had 7% urethroplasty complications (Wilkinson et al, 2012). A long-term study used uroflowmetry at periodic intervals to *at least 10 years* postoperatively to compare these 2 operations, reporting no difference in either Qmax, or percent with Qmax < 5%, in those who had Mathieu versus TIP, as shown in Figure 25 (Hueber et al, 2015).

TIP vs Mathieu Aesthetic Results

Although distal TIP and Mathieu repairs have similar functional outcomes and complication rates, there are differences in the aesthetic results of these 2 procedures. The 'hinging' maneuver Rich et al described which led to TIP was done specifically to make the rounded meatus of a Mathieu more vertical and slit-like. Studies comparing the meatal appearance of TIP versus Mathieu universally report TIP creates a more natural appearance. Two of these used standardized photographs scored blindly, while a third had a blinded urologist who was not the surgeon judge the outcome (Ververidis et al, 2005; Scarpa et al, 2009; El Ganainy et al, 2010).

It was the improved, more normal appearance after TIP that led to the rapid and widespread change by surgeons from Mathieu to TIP.

Rather than hinge the urethral plate dorsally, Hadidi recommended a ventral V-shaped incision into the flap-flap to improve appearance after Mathieu repair (Hadidi, 2012). He has not published results for this modification. However, a previous study found that this same V incision successfully created a vertical slit meatus in less than 50% of patients repaired with onlay flaps. A photograph from that article shows the V incision into a flap resulted in abnormally short glans fusion, seen in Figure 26 (Hayashi et al, 2007), which increases risk for urine spraying.

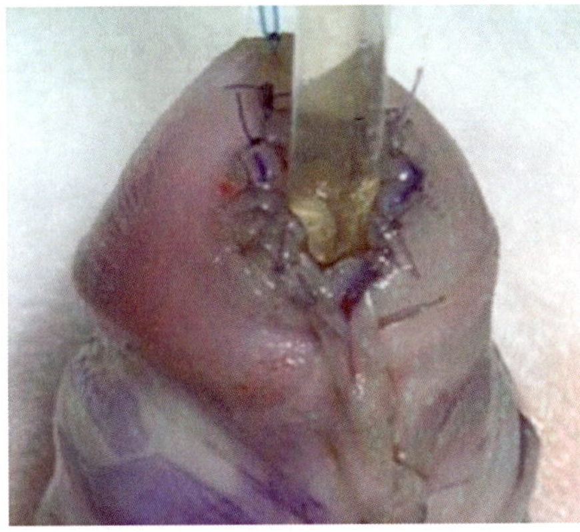

Figure 26. Appearance after V-incision of a flap repair showing subnormal glans fusion below the meatus. The goal of hypospadias repair is to create a normal penis, which includes a vertical slit meatus enclosed by glans fusion ≥ 2.5mm, averaging 4.5mm (Hutton and Babu, 2007). This photograph taken from Hayashi et al clearly shows glans fusion below the meatus less than normal after making a V incision into an onlay flap. Inadequate glans fusion increases risk for urine spraying in older children and adults.

Urethral Advancement

This procedure was first described by Beck in the late 1800s. The main problem using this technique is defining when it can be done and when it should be avoided. This recalls again the 1980s with its emphasis on studying the anatomy and then choosing an appropriate repair. Inevitably, mistakes will be made and urethral advancement will be done when it should not be, resulting in complications that likely would not have occurred had TIP been used instead.

Proponents state this operation should not be done when the distal urethra is "atretic", or the urethra is not "appropriately mobile" (Hammouda et al, 2008; Seibold et al, 2010). How these determinations were made by these authors was not described, and such subjective assessments almost certainly would result in different surgeons choosing different patients as candidates for this repair.

Urethral advancement can cause penile curvature if the urethra is not sufficiently mobilized or contracts somewhat postoperatively. One author stated the urethra needed to be mobilized 4-5 times the length measured from the meatus to the tip of the glans (Atala, 2011).

Although most authors split open the glans to secure the urethra to the tip rather than tunneling it as Beck did, 1 study reported 13% of patients had urine spraying (Seibold et al, 2010). That usually indicates glans dehiscence, which could be a risk after urethral advancement if proximal mobilization of the urethra was not sufficient to then place the meatus in the orthotopic location without tension. Future studies of this method should prospectively define glans dehiscence and report it.

Results of Skin Closure

Reviews of hypospadias surgery usually focus on urethroplasty complications and rarely mention outcomes of skin management. Yet successful hypospadias repair includes redistributing the penile skin to cover the shaft symmetrically. It also requires the skin to be closed without tension, leaving no tracts or scars outside the median raphe and circumcision lines.

These are difficult outcomes to objectively measure. The Dutch Hypospadias Study included postoperative skin assessment using standardized photographs scored on a scale they developed. They defined a skin complication as either excess skin after circumcision resulting in revision, or prepucial fistula or dehiscence when foreskin reconstruction was done. They reported skin surplus in 6%. Prepucioplasty complications occurred in 14.5% (Van der Toorn, 2015).

We also reported outcomes from skin management, comparing distal repairs with circumcision versus prepucioplasty. Revisions were done in 2% following either circumcision or prepucioplasty. Those after circumcision were mostly for redundant skin and once for left penile torsion (Snodgrass and Bush et al, 2013). We believe the skin was correctly sized in these during surgery with the penis on stretch to its full length. However, postoperative swelling is common following penile surgery, and if that distention of the skin does not completely resolve, unsightly excess remains. This process can also create secondary phimosis, or the appearance of lymphedema in the mucosal collar.

Skin complications after prepucioplasty were an unsightly dorsal whirl in 1 patient that was later excised, and the late development of BXO in another. We have also seen foreskin fistulas and dehiscences in other series of boys after foreskin reconstruction. Nevertheless, most do not develop complications.

It could be that body habitus influences likelihood for skin complications, with increasing risk when there is a large peripenile fat pad. We did not record any description of the fat pad or determine BMI in our series. Tacking the skin to the corpora at the penoscrotal junction on either side of the urethra in cases thought to have this risk probably reduces secondary phimosis.

Finally, we have seen that concomitant hypospadias plus significant penile torsion can increase the risk for skin complications, both in patients undergoing circumcision as well as foreskin reconstruction. Because this is a relatively uncommon finding in boys with hypospadias, we do not have prevalence data as of yet or know the percentage that will experience skin complications when it is present. In these patients, we hypothesize that either the missing left-sided penile skin creates tension on skin closure, leading to increased problems with skin healing, and/or that there is intrinsic differences in blood supply to the ventral and left penile skin which may contribute to poor wound healing.

When should distal TIP not be done?

The main contraindication to TIP repair is VC ≥ 30°. It is a change in traditional decision-making to choose the operation based on the extent of curvature after degloving rather than by the meatal location. Our emphasis on curvature grew partly from the tsunami of patients we encounter in our tertiary practice with urethroplasty complications – fistulas, dehiscences, meatal stenoses, neourethra strictures – who most often also have recurrent or persistent VC (Snodgrass and Bush, 2019). Plication for more than 30° VC just because the meatus is distal can lead to recurrent bending, urethroplasty and skin complications, and need for the staged repair that should have been done in the first place. A 2-stage STAC-TIP repair for these is described in Chapter 10.

An example of a distal meatus with ventral curvature is shown above in Figure 2. Because of the curvature, this and similar patients should be considered proximal hypospadias variants and managed accordingly.

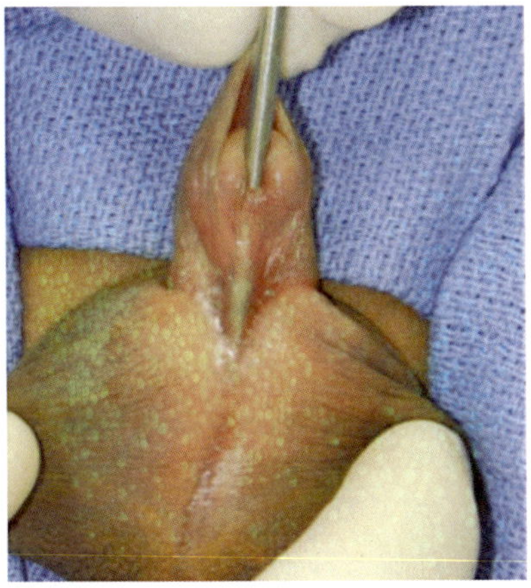

Figure 27. Proximal variant with a distal meatus. This anomaly is usually suspected from the abnormal appearance of the ventral skin, and confirmed when a sound shows a "thin" urethra - actually a lack of dartos and spongiosum between the skin and urethra. These also are likely to have VC of 30° or more, and for all these reasons such cases represent proximal hypospadias variants despite the distal meatus.

Other less common proximal variants with a distal meatus are recognized by the "thin" urethra shown in Figure 27. These also likely have VC ≥ 30°, but the realization that it is not a typical distal hypospadias is made before artificial erection because of abnormal appearing ventral skin with no dartos or spongiosum between it and the distal urethra.

Key Points

The algorithm we present liberates surgeons from subjective assessments of patient anatomy to select the technique for distal hypospadias repair. Instead, surgeons can determine that there is less than 30° ventral curvature after degloving and then perform distal TIP regardless of the width or depth or shape of the urethral plate. Consequently, the surgeon can then focus on doing the steps of TIP repair in the best way, to achieve success in over 90% of cases.

Conversely, surgeons should *not* perform dorsal plications and TIP repair when there is VC measuring ≥ 30°. It is important to emphasize that this occurs in at least 1 of every 10 boys presenting with a distal meatus. Plication in that circumstance is likely to fail, and tension generated by spontaneous erections in a bent penis then cause urethroplasty complications, which often recur if the surgeon tries to correct them without recognizing and straightening the underlying VC. These patients usually need a STAC-type repair which should have been done in the first place.

Since numerous studies show that distal TIP can be done with < 10% complications, this should be considered the standard for all surgeons performing distal hypospadias surgery. Those with more complications are encouraged to carefully review their decision-making and surgical technique to bring their results into that range.

Proximal TIP Repair

Most boys with proximal hypospadias have VC that is ≥ 30°. Consequently, few should have a long TIP repair. Today our practice is mostly proximal repairs, and we rarely do a proximal TIP.

*We cannot over-emphasize that surgeons should **not** plicate curvature ≥ 30° and then do a TIP repair.*

Surgical Technique

While the basic principles of TIP repair - urethral plate incision and tubularization, barrier layer coverage over the neourethra, glansplasty and skin closure - are the same whether the meatus is distal or proximal, these key steps are done differently when it is proximal. Each of these modifications was evidence-based when review of our outcomes showed complication rates that needed to be reduced, and all of them have been published for others to avoid our mistakes.

Skin Incision

Since most boys with a proximal meatus will have ventral curvature ≥ 30°, the initial skin incision has changed since the last edition of this textbook. We no longer begin the operation by completely degloving the penis, because when there is curvature ≥ 30° a STAC repair is needed and the foreskin can be preserved for the urethroplasty graft at the second stage if the initial degloving incision is made ventrally as shown in Figure 28.

Before incising, 1:100,000 epinephrine is injected alongside the urethral plate. In proximal hypospadias there often is little or no dartos between the skin and spongiosum, and this injection hydro-distends the tissues and facilitates dissection in the plane under

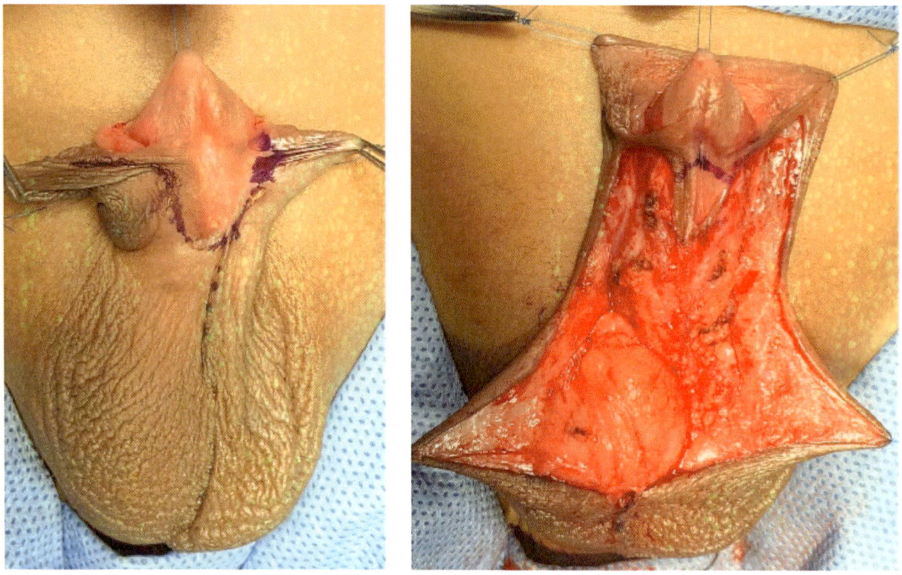

Figure 28. Ventral skin incision and exposure to begin proximal repairs.
A, initial skin incision is made ventrally, from near the corners of the prepuce, within 3mm of the edge of the glans, alongside the urethral plate, and then down the midline of the scrotum. B, excellent exposure gained by dissection done without complete degloving. The dorsal skin is not degloved to preserve the foreskin for the next operation should STAC be done. However, dissection goes under the dorsal skin so that the entire shaft below the mucosal collar is freed and accessible.

the skin while helping avoid troublesome bleeding from the spongiosum.

The incision runs alongside the urethral plate, but wider than we previously recommended to save some shaft skin next to the meatus to use in the proximal urethrostomy if the repair is staged. Distally, 3mm of the mucosal collar is preserved as the skin incisions extend near the ventral corners of the glans before continuing towards the dorsal prepuce. The intent is to gain sufficient exposure for a thorough dissection while minimally disturbing the foreskin.

Below the meatus the incision extends down the scrotum in the midline to near the perineum. In proximal hypospadias the native urethra often runs superficially under the skin towards the anus, and dissection releasing it from proximal attachments moves it into a normal position and reduces downward tension on it.

Scrotal dartos usually is found encroaching up the penile shaft and this is all released to drop it proximally. We then continue dissection circumferentially around the penile shaft from below the attachment of the mucosal collar down to the base, working under the shaft skin on the dorsal side and leaving the preputial skin intact along the mucosal collar and distal to it.

Artificial Erection

Next, artificial erection is performed and the extent of curvature determined using a goniometer as described in Chapter 3. If there is VC ≥ 30°, STAC repair is done as explained in Chapter 8.

VC measuring < 30° next leads to complete degloving. The curvature is straightened using a Heineke-Mikulicz dorsal plication described in Chapter 2. Artificial erection is then repeated to confirm the penis is straight.

Because eye-balling curvature up to 40° is inaccurate, and TIP should never be done when there is VC ≥ 30°, any curvature should be measured objectively.

Urethroplasty

Key steps in proximal TIP urethroplasty are diagramed in Figure 29.

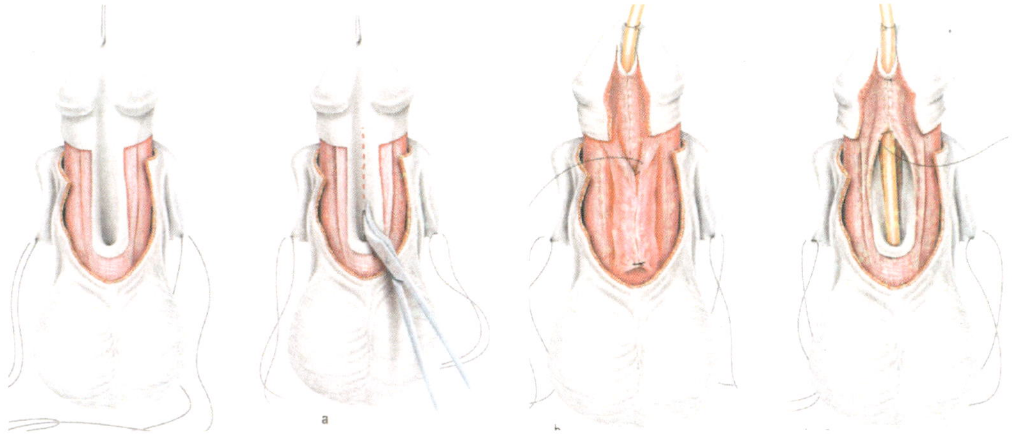

Figure 29. Proximal TIP urethroplasty.
A, the penis is degloved once it is verified curvature is less than 30°. A single dorsal Heineke-Mikulicz plication is done to correct curvature measuring less than 30°. B, the urethral plate is incised down to the corpora, from within the meatus distally to its end. C, tubularization begins distally in the midglans, as described for distal TIP. In contrast to distal TIP, where the first layer is run as a continuous layer, patients with proximal TIP have interrupted sutures for the first layer, which continues proximally, using 7-0 Vicryl sutures. Then a second running layer is placed subepithelially from proximal to distal using 6-0 or 7-0 PDS. D, spongioplasty is done to provide a 3rd layer of closure, extending up to the corona. Next, the neourethra will be covered with a tunica vaginalis flap. Glansplasty is done as described above for distal TIP, and skin closure is completed.

Glans Wings Dissection

Glans wings are created and dissected laterally (Figure 30). The lines for incision are the same as described above for distal TIP, extending from the end of the plate and along its visible junction to the glans. We first inject 1:100,000 epinephrine and also apply a tourniquet to optimally visualize the planes for dissection.

Because the glans in proximal hypospadias is typically smaller than in distal hypospadias (Bush and Snodgrass et al, 2013), additional dissection superiorly along the corpora at 3 and 9 o'clock further releases the wings until it is determined their later approximation will be without tension (Snodgrass and Bush, 2016).

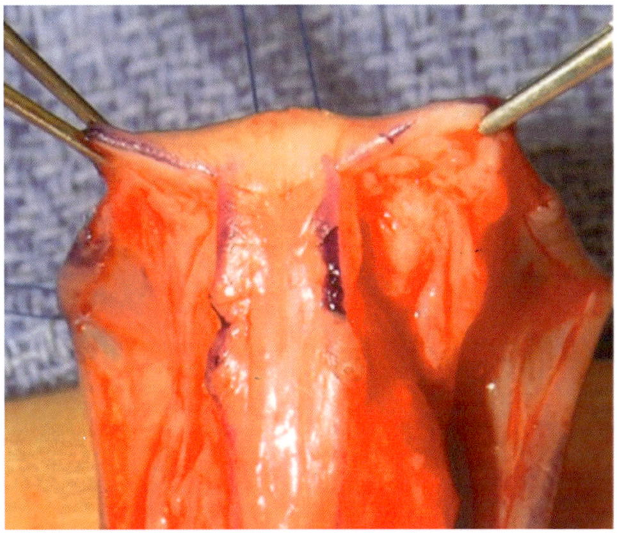

Figure 30. Extended glans wings dissection for proximal hypospadias repairs.
The glans wings are created along the visible junction of glans to urethral plate as in distal TIP. After dissection laterally to 3 and 9 o'clock, the wings are additionally freed off the corpora superiorly as shown. The exposed distal coropora are clearly seen after this dissection.

TIP Incision

With the surgeon and assistant retracting the edges laterally, the urethral plate is incised in the midline using tenotomy scissors. As in distal TIP, the incision begins in the middle of the glans and then continues both distally to the end of the plate and proximally to within the meatus. It extends from the surface epithelium down to the corpora, significantly widening the plate (Figure 31).

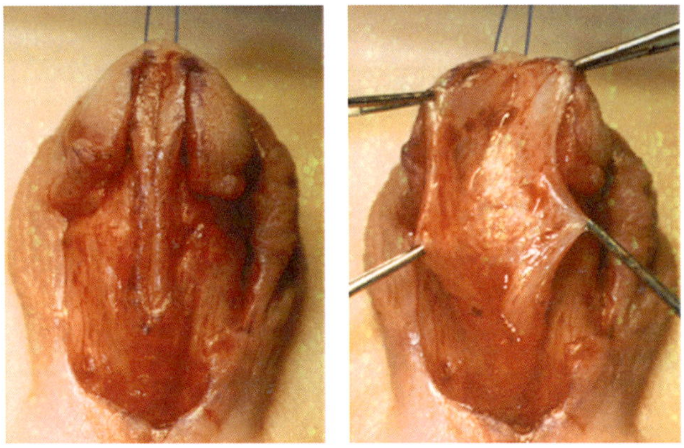

Figure 31. Proximal TIP urethral plate incision. A, urethral plate before TIP incision. B, plate after incision from within the meatus to the end of the plate. This will create a normal caliber neourethra.

Tubularizing the Urethral Plate

A 6Fr stent is passed into the bladder and secured to the glans traction suture. When the glans measures < 14mm wide a 5Fr feeding tube is used for urine diversion to reduce pressure on the later glansplasty that might promote dehiscence. As in distal TIP, the first stitch tubularizing the urethral plate is placed distally, in the midglans at least 3mm from its end. The resulting opening should be oval, and not round.

We published that 2-layer tubularization using interrupted subepithelial stitches for the first and a continuous stitch for the second layer, significantly reduces likelihood for fistulas (Snodgrass and Bush, 2011). While it is faster for the surgeon to run both layers, or to run the first layer and buttress it with some interrupted stitches in a second layer, it is impossible to reliably align the edges symmetrically and with even tension when the neourethra extends down the proximal shaft using these shortcuts. As discussed below, published results show significantly more fistulas when the first layer is closed with continuous suturing.

The first layer is sewn using 7-0 Vicryl, while the second is 6-0 or 7-0 PDS (Figure 32).

Tunica Vaginalis Flap

Next, one testicle is exposed through the midline scrotal incision and the tunica vaginalis is opened transversely near the inferior pole. A stay stitch of

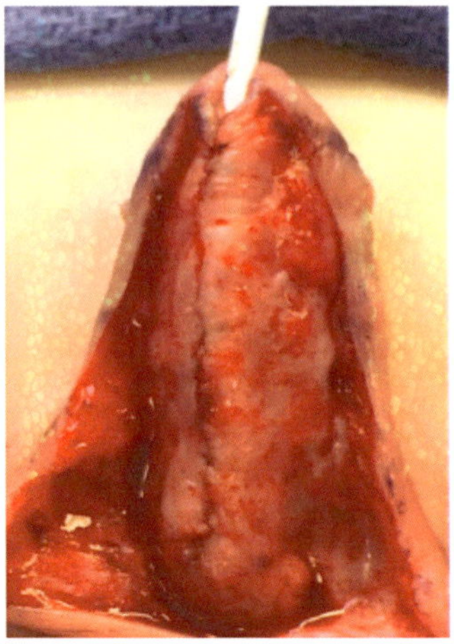

Figure 32. 2-layer urethral plate tubularization. As in distal TIP, the first stitch is placed distally, at least 3mm from the end of the plate at approximately the midglans level so that the resulting opening is oval and not round. The first layer is closed with interrupted subepithelial stitches. We prefer the TG 180 needle on 7-0 Vicryl. The second layer runs a 6-0 or 7-0 PDS suture proximally to distally.

5-0 absorbable suture is then placed superficially at the inferior pole, and an additional 2 traction sutures are placed into the corners of the flap. With the scrub tech holding the testicular traction stitch taut and an assistant holding the other 2 flap stays, a rectangle of tunica vaginalis is dissected off the spermatic cord to near the external ring. An army/navy retractor provides exposure superiorly to release bands tethering the flap. Medially and inferiorly a sheet of scrotal fat connects to the flap, and this is also released (Figure 33). It is important that there is sufficient length on the flap to easily cover the entire neourethra without exerting tension on the penis.

If the flap is not adequately freed it can pull the penis laterally during erections. If the blood supply to the flap is not protected it can contract postoperatively and cause glans dehiscence, a fistula, or recurrent VC.

Sometimes dartos muscular contraction is noted in the flap. We incise transversely through the muscle avoiding damage to the pedicle as otherwise these contractions postoperatively can cause the penis to intermittently torse.

The tunica vaginalis flap is spread out and first secured over the neourethra distally on either side of

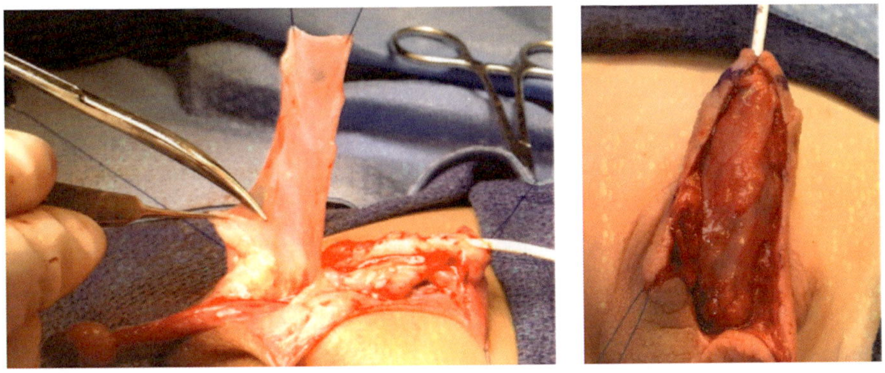

Figure 33. Tunica vaginalis flap.
A, a flap of tunica vaginalis is harvested from one testicle up to the external ring, and then used to cover the neourethra. In the photo scrotal fat adhering to the inferior medial aspect of the flap is stripped off. When the neourethra extends deep within the scrotum this scrotal fat is kept with the flap to cover the proximal suture line. B, the flap covers the entire neourethra without tension.

the suture line just below the meatus using 7-0 PDS. Additional sutures hold the flap to the corpora at intervals proximally. The penis is stretched taut as these stitches are placed as another maneuver to avoid tension from the flap.

Next, the testicle is suture pexed back to the scrotal wall, and then the hemiscrotal compartment is sewn closed. These are important steps, and we have seen testicles that migrated medially when they were not done, adhering to the urethra during healing and causing discomfort sitting.

Glansplasty

Glansplasty is done next (Figure 34). First, the glans wings are lifted and stretched again to be certain there is no tension. This is a critical second check to reduce glans dehiscence, as sometimes tissue can become edematous while the urethroplasty is sewn and the tunica vaginalis flap harvested. The glans wings are approximated as described above for distal TIP. They are first aligned with a 9-0 Vicryl epithelial suture in the midglans. Then 3 interrupted 6-0 Vicryl stitches are placed subepithelially from under that alignment stitch to the corona, the second also catching a bite of the tunica vaginalis to hold it in place. Glans fusion should be 3-4mm even in small glans with a preoperative width < 14 mm.

The glans epithelium is never sutured. Although we have not sutured the glans epithelium in more than 20 years, it seems many surgeons still do despite the fact that this layer is not needed and epithelial stitches create visible scars.

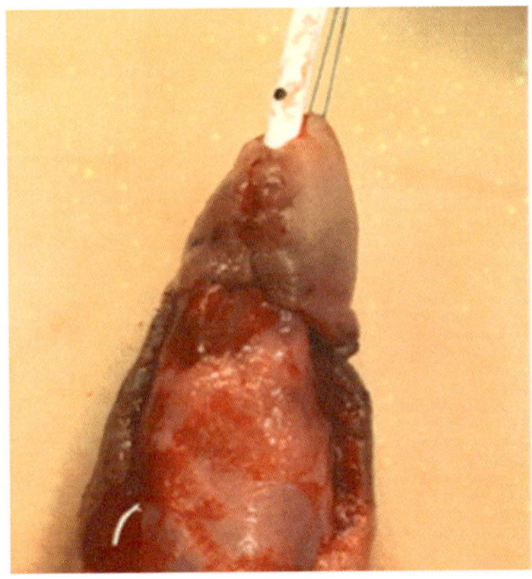

Figure 34. Glansplasty.
As in distal TIP, the glans wings are approximated with 3 interrupted subepithelial 6-0 Vicryl stitches. The 1st is at approximately the midglans, which creates the neomeatus. The 2nd is midway between the first stitch and the corona, and catches a small bite of tunica vaginalis to hold it in place. The 3rd approximates the coronal. No epithelial stitches are used. Note the glans fusion is normal after glansplasty.

Approximating the Mucosal Collar

Next, the mucosal collar is sewn together in the midline with interrupted subepithelial 7-0 Vicryl. An epithelial 9-0 stitch is often used to close the skin at the corona, which may be too thin for subepithelial suturing. The remainder of the collar is sewn with interrupted subepithelial 7-0 Vicryl. As mentioned above, the mucosal collar should not exert any tension onto the glansplasty.

Shaft Skin Closure and Scrotoplasty

Ventral skin closure is more complex in proximal hypospadias since it is more deficient than in distal cases. It is important that the skin be arranged so that it is symmetric in length from the base of the penis to the corona circumferentially and does not exert tension on the urethroplasty or glansplasty. We have noticed that the left-sided skin is often shorter ventrally than the right side, which the surgeon must recognize and correct.

The scrotum usually is higher on the penile shaft in proximal hypospadias. This transposition decreases when scrotal dartos is dissected off the shaft. Scrotal dartos bands also run from the scrotum alongside the penis towards the pubis, and we have learned that even the most extreme cases of penoscrotal transposition can be corrected by cutting into these bands transversely from within the midline scrotal incision, which also moves the scrotum down (Figure 35). We *never* make skin incisions around the scrotum to create scrotal flaps, because this is both unnecessary and leaves visible scars beside the penis which are *not* reliably concealed by pubic hair after puberty (Chapter 20).

Complex skin closure is discussed in Chapter 21. In general, we first align the penoscrotal junction to be even between the left and right, and the ventral skin the same length as from the penopubic junction to corona dorsally. Then 5-0 PDS anchors the penile shaft skin at the penoscrotal junction to the corpora on either side of the urethra at the 3 and 9 o'clock positions. These 2 tacking stitches also prevent acquired buried penis.

After creating the penoscrotal junction, any scrotal cleft is excised and the scrotal incision closed with a continuous subepithelial 6-0 PDS. It helps to place a stay stitch through the scrotal midline to hold it taut while closing this incision as can be seen in our You Tube videos.

Dorsal foreskin is incised laterally to transpose needed skin ventrally for shaft coverage. We always seek to close the skin into a median raphe, mimicking normal appearance. Should contraction occur postoperatively, which sometimes happens at the penoscrotal junction, a 6 to 12-week course of 0.1% betamethasone cream and skin massage will correct or significantly reduce it.

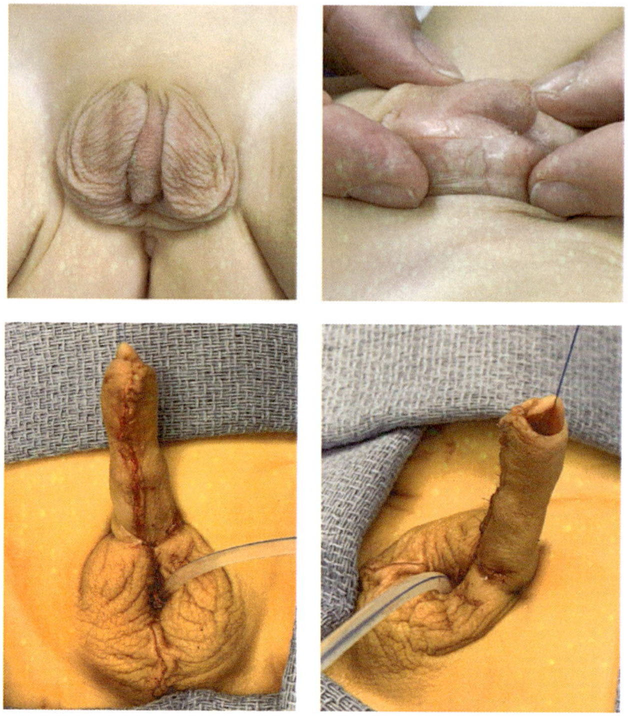

Figure 35. Correcting penoscrotal transposition without scrotal skin flaps.
A,B, preoperative photos showing proximal scrotal hypospadias with penoscrotal transposition. There is almost no ventral penile skin. C,D after STAC the penis is straight with a clearly delineated penoscrotal junction. The scrotal transposition was corrected without making scrotal skin flaps by releasing dartos extending from the scrotum to the pubis.

Boys with proximal hypospadias often have “humps” of skin dorsally. These serve as tissue repositories for the skin needed for shaft coverage, but they also require attention because, left alone, they are unsightly. Use and correction of these are discussed in Chapter 21.

Excess skin is removed after checking again that the shaft skin is the same length circumferentially. All skin edges are closed with interrupted subepithelial 7-0 Vicryl.

Postoperative Care

Medications

Pain management and control of bladder spasms are the same as described above for distal TIP.

Bandage

We use a similar bandage as for distal TIP. A medium Tegaderm is wrapped around the penis, folded gauzes are laid over its ventral aspect, and then a larger Tegaderm is placed over the gauzes to gently compress the penis against the abdomen. This bandage falls off spontaneously and is not replaced.

Stent

The stent provides urinary diversion for 2 weeks. If it comes out prematurely it rarely needs to be re-inserted because the neourethra suture line is watertight. Should it need to be replaced because of extravasation or retention, we always do that under general anesthesia to gently insert a new stent. If any resistance is encountered, we pass a glide wire into the bladder and feed the stent over it. On rare occasion we have used a 7Fr cystoscope to pass the wire when these other attempts were not successful, usually because of a utricle.

Helpful Explanations for Parents Regarding the Longer Neourethra

The longer neourethra created by proximal hypospadias repairs behaves in ways that are noticeable, and sometimes worrying, to parents. We discuss the following points preoperatively and then refer back to them after surgery if questions arise.

Postoperative edema temporarily reduces the lumen of the neourethra after proximal TIP repair. When the stent is removed the parents may notice the stream is thin and/or deflected. This does not indicate meatal stenosis, and neither calibration nor dilation should be done.

During this phase of postoperative edema and related turbulent urine flow urinary infection may occur, which almost never happens after distal repairs. In the few who develop an infection, the first typically happens soon after the stent is removed and is often febrile. We simply treat with a 1-week course of oral antibiotic, and do not pursue any other diagnostic tests such as renal sonography or VCUG. These few boys sometimes go on to experience additional episodes of cystitis, which we treat with a 3-day course of antibiotic. We cannot recall a patient who continued this pattern beyond 1 year following surgery. In contrast, UTIs that occur well after healing and resolution of edema are more likely to indicate a complication.

The stream strengthens and straightens over the first several postoperative months. But the stream after proximal repairs remains slower and prolonged compared to other boys. Parents notice this when they watch their son with hypospadias repair urinate at the same time as his brother or a friend. Uroflowmetry also commonly demonstrates a decreased Qmax and flattened curve. Interestingly, this difference in voiding is rarely noticed by patients, either as children or adults, or their friends. We routinely ask older boys if their friends ever comment that they take longer to urinate, and the answer is invariably no. Teens and adults with hypospadias seen in follow up who completed the International Prostate System Score (IPSS) to assess obstructive voiding symptoms did not indicate obstruction despite low Qmax and/or plateau-shaped uroflow curves (unpublished data).

The neourethra is not a natural urethra, regardless of the technique used to create it. It is less elastic, which likely accounts for the slower flow rate and flattened curve. In addition, decreased elasticity explains the postvoid dribbling most patients experience after proximal repair. Similar to how a stiff garden hose dribbles when the faucet is turned off, the neourethra does not collapse like the normal urethra does as bladder emptying finishes, leaving a few drops to expel when urination is otherwise complete. The amount of leakage is small, producing a wet spot smaller than a nickel on the underwear. Older boys and men learn to easily manage it, but should be aware this is a common finding after proximal hypospadias urethroplasty.

Results After Proximal TIP Repair

We reported 13% complications after proximal TIP repair in 26 consecutive boys undergoing surgery for proximal hypospadias. Those comprised 2 glans dehiscences and 1 neourethral stricture, with no fistulas or meatal stenosis. TIP was done when VC was estimated to be < 30° after a series of stepwise maneuvers which included elevating the urethral plate off the corpora and making 3 corporotomies underneath it in addition to dorsal plications (Snodgrass and Bush, 2011). However, we stopped elevating the plate when we realized it resulted in focal neourethral strictures in nearly 20% of patients (Snodgrass and Bush et al, 2013).

The meta-analysis of TIP repairs by Pfistermuller et al (2015) analyzed 625 primary proximal TIPs, finding a reoperation rate of 12%: 10% fistulas, 4% meatal stenosis and 2% strictures. Glans dehiscence was not reported.

A most recent evaluation of proximal repairs included 60 consecutive patients whose ventral curvature was measured objectively using the goniometer. Of these, only 8 (13%) had less than 30° bending and underwent TIP repair. Complications developed in 14% of those, all glans dehiscences (Snodgrass and Bush, 2017).

Together, these data indicate that proximal TIP remains a good option when VC measures < 30°. As we have emphasized, dorsal plication should *not* be done when the penis is bent ≥ 30°, which restricts TIP to a minority of patients with proximal hypospadias, and emphasizes again that VC should be objectively measured rather than eyeballed.

WS recently reviewed outcomes for all 90 proximal TIPs he did between 1993 and 2019, of which 77 had follow up averaging 44 months. There was no VC at operation in 25%, while a third had dorsal plication alone and another third had plication plus additional maneuvers for straightening. Recurrent VC was identified in 1 out of every 4 of these patients, and suspected in hindsight in 1 out of every 3. Those diagnosed with recurrent VC were measured intraoperatively to have an average 50° (30-75) curvature. Reoperation to correct this curvature required transecting the neourethra, ventral corporotomies, and a STAC repair, supplemented with hyperbaric oxygen therapy (Snodgrass and Bush, 2021).

We state again that hypospadias repair should be done right the first time, which means ***not*** relying on dorsal plications to straighten 30° or more curvature and then doing a proximal TIP. Snodgrass rarely does a "long Snodgrass" anymore!

Reducing Fistulas

WS initially did a single-layer running tubularization of the urethral plate, extrapolating what he learned in residency doing tubularized prepucial flap repairs to TIP. Covering every one of those with a dartos flap did not prevent a 33% fistula rate (Snodgrass and Yucel, 2007). Changing to a 2-layer tubularization did – but with the caveat that the first layer is closed with interrupted subepithelial stitches, while the second is a continuous stitch – which reduced fistulas to 11% (Snodgrass and Yucel, 2007).

Braga et al (2007) reported urethroplasty with a running suture resulted in 43% fistulas, similar to the 33% noted by WS. Recently, he described 2-layer tubularization done by running the first layer and then interrupting the second. That resulted in 18% fistulas (Braga, 2022).

The coverage layer matters, too. Although WS initially used dartos flaps, he changed to tunica vaginalis for all proximal repairs. This reduced the fistula rate further, with none in the subsequent 2 series (Snodgrass and Bush, 2011; Snodgrass and Bush, 2017).

Reducing Glans Dehiscence

Once we decreased fistulas, glans dehiscence became our primary complication. We first thought that enlarging the glans with preoperative testosterone would facilitate better glans closure, but found that successful increase in glans width did not decrease dehiscence (Snodgrass and Bush, 2016). More extensive glans wings mobilization until there is no tension, as described above, decreases glans dehiscence (Snodgrass and Bush, 2016). This is yet another example showing that complications most often result from technical factors rather than patient anatomy.

TIP versus Onlay Prepucial Flap

TIP incises the urethral plate to make a neourethra with a normal caliber. The onlay flap adds prepucial skin to the urethral plate to achieve a normal caliber. Both require the urethral plate to remain intact after straightening VC, and so neither should be used when curvature is ≥ 30°. Dorsal plication used to correct curvature of that extent appears effective intraoperatively, but does not reliably keep the penis straight. This limits both operations to only a minority of proximal hypospadias.

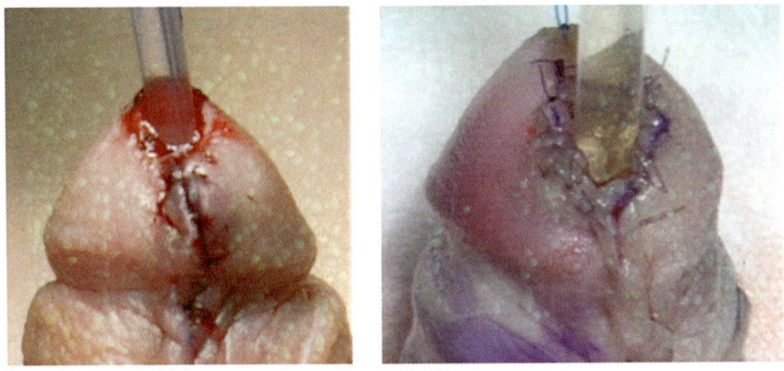

Figure 36. Glans fusion in TIP versus Onlay flap repairs. A, the length of glans fusion in TIP is greater than in B, onlay flap. The risk for urine spraying after toilet training is therefore greater after onlay flaps.

A systemic literature review and meta-analysis compared these two techniques, comprising a total of 6 articles describing 309 onlay and 262 TIP operations. Overall complication rates were similar. Two studies examined uroflowmetry, one finding no functional differences between the two operations, while the other reported relatively decreased peak and mean flow rates after TIP (Xiao et al, 2014).

These differences in uroflows are likely explained by the differing glansplasty in these techniques. In TIP, the glans wings are approximated together over the neourethra, achieving normal glans fusion and a compact urine stream. For onlay, the distal end of the flap is sutured to the glans wings, which can result in little or no glans fusion (Figure 36). That decreases resistance to urine flow, but increases risk for urine spraying.

The goal of hypospadias repair is to make the penis normal. Therefore, TIP is the superior choice for primary proximal repairs when VC is < 30°.

Key Points

When artificial erection demonstrates < 30° VC after degloving, TIP repair is the best option to make a normal penis - without concern regarding the depth or width or "quality" or other characterizations of the urethral plate. However, the curvature must be measured objectively, because surgeons can easily encounter 30° and judge it to be less. Surgeons should resist the temptation to do dorsal plications and TIP repairs when VC is 30° or more.

How the various steps in TIP are done is also important to achieve the best results, as reviewed in this chapter.

Based on published data, all surgeons repairing distal hypospadias should encounter complications in less than 10% of their patients, and the penis should look normal afterwards. Similarly, there should be complications in < 25% of proximal TIP repairs. Urologists who have higher rates of complications are making technical errors which can, and should, be corrected to improve their results to within these standards.

References

Abbas TO, Adnan I, Hatem J, Boyko A, Zorkin S, Plate Objective Scoring Tool (POST) in distal hypospadias: correlation with post-repair complications, *J Pediatr Urol* e-pub, 2023

Abbas TO and Pippi Salle JL: When to graft the incised plate during TIP repair? A suggested algorithm that might help in the decision-making process. *Front Pediatr*, 2018

Atala A: Urethral advancement for midshaft to distal hypospadias. *J Urol* 168: 1738, 2002

Beck C: Hypospadias and its treatment. *SGO* 24: 511, 1917

Braga LH, Pippi Salle JL, Lorenzo AJ, Skeldon S, Dave S, Farhat WA, Koury AE and Bagli DJ: Comparative analysis of tubularized incised plate versus onlay island flap urethroplasty for penoscrotal hypospadias. *J Urol* 178: 1451, 2007

Braga LH: presented data, 2022

Bush N, DaJusta D, and Snodgrass W: Glans penis width in patients with hypospadias compared to normal controls. *J Pediatr Urol* 9:1188, 2013

Bush N and Snodgrass W: Pre-incision urethral plate width does not impact short-term tubularized incised plate urethroplasty outcomes. *J Pediatr Urol* 13: 625e1, 2017

Bush N and Snodgrass W: Functional and aesthetic concerns of men with uncorrected hypospadias. Abstract presented to AUA, 2021

Doersch KM, Logvinenka T, Nelson CP, Venna AM, Masoom SN and Diamond DA: Is parenteral antibiotic prophylaxis associated with fewer infectious complications in stented, distal hypospadias repair? *J Pediatr Urol* published online, 2022.

El Ganainy EO, Abdelsalam YM, Gadelmoula MM, and Shalaby MM: Combined Mathieu and Snodgrass urethroplasty for hypospadias repair: a prospective randomized trial. *Int J Urol* 17: 661, 2010

El-Hout Y, Braga LH, Pippi Salle JL, Moore K, Bagli DJ, and Lorenza AJ: Assessment of urethral plate appearance through digital photography: do pediatric urologist agree in their visual impressions of the urethral plate in children with hypospadias? *J Pediatr Urol* 6: 294, 2010

Gibbons MD and Gonzales ET, Jr: The subcoronal meatus. *J Urol* 130: 739, 1983

Hadidi, AT: Functional urethral obstruction following tubularized incised plate repair of hypospadias. *J Pediatr Surg* 48: 1778, 2013

Holland AJA and Smith GHH: Effect of the depth and width of the urethral plate on tubularized incised plate urethroplasty. *J Urol* 164: 489, 2000

Holmdahl G, Karstrom L, Abrahamsson K, Doroszkiewicz M, and Sillen U: Hypospadias repair with tubularized incised plate. Is uroflowmetry necessary postoperatively? *J Pediatri Urol* 2: 304, 2006

Hammouda HM, Hassan YS, Abdelateef AM and Elgammal MA: New concept in urethral advancement for anterior hypospadias. *J Pediatr Urol* 4: 289, 2008

Hueber PA, Antczac C, Abdo A, Franc-Guimond J, Barrieras D, and Houle AM: Long-term functional outcomes of distal hypospadias repair: a single center retrospective comparative study of TIPs, Mathieu and MAGPI. *J Pediatr Urol* 11: 68, 2015

Hutton KA and Babu R. Normal anatomy of the external urethral meatus in boys: implications for hypospadias repair. *BJU Int* 100: 161, 2007.

Keating MA and Duckett JW: Failed hypospadias repair. In Cohen MS and Resnick M (Eds): **Reoperative Urology.** Boston, Little Brown and Co, 1995, p. 188

Mouravas V, Filippopoupos A and Sfoungaris D: Urethral plate grafting improves the results of tubularized incised plate urethroplasty in primary hypospadias. *J Pediatr Urol* 10: 463, 2010

Pfistermuller KL, McArdle J and Cuckow PM: Meta-analysis of complication rates of the tubularized incised plate (TIP) repair. *J Pediatr Urol* 11: 54, 2015

Sarhan O, Saad M, Helmy T, Hafez A. Effect of suturing technique and urethral plate characteristics on complication rate following hypospadias repair: a prospective randomized study. *J Urol* 2009; 182: 682.

Scarpa MG, Castagnetti M, Berrettini R, RIgamonti W and Musi L: Urinary function after Snodgrass repair of distal hypospadias: comparison with the Mathieu repair. *Pediatr Surg Int* 26: 519, 2010

Seibold J, Werther M, Allousi S, Gakis G, Schilling D, Colleselli D, Stenzl A and Schwenter C: Objective long-term evaluation after distal hypospadias repair using the meatal mobilization technique. *Scand J Urol Nephrol* 44: 298, 2010

Shimotakahara A, Nakazawa N, Wada A, Nagata S, Koga H, Takahashi T, Miyano G, Lane GL and Yamataka A: Tubiularized incised plate urethroplasty with doral inlay graft prevents meatal/ neourethral stenosis: a single surgeon's experience. *J Pediatr Surg* 46: 2370, 2011

Snodgrass W: Tubularized incised plate urethroplasty for distal hyposapadias. J Urol, 151: 464, 1994

Snodgrass WT, Bush N and Cost N: Tubularized incised plate hypospadias repair for distal hypospadias. *J Pediatr Urol* 6: 408, 2010

Snodgrass W and Bush N: Tubularized incised plate proximal hypospadias repair: continued evolution and extended applications. *J Pediatr Urol* 7: 2, 2011

Snodgrass W and Bush N: Hypospadias. In Wein A (Ed) **Campbell's Urology**, 10th Ed, 2011, pp

Snodgrass W and Bush N: Extensive glans wings mobilization reduces hypospadias repair complications. Abstract presented to SPU, 2016

Snodgrass W and Bush N: TIP hypospadias repair: a pediatric urology indicator operation. *J Pediatr Urol* 12:11, 2016

Snodgrass W and Bush N: Staged tubularized autograft repair for primary proximal hypospadias with 30-degree or greater ventral curvature. *J Urol* 198: 680, 2017

Snodgrass W and Bush N: Persistent or recurrent ventral curvature after failed proximal hypospadias repair. *J Pediatr Urol* 15: 344, 2019

Snodgrass W and Bush N: Recurrent ventral curvature after proximal TIP hypospadias repair. *J Pediatr Urol*, 17: epub, 2021

Snodgrass W and Bush N: Letter to editor re: Abbas et al, Plate Objective Scoring Tool (POST) in distal hypospadias: correlation with post-repair complications. J Pediatr Urol, 2024

Snodgrass W, DaJusta D, Villaneuva C, and Bush N: Foreskin reconstruction does not increase urethroplasty or skin complications after distal TIP hypospadias repair. *J Pediatr Urol*, 9:401, 2013

Snodgrass W, Granberg C and Bush NC: Urethral strictures following urethral plate and proximal urethral elevation during proximal TIP hypospadias repair. *J Pediatr Urol* 9: 990, 2013

Snodgrass W and Yucel S: Tubularized incised plate for mid shaft and proximal hypospadias. *J Urol* 177: 698, 2007

Stojanovic B, Bizic M, Majstorovic M, Kojovic V, and Djordjevic M: Penile curvature incidence in hypospadias: can it be determined? *Adv Urol*, epub 2011,

Van der Toorn F, de Mooij K, Nijman R et al. The Dutch hypospadias study: complications and prognostic factors after distal and mid-type hypospadias repair. Abstract presented to ESPU, Prague, 2015.

Ververidis M, Dickson AP and Gough DC: An objective assessment of the results of hypospadias surgery. *BJU Int* 96: 135, 2005

Wilkinson DJ, Farrelly P and Kenny SE: Outcomes in distal hypospadias: a systematic review of the Mathieu and tubularized incised plate repairs. *J Pediatr Urol* 8: 307, 2012

Xiao D, Nie X, Wang W, Zhou J, Zhang M, Zhou Z, Zhao Y, Gu M, Wang Z and Lu M: Comparison of transverse island onlay and tubularized incised-plate urethroplasties for primary proximal hypospadias: a systematic review and meta-analysis. *PLOS One* 9, 2014

Chapter 7

Urethral Plate "Quality"

We repaired distal hypospadias in 426 consecutive boys using only TIP. We found no contraindications to the procedure (except ventral curvature 30° or more), and complications developed afterwards in 4% (Snodgrass and Bush et al, 2010). The editors of the *Journal of Pediatric Urology* wrote that TIP had become the "gold standard" for distal hypospadias repair.

Earlier, Cheng et al performed 414 distal TIP repairs with an even lower complication rate. They did not report any contraindications either, but rather called TIP "the perfect repair for virgin cases of hypospadias". Pfistermuller et al did a meta-analysis of published results that included 3621 primary distal hypospadias repaired by TIP, finding the mean percentage of reoperations was 4.5%. They also did not identify a contraindication to TIP for distal hypospadias.

One Repair for Distal Hypospadias

These data make clear that TIP can be done by many different surgeons achieving success in over 90% of cases. That observation is incredibly important, because instead of worrying about what operation is best for the anatomy of a specific patient, a surgeon can use TIP for all distal repairs (with ventral curvature < 30°) *and focus on doing each step optimally.*

Data from the Board of Urology emphasizes this need, finding that the median number of distal hypospadias repairs by certified US pediatric urologists was only 1 a month when there were 230 pediatric urologists (Kogan and Feustel, 2011). Today with more than 1000 US pediatric urologists (AUA, 2023), the median number of distal repairs is undoubtedly less.

Dissenting Views

However, some disagree. For example, White and Hanna (2018) wrote that "urethral plate characterization is critical to proper treatment". Two reports warned that pre-incision urethral plate width <8mm was a contraindication because the final neourethra was too small (Holland and Smith, 2000; Sarhan et al, 2008). Abbas and Pippi-Salle (2018) thought TIP could be used in most distal hypospadias, but not when there is an "unfavorable urethral plate".

If there is unfavorable anatomy which increases complications when TIP is done for distal hypospadias, it is important that it be identified and clearly defined so that all surgeons can recognize that anatomy and perform an alternative repair.

Urethral Plate "Characteristics"

In his original TIP report, WS described the patients as having either a "flat" or "cleft" urethral plate groove, with none having a "deep" groove. However, incision of the plate down to the surface of the corpora enlarged it to a diameter exceeding 10 to 12Fr – proven by postoperative calibration done in every case during median follow up of 22 months (Snodgrass, 1994). A figure from that article showed a "flat" urethral plate before and after TIP incision.

Our last distal TIP report described the configuration of the urethral plate in 468 patients as "flat" in 35%, "cleft" in 38% and "deep" in 22%. Statistical analysis showed that these designations did *not* predict complications (Snodgrass and Bush et al, 2010). Others similarly reported these urethral plate characterizations do not correlate with urethroplasty complications after TIP repair (Holland and Smith, 2000; Sarhan et al, 2008). Nevertheless, some urologists still believe a "flat" urethral plate should be managed using an alternative method.

Urethral Plate < 8mm

Six years after TIP was first described, Holland and Smith wrote that pre-incision urethral plate width <8mm increased risk for complications. The authors stated they incised the plate "deeply down to the corporal bodies, as described by Snodgrass".

Subsequently, Sarhan et al also reported increased complications in those whose pre-incision plate width was <8mm, concluding that width 8mm or greater was "essential for successful TIP". Like Holland and Smith, they described incising the urethral plate "deeply down to the corporal bodies". Anticipating our response, the authors wrote there was no doubt that urethral plate anatomy affected results and disagreed that most TIP complications resulted from technical errors.

Half of the patients studied by Sarhan et al had a pre-incision width <8mm, which their TIP incision increased by 57%. We subsequently measured pre- and post-incision widths in 224 consecutive patients with distal hypospadias. 86% measured <8mm before TIP incision increased the width by 116%, double that achieved by Sarhan et al (Bush and Snodgrass, 2017). This difference is readily apparent from post-incision photographs in these 2 articles shown in Figure 1. The inadequate incision made by Sarhan et al resulted in twice as many urethroplasty complications, 14% versus our 6%.

Similarly, years after his report Smith watched us perform a distal TIP repair at a surgical workshop, and commented that our incision was much deeper than his.

Therefore, it *was* technical error, and not patient anatomy, which explains the complications that Holland and Smith and Sarhan et al experienced. Surgeons who visit our center worried about the meatal stenosis or fistulas that they are encountering universally tell us that the TIP incision they watch us make is longer and deeper than theirs. Similarly, the operative reports from other pediatric urologists that we review in patients with complications after distal TIP most often indicate a partial and less deep incision was done only "as needed to tubularize over an 8Fr catheter". Articles about distal TIP that we have reviewed commonly report a substantial number of patients who did not "require" a urethral plate incision. This finding in articles almost certainly indicates an inadequate incision in the remainder.

Incision of the urethral plate from within the meatus to the end of the plate which extends down to the underlying corpora is the most important step in TIP

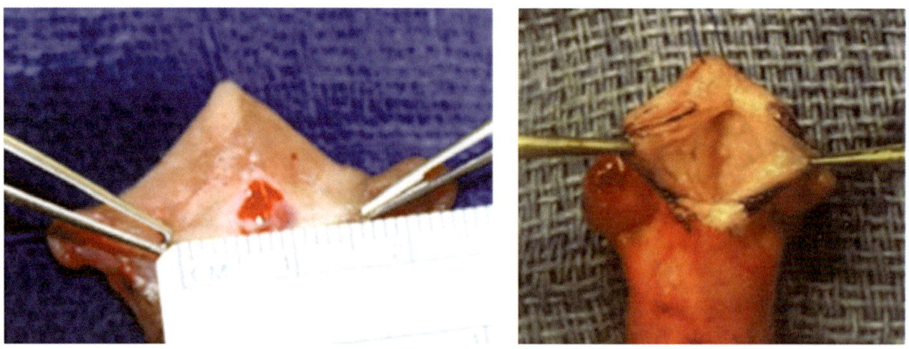

Figure 1. Difference in appearance after TIP incision by Sarhan et al versus Bush and Snodgrass.
A, clearly, the urethral plate incision made by Sarhan et al was not as deep as that made by Bush and Snodgrass in B. Their *shallow incision* explains how urethral plates with a width < 8mm had a greater risk for complications. So it was a technical error, and not the fault of anatomy, which led to complications.

repair and should be done *in every case*. It is not a TIP repair without this incision.

'Unfavorable' Urethral Plate

For several years Pippi Salle has said that an "unfavorable" urethral plate might account for some of the patients who have complications after TIP repair when the operation appears to have been done correctly. He described "unfavorable" as a "narrow plate with poor spongiosum" (Abbas and Pippi Salle, 2008), although the article did not include any photographs to illustrate that for readers. He also linked his own concern for a "narrow plate" to Holland and Smith and to Sarhan et al, which were discussed above.

Subsequently, Abbas et al (2024) reported a score derived from urethral plate measurements distinguished "favorable" from "unfavorable" plates, and wrote that complications after distal TIP were greater when the score was unfavorable. However, fistulas were not included among those complications and 25% of his patients had midshaft, rather than distal, hypospadias which has higher complications. Furthermore, only 13% of their distal hypospadias were coronal/subcoronal, which accounted for 80% of our cases in a series of 551 consecutive patients (Snodgrass and Bush et al, 2010). Therefore it is likely that selection biases, rather than anatomy, explains the findings by Abbas et al.

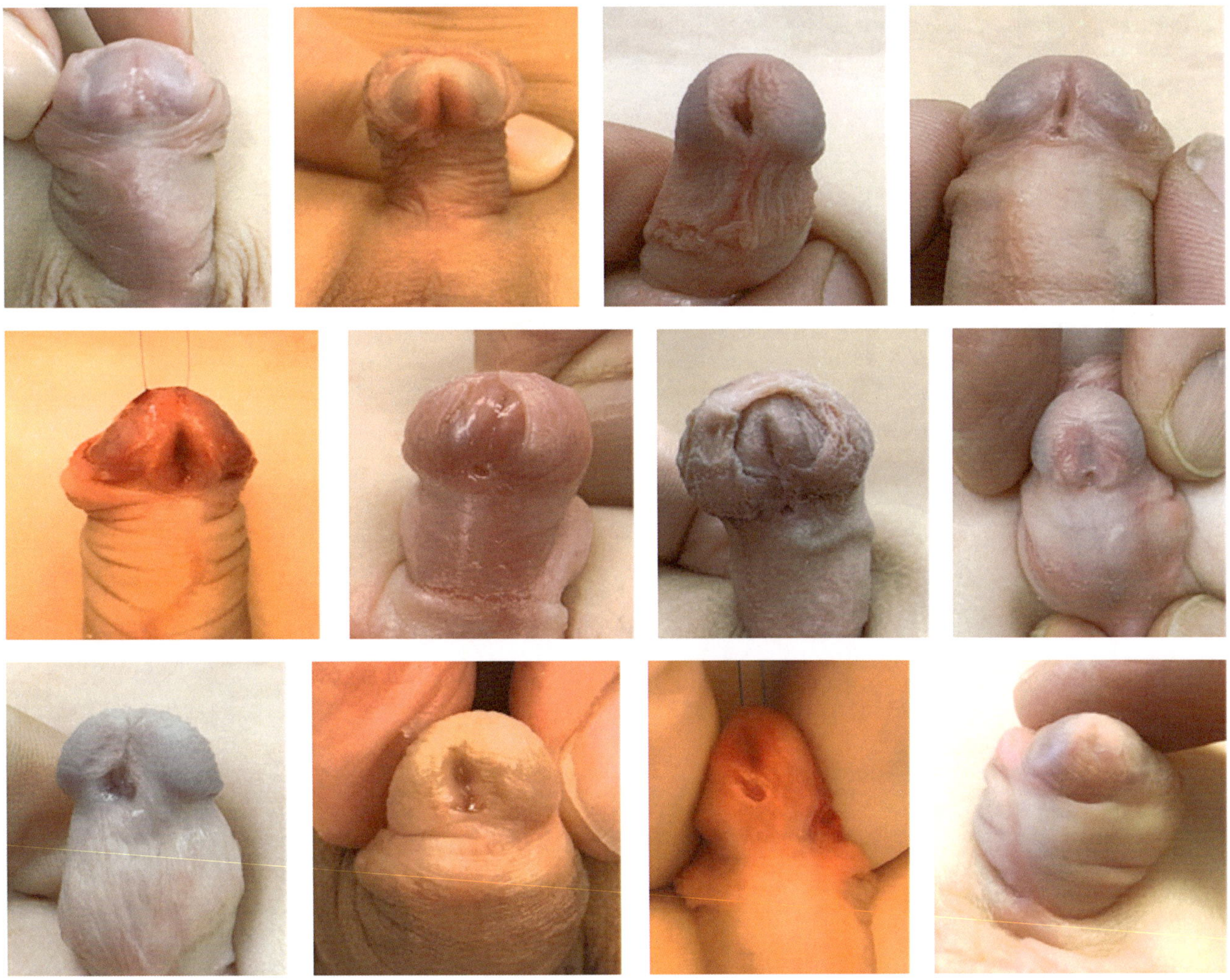

Figure 2. Varying anatomy in distal hypospadias.
Do any of these have an "unfavorable" urethral plate? We repaired all of them using TIP.

Abbas and Pippi Salle (2018) wrote the "unfavorable" plate should be managed by a G-TIP repair. However, as discussed in Chapter 6, no study has shown that grafting the incised plate gives fewer complications than TIP. We have noticed how the urethra can exert downward tension on the urethral plate, and how TIP incision releases that pull and visibly lengthens the plate. A shallow incision would not accomplish this, and the benefit of G-TIP could be to convince surgeons to incise the plate deeply, knowing they are going to graft the defect.

While measurement of the urethral plate is objective, descriptions like "narrow" and "poor spongiosum" are not, recalling an earlier time when the surgical technique had to be matched to the patient's anatomy. For example, Gibbons and Gonzales warned that a "patulous fish-mouth" meatus, a "non-compliant" meatus, and a "hyposplastic" meatus should each be considered contraindications to MAGPI repair. On the other hand, Zaontz wrote that the GAP procedure was specifically designed for the "non-compliant" or "patulous fish-mouth" meatus with an "excessively deep" urethral plate. Duckett and Keating advised the Pyramid repair be limited to MIP having a "widely splayed blunderbuss" meatus.

Although these specific authors might have been able to reproducibly identify patients with and without these characteristics, it is certain that other surgeons would not reliably draw the same conclusions when they assessed their own patients. Duckett blamed complications on surgeons choosing the wrong surgical technique for the anatomy, and ran a postgraduate course during the annual AUA meeting where "experts" argued which types of a meatus they were seeing in photographs he showed. WS recalls watching Gibbons begin every distal hypospadias repair sketching his interpretation of the anatomy and the options it presented for repair, which the young urologist in training found to be utterly confusing.

Figure 2 illustrates the variation in phenotype present in distal hypospadias. Pippi Salle showed similar photographs to pediatric urologists asking if the hypospadias was suitable for TIP repair, using a Likert scale ranking favorability. He reported poor agreement in their assessments, kappa = 0.6 (El Hout et al, 2010). If surgeons have to select "favorable" anatomy for TIP, then some will at least occasionally use TIP when they should not, and not use TIP when they could.

"Large Raw Area"

A related concern for some surgeons is the "raw area" made by TIP incision, which is larger when the plate is flat than when it is deeply grooved. They worry this area will stenose during healing, creating meatal stenosis or a neourethral stricture, and therefore choose another surgical technique or graft the TIP incision (Kolon and Gonzales, 2000).

However, as stated above, the flat plates we found in a third of patients did not increase our complications (Snodgrass & Bush et al, 2010), or those of others (Holland and Smith, 2000; Sarhan et al, 2008). Furthermore, Pfistermuller found only a 3.6% mean incidence of meatal stenosis and 1.3% urethral strictures after primary distal TIP, while we reported only 1 case of meatal stenosis from BXO a few years after a TIP repair and no neourethral strictures (Snodgrass and Bush et al, 2010). In addition, no report has shown decreased complications after G-TIP versus TIP. From these data is is clear that surgeons encountering more meatal stenosis or strictures are making technical errors, rather than using the operation for unsuitable anatomy. In fact, the irony is that most of these obstructions occur because a surgeon does not make the TIP incision deeply through the entire plate because he or she is afraid of creating an obstruction!

We have published these observations several times (Snodgrass, 1994; Lorenzo and Snodgrass, 2002; Nguyen and Snodgrass, 2004; Bush and Snodgrass, 2017), yet some refuse to accept these conclusions. We have no issue when a surgeon chooses to graft the TIP incision with foreskin that otherwise would be discarded, since outcomes from TIP and G-TIP are the same. But surgeons should not use the excuse that the TIP incision could stricture to justify using other repairs, such as the Mathieu which does not reliably achieve the same aesthetic results. Nor should they teach fellows that TIP is prone to stricture since there are no published data supporting that. And foreskin should not be used to graft a TIP incision when the family desires foreskin reconstruction, unless data is presented that this does not increase the rate of foreskin complications.

Key Points

While some older surgical techniques for distal hypospadias were limited to patients with specific anatomy, TIP is not. Rather, TIP can be used whether the plate has a deep groove or is flat, and whether it is narrow measuring < 8mm, or wider.

The 426 consecutive patients we repaired using only TIP certainly represented every variation in anatomy, yet our complication rate was only 4% (Snodgrass and Bush et al, 2010). More importantly, the meta-analysis by Pfistermuller et al evaluated 49 studies done worldwide in 3621 patients with distal hypospadias and also reported reoperations in only 4.4% after TIP repair.

These data prove that surgeons do not need to worry if TIP can be used for a specific distal hypospadias repair. Instead, they can focus on performing TIP optimally in every patient to similarly achieve > 90% success. Given that many surgeons do not currently meet that standard, debates regarding urethral plate suitability for TIP repair should end, and give way to an emphasis on doing the operation in the best known way everytime.

References

Abbas TO and Pippi-Salle JL: When to graft the incised plate during TIP repair? A suggested algorithm that may help in the decision-making process. *Front Pediatr* 6: 326, 2018

Abbas TO, Adnan I, Hatem J, Boyko A, Zorkin S, Plate Objective Scoring Tool (POST) in distal hypospadias: correlation with post-repair complications, *J Pediatr Urol* e-pub, 2023

AUA: Practicing urologists in the United States 2022.

Bush N and Snodgrass W: Pre-incision urethral plate width does not impact short-term tubularized incised plate urethroplasty outcomes. *J Pediatr Urol* 13:625, 2017

Cheng EY, Vemulapalli SN, Kropp BP, Pope JC, IV, Furness PD, III, Kaplan WE and Smith DP: Snodgrass repair with vascularized dartos flap: the perfect repair for virgin cases of hypospadias? *J Urol* 168: 1723, 2002

Duckett JW and Keating MA: Technical challenge of the megameatus intact prepuce hypospadias variant: the pyramid procedure. *J Urol* 141: 1407, 1989

El-Hout Y, Braga LHP, Pippi Salle JL, Moore K, Bägli DJ, Lorenzo AJ: Assessment of urethral plate appearance through digital photography: do pediatric urologists agree in their visual impressions of the urethral plate in children with hypospadias? *J Pediatr Urol* 6:294, 2010

Gibbons MD and Gonzales ET, Jr: The subcoronal meatus. *J Urol* 130:739, 1983

Holland AJA and Smith GHH: Effect of the depth and width of the urethral plate on tubularized incised plate urethroplasty. *J Urol* 164: 489, 2000

Kogan BA and Feustel PJ: What can we learn from pediatric urology certification logs? *Urology* 78: 147, 2011

Kolon TF and Gonzales ET Jr: The dorsal inlay graft for hypospadias repair. *J Urol* 163:1941, 2000

Lorenzo AJ and Snodgrass W: Regular dilation is unnecessary after tubularized incised plate repair. *BJU Int* 89: 94, 2002

Nguyen MT and Snodgrass W: Effect of urethral plate characteristics on tubularized incised plate urethroplasty. *J Urol* 171: 1260, 2004

Pfistermuller KLM, McArdle AJ and Cuckow PM: Meta-analysis of complication rates of the tubularized incised plate (TIP) repair. *J Pediatr Urol* 11:54, 2015

Sarhan O, Saad M, Helmy T, and Hafez A: Effect of suturing technique and urethral plate characteristics on complication rate following hypospadias repair: a prospective randomized study. *J Urol* 182: 682, 2009

Snodgrass W: Tubularized incised plate urethroplasty for distal hypospadias. *J Urol* 151: 464, 1994

Snodgrass W and Bush N: Hypospadias. In Wein A (Ed) **Campbell's Urology**, 10th Ed, 2011, pp

Snodgrass WT, Bush N and Cost N: Tubularized incised plate hypospadias repair for distal hypospadias. *J Pediatr Urol* 6: 408, 2010

White CM and Hanna MK: Salvaging the dehisced glans penis. *J Pediatr Urol* 14: 422, 2018

Zaontz MR: The GAP (glans approximation procedure) for glanular/coronal hypospadias. J Urol 141: 359, 1989

Repair When Ventral Curvature is 30° Or More

Chapter 8

Urethroplasty When Ventral Curvature Is ≥ 30°

30° or more VC defines severe hypospadias, regardless of the meatal location. This extent of bending is most reliably and durably straightened by transecting the urethral plate and making 3 ventral corporotomies. Those corporotomies also lengthen the penis an average of 30%, which is an additional advantage for boys with proximal hypospadias whose length is often less than the mean.

Technically, all hypospadias can be repaired in a single operation and the push to do so reached its apex with John Duckett, who wrote the transverse island flap achieved 90% *success* (Duckett, 1980). However, his successors reported 87% *complications* using that procedure for proximal hypospadias and said they no longer do it (Long et al, 2017).

Similarly, WS tried to extend TIP indications to include patients with VC greater than 30°. Straightening their curvature while preserving the urethral plate relies on dorsal plication, but it is clear that plications done using whatever technique or sutures cannot reliably withstand the ventral tension generated by spontaneous erections when there is more than 30 degrees of VC. So, while WS had some successes, these came with an unacceptable price of complications for others which included neourethra strictures (Snodgrass and Bush et al, 2013) and recurrent VC (Snodgrass and Bush, 2021) requiring reoperations.

The trend since the 1990s has returned to staged repairs for proximal hypospadias. In the US, these have mostly been Byars flaps. Early reports said this operation also had few complications, but 3 recent series each found they developed in over 50% of patients (Stanasel et al, 2015; McNamara et al, 2015; Long et al, 2017).

An ironic consequence of these 3 publications is nihilism that proximal hypospadias can be repaired to make a normal penis. Increasingly, surgeons recommend extending the neourethra only to the corona—essentially making proximal hypospadias into distal hypospadias. Those boys are at increased risk for a lifetime of urine spraying, and the myriad of social concerns that abnormal urination, and their different appearance, creates.

Our profession can do better.

Graft repairs popularized by Bracka have fewer than half the complications of flaps. However, Bracka did not reliably straighten the penis, and doing so impacts both grafting and ventral skin management. We refined staged graft repairs taking these factors into account, which led first to STAG (STraighten and Graft) that then evolved into STAC (STraighten And Close). The reliability of STAC to repair even the most severe hypospadias into a normal penis has made it the default operation when VC is 30° or more.

This chapter explains how to perform the key steps in STAC in the best way that we have found to date.

Goal of Proximal Hypospadias Repair

The goal is to make the abnormal anatomy of the penis with proximal hypospadias normal. That means the penile shaft must be straight. The meatus should be vertical and slit, and located at the tip of the glans with normal glans fusion. Penis skin should cover the shaft symmetrically with no visible scars outside the circumcision line and/or median raphe. There should be no lingering or recurring complications.

No other current approach achieves this goal better than STAC.

Straightening Ventral Curvature

This topic is discussed in Chapter 2. We begin this chapter on urethroplasty when there is VC ≥ 30° emphasizing again that the penis *must be straight* before urethroplasty, and that persistent or recurrent VC is the main underlying cause of complications after proximal repairs. Chordee excision and dorsal plication are *not* reliable means to straighten VC ≥ 30°. Neither is a single ventral corporotomy with corporal grafting, which may not be sufficient for the higher degrees of curvature commonly found in proximal hypospadias (Snodgrass and Bush, 2019).

The 3 corporotomies we use to straighten VC ≥ 30° reliably and durably correct any extent of curvature - which makes it superior to single corporotomy with corporal grafting. Some have questioned if ventral corporotomy(ies) cause erectile dysfunction, but our experience in older teens and adults shows 3 corporotomies do not.

Skin incision

Many surgeons begin every hypospadias repair by completely degloving the penis through a circumcision incision. This traditional step limits STAC since the circumcision incision does not preserve foreskin for urethroplasty grafting at the second operation. Traditional degloving also limits visualization and access to the penoscrotal region and below compared to opening the ventral skin down the median raphe.

Because the etiology and extent of VC cannot be accurately determined preoperatively, we begin *every* repair by degloving ventrally through the incision shown in Figure 1, *whether the meatus is distal or proximal*. Penile and scrotal dartos are released, and dissection can continue around the shaft under the dorsal skin without circumferential degloving.

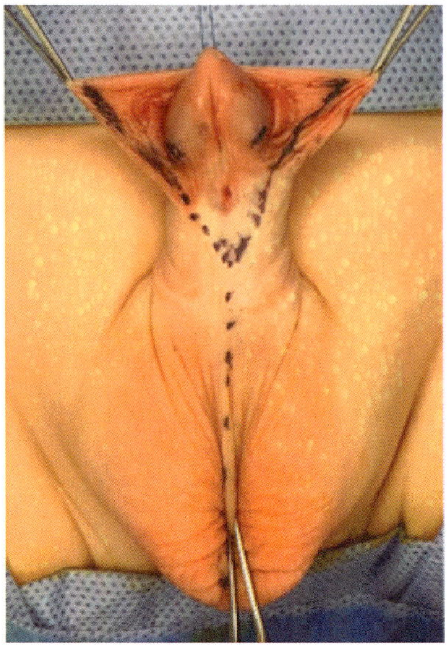

Figure 1. Initial skin incision for hypospadias. This skin incision begins distally into the ventral junction of inner and outer prepuce at least 3mm away from the glans. It continues alongside the urethral plate onto the proximal shaft to the penoscrotal junction, or lower as needed. Then ventral dartos is released and an artificial erection done. If VC measures < 30° then degloving is completed and TIP repair done. If VC ≥ 30° is found, then STAC is done with prepucioplasty as described in the following sections. In either situation the incision can be extended into the scrotum to correct transposition or gain additional exposure to the urethra.

Once the situation is determined, dorsal degloving is completed for TIP when VC is less than 30° and the family desires circumcision. When VC is 30° or more STAC is done, which includes prepucioplasty to preserve and enlarge the foreskin for use during the next operation.

Because most patients with hypospadias have ventral curvature during preoperative examination, today we no longer begin surgery with a circumferential incision - since it cannot be determined whether a bend is due to short ventral skin or a short ventral corporal sheath until the operation is underway.

STAC Repair

STAC 1

The typical patient with proximal hypospadias has ventral curvature and deficient, often near absent, ventral penile skin. The aim of STAC 1 is to straighten the penis and adjust the penile shaft skin so that it is symmetric circumferentially. Skin management includes prepucioplasty so that there is sufficient penile skin at the next operation to maintain symmetric shaft coverage and prepuce to provide the graft for urethroplasty.

Ventral Degloving

The dorsal corners of the foreskin are identified and short 5-0 Prolene stays are placed on each side. They are tied so that hemostats holding them can be removed at various times during the operation, such as during artificial erection.

The lines for incision shown in Figure 2 are first injected with 1:100,000 epinephrine (or 1:200,000, depending on which is available). Typically, the skin in these cases is close to, or adheres to, the underlying wings of corpus spongiosum, and troublesome bleeding can result despite a careful, superficial skin

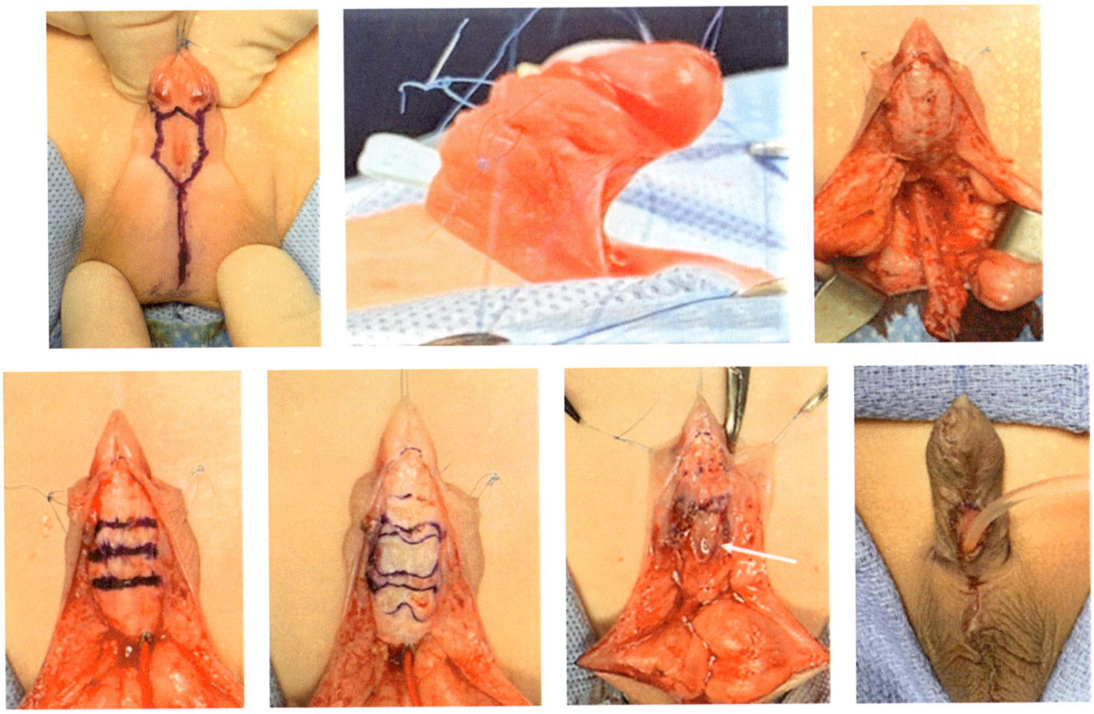

Figure 2. Key steps in STAC 1 repair.
A, ventral degloving incision. The location for the anticipated cut across the urethral plate near the coronal is marked, but is not made until later in the operation after VC ≥ 30° is confirmed. B, artificial erection demonstrates ventral curvature, which is objectively measured using a goniometer. C, when VC 30° or more is measured, as in this case, the urethral plate is transected distally and then dissected along with the native urethra off the corpora down into the scrotum. D, lines for the 3 corporotomy incisions are marked across the arc where the penis is bent, with the middle incision through the area of greatest curvature. E, with a tourniquet applied, the corporotomy incisions are cut through the tunica albuginea but not into erectile tissues. F, the corporotomy incisions are covered with dartos tacked to the tunica albuginea around the perimeter and along the isthmuses to contain bleeding. The proximal urethrostomy (arrow) is made where the meatus reaches without tension. G, shaft skin at the penoscrotal junction has been tacked to the corpora on each side lateral to the urethra. Ventral skin has been sized to cover the shaft, without splitting the dorsal foreskin, and sewn to the meatus to complete the urethrostomy. Prepucioplasty was done to encircle the glans with the dorsal foreskin hood. Shiny midline scrotal skin has been excised and the median raphe approximated.

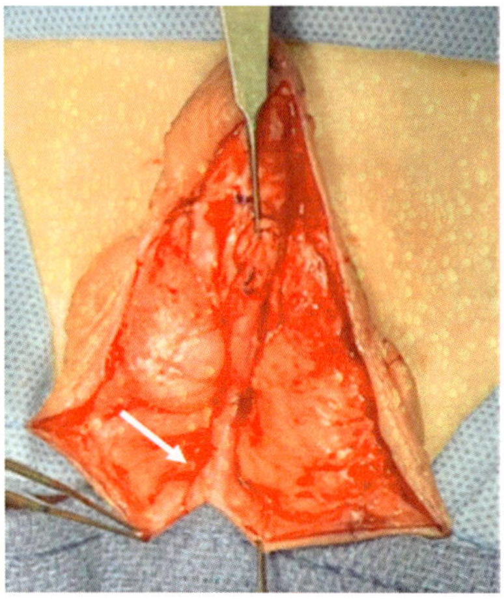

Figure 3. Proximal urethra running superficially within the scrotum towards the anus.
Note that the course of the urethra below the penoscrotal junction is horizontal rather than the normal vertical path towards the external sphincter. In addition, it adheres to perineal skin (arrow). These skin attachments are released so that the urethra can move into a normal position, which also adds length to it.

incision. Epinephrine injection vasoconstricts the spongiosum and hydrodistends the space under the skin, making injury less likely.

Then superficial incision is made just through the skin using the 69 Beaver blade. Next, scissor dissection begins in the scrotum and moves distally, initially staying immediately under the penile skin to avoid injuring the spongiosum. Lateral to the spongiosum dissection moves to a deeper plane against the corpora to preserve dartos on the shaft skin. Scrotal dartos is released, and penile shaft dissection continues circumferentially under the intact dorsal skin.

The scrotum typically encroaches up the penile shaft in proximal hypospadias, creating penoscrotal transposition. As discussed in Chapter 6, scrotal dartos contributing to this transposition runs from the scrotal skin alongside the penile shaft to insert on the pubis. Identifying and transecting these bands of dartos resolves transposition without needing to create rotational scrotal flaps.

Frequently, the urethra proximal to the meatus runs superficially under the scrotal raphe a variable distance towards the anus (Figure 3). Dissection frees its lateral edges and continues proximally to release it from perineal skin attachments. These are often dense, with only a millimeter distance between urethral spongiosum and the perineal epithelium, and this dissection is best done keeping taut countertraction to expose the correct plane. As the urethra is mobilized cephalad, it is additionally dissected from the rectum dorsally. This allows it to move to a natural position and helps gains length to later move the meatus farther distally.

Artificial Erection

Next, artificial erection is performed. The first test is done without a tourniquet, since bending can occur at or just below the penoscrotal junction and a tourniquet placed there can obscure it. Once it is determined the curvature is farther distally a tourniquet is placed.

The degree of curvature is measured using a goniometer as described in Chapter 3.

In some cases the ventral penile skin is so short that accurate assessment of the VC requires it to first be lengthened by oblique incisions as described below.

Dissecting the urethral plate and urethra

When goniometry measures curvature ≥ 30°, the next step is to dissect the urethral plate and urethra off the corpora. It is usually easiest to find the correct plane in approximately the midshaft. Once a space is developed completely under the plate, dissection continues in that plane to the corona, where the urethral plate is transected with an inverted V cut, which makes later skin closure at the urethrostomy easier.

Then dissection moves proximally, freeing the urethral plate and native urethra, as well as dartos and spongiosum alongside them, as one unit off the corpora to within the scrotum. The urethra is most adherent in the midline, where upward traction by the assistant slightly lifts the tunica albuginea with it. With the surgeon creating countertraction by pressing down on the corpora, the correct plane between urethra and corpora can be seen and developed by small snips of fine-tipped tenotomy scissors.

The goal is to accomplish this dissection of the urethral plate and urethra without entering the tunica albuginea of the corpora, which otherwise makes it more difficult to achieve firmness during the

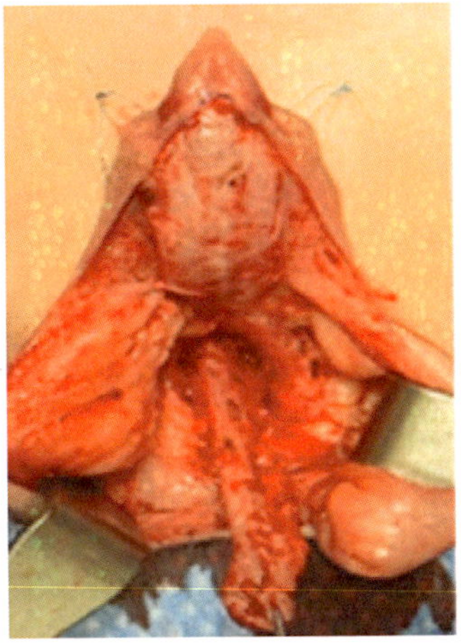

Figure 4. Mobilization of the urethral plate/urethra down to near the membraneous portion.

subsequent artificial erection. If a leak occurs, it can be oversewn with 6-0 PDS.

When the meatus is located on the penile shaft, urethral mobilization into the distal scrotum suffices and will result in a urethrostomy beyond the penoscrotal junction. That reduces the length of urethroplasty graft needed at the 2nd stage and minimizes likelihood of introducing hair follicles into the urethrostomy. However, in the most severe cases with the meatus within or below the scrotum (Figure 4), urethral dissection continues until the membraneous segment so that the urethrostomy will lie closer to, or at, the penoscrotal junction.

Further length on the urethra is gained by also releasing fibrovascular tissues tethering it ventrally to dartos within the scrotum.

Repeat Artificial Erection and 3 Corporotomies

Next, artificial erection is repeated to accurately determine the point of greatest curvature. Then 3 lines are marked transversely, the first across the greatest bend, then another 3-4mm proximally and a third 3-4mm distally. With a tourniquet secured, incision is made through the tunica albuginea along each line from 3 to 9 o'clock, starting with the middle line, as described in more detail and shown in Figure 5.

Buck's fascia is also short ventrally, and it too is incised laterally at 3 and 9 o'clock adjacent to the incisions into tunica albuginea.

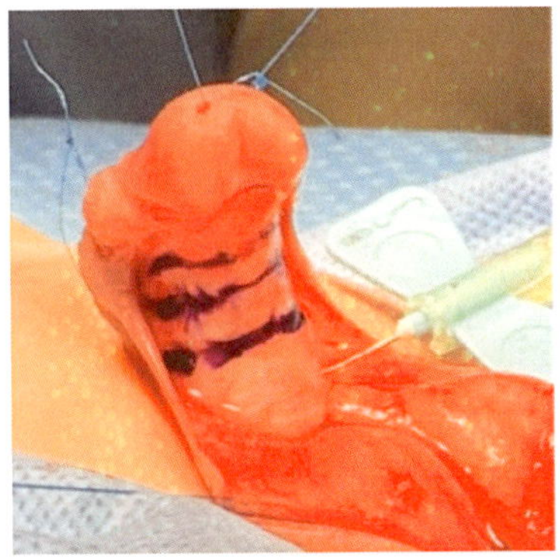

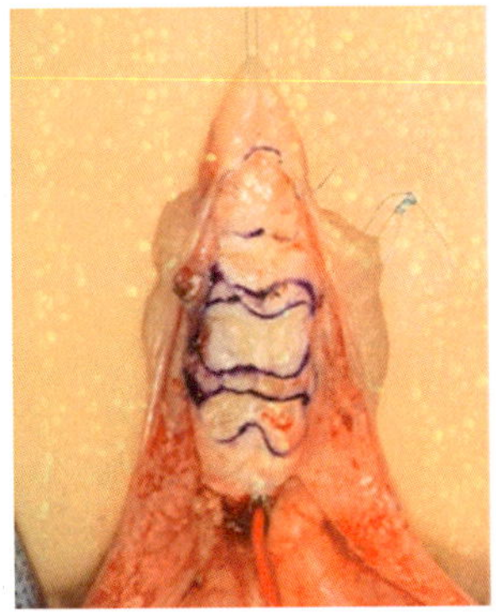

Figure 5. 3 transverse corporotomies.
A, lines have been drawn across the arc of curvature, the middle line through the greatest bend and the others, 3-4mm distally and proximally. B, a tourniquet was placed, and then incisions made starting with the middle line, from 3 to 9 o'clock through the tunica abuginea, which expose but do not enter the erectile tissues. Buck's fascia is also incised adjacent to the tunica albuginea incisions. These corporotomies straighten the curvature, release ventral tension from the tunica albuginea, and lengthen the penis an average of 30%.

Covering the corporotomies with dartos

One of the most important steps in STAC 1 is to cover the corporporotomies with a dartos flap to contain any bleeding that might occur when the tourniquet is released. This dartos flap is raised from the shaft skin on one side or the other, mobilizing tissues preserved with the skin during its initial dissection (Figure 6). This is why the correct plane of dissection against the tunica albugenia during degloving is important, so that this dartos will be available. The flap is advanced medially to cover the 3 incisions without tension and sutured around the perimeter using interrupted 6-0 PDS. These horizontal mattress stitches are placed

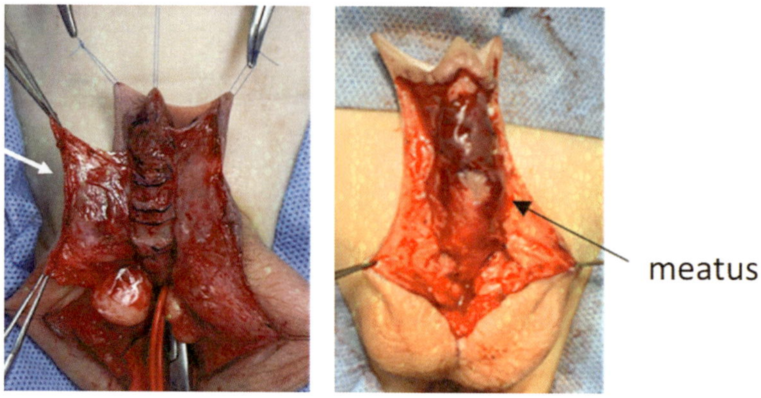

Figure 6. Dartos flap covering the corporotomy incisions.
A, dartos flap (arrow) has been harvested from the right shaft skin. B, dartos is used to cover the 3 corporotomy incisions, and sewn to the tunica albuginea around the perimeter and the isthmuses between incision to contain bleeding. The urethral meatus was secured where it reached without tension, in this case on the isthmus between the most poximal and middle corporotomy. A typical small volume of blood is seen under the flap.

transversely through the edge of the flap, then into the tunica albuginea just beyond the cut edges of the corporotomies, and back out through the flap to best contain any bleeding. The flap is also sutured in 3 places to each isthmus of tunica albuginea between the incisions: in the midline and to either side.

Making the proximal urethrostomy

Next we drizzle 1:1000 epinephrine over the dartos flap and then the assistant holds firm pressure onto a gauze laid on top of the now covered corporotomy incisions with one hand, and lifts the urethra with the other. The surgeon releases the tourniquet, and then stitches the uretha back onto the midline of the corpora at approximately 1cm intervals using 6-0 PDS. The urethra is gently advanced distally, taking care not to stretch it tight or create downward tension onto the penis. It is important to keep the penis stretched taut to its full length as the urethra is sewn to the corpora.

The meatus is spatulated and the floor of the urethra sewn to the corpora or onto one of the isthmuses using 7-0 Vicryl. Two more stitches are used to either side to complete the dorsal aspect of the urethrostomy, maintaining its inverted V shape. The urethrostomy is completed later in the procedure, after the penile skin is adjusted to cover the ventral shaft.

Meanwhile, additional 6-0 PDS sutures are placed to further anchor the distal urethra to the corpora on each side and reduce downward tension.

The site of the corporotomies is then inspected again for bleeding, and additional 6-0 PDS sutures placed as needed to contain it. Full-strength epinephrine can also be applied topically again, and, in rare cases of continuing, bothersome bleeding, the tourniquet can be reapplied proximally under the urethra while work continues.

If bleeding is not contained by the dartos flap it can create a scrotal hematoma. Blood collecting under the thin penile skin of proximal hypospadias can also cause irritation and reaction that contracts it. These steps to minimize bleeding, plus a snug, but not tight, compression bandage when the operation is complete, prevent these complications.

Ventral skin lengthening

Patients with proximal hypospadias and VC $\geq 30°$ nearly always have little or no penile skin on the ventral shaft. Once scrotal dartos is released to lower the scrotum down off the penile shaft, and the curvature is straightened by 3 corporotomies, the relative deficiency of ventral skin has increased. It is important that available skin be apportioned symmetrically around the penis, meaning there is the same length of penile skin covering the dorsal and ventral shaft. This

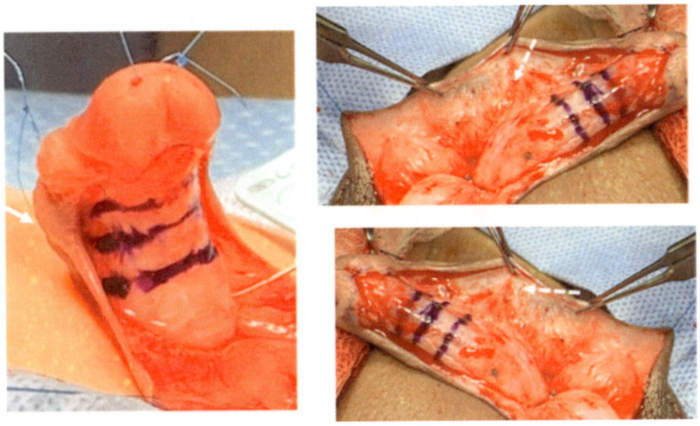

Figure 7. Lengthening the ventral skin *without* using Byars flaps.
A, the short ventral skin is taut. The arrow indicates a skin hump, which releases extra skin when an incision is made into it. Most often these are found bilaterally on the dorsal mid- to distal shaft. B, oblique incision is made towards the skin hump to lenthen the ventral skin edge. C, a similar incision is made in the opposite direction on the contralateral side to lengthen it. Direct transverse cuts, and bilateral oblique cuts at the same angle, are avoided as they can tighten the skin horizontally.

is accomplished by judicious oblique cuts to lengthen the skin along the ventral degloving incision as shown in Figure 7 and further discussed in Chapter 21.

It is important to emphasize that the traditional splitting of the dorsal prepuce into 2 Byars flaps rotated ventrally to cover the shaft is *not* done in STAC. Instead, the dorsal foreskin is left undisturbed to use during STAC 2 as a graft for the neourethra.

Pexing the penoscrotal junction

It is also important to provide fixed points at the penoscrotal junction so that postoperative erections can stretch the newly lengthened ventral skin (Figure 8). This is the same maneuver done by many surgeons at the final stage to establish the penoscrotal junction, but we have learned that it should also be used during STAC 1 to help correct the ventral skin deficiency.

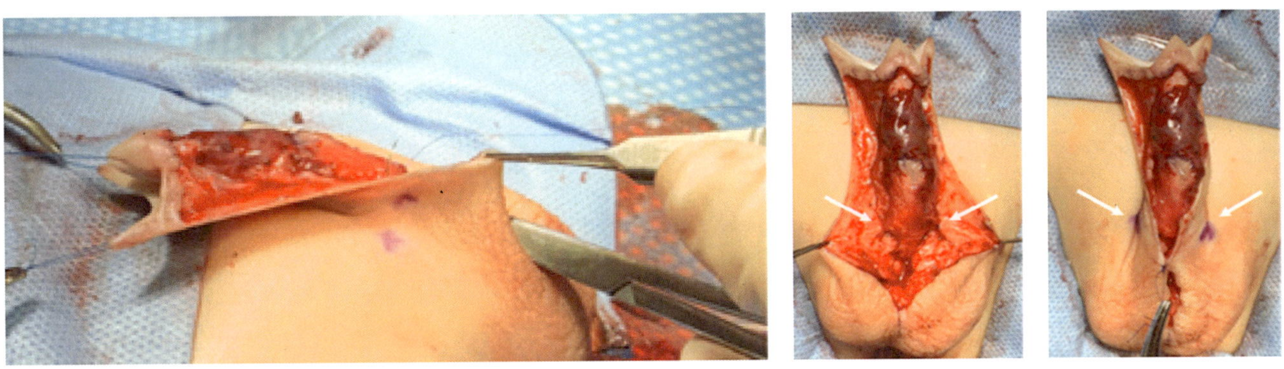

Figure 8. Pexing the penoscrotal junction.
A, the skin has been marked at the penoscrotal junction and a 5-0 PDS suture is being placed there to anchor it to the corpora. B, arrows indicate where the 2 stitches have been placed, 1 on each side. C. external skin marks where the stitches were taken can be seen, and the skin has been approximated in the midline, temporarily, with another suture which is held in the hemostat. This stay helps with sizing the ventral shaft skin, reducing the possibility for it to be pulled too far distally and cut too short. Failing to properly size the ventral shaft skin is one of the most common technical errors made in proximal repairs.

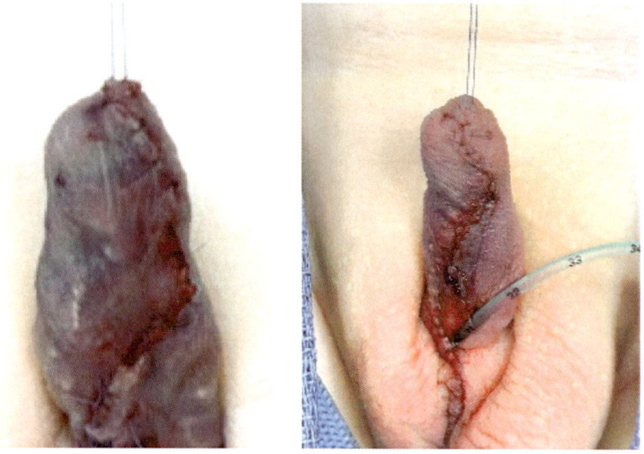

Figure 9. Prepucioplasty.
Two example of prepucioplasty in STAC patients. The ventral edges of the foreskin hood have been sutured together to encompass the glans. Iatrogenic phimosis is acceptable and possibly desireable so that postoperative erections can stretch the foreskin larger.

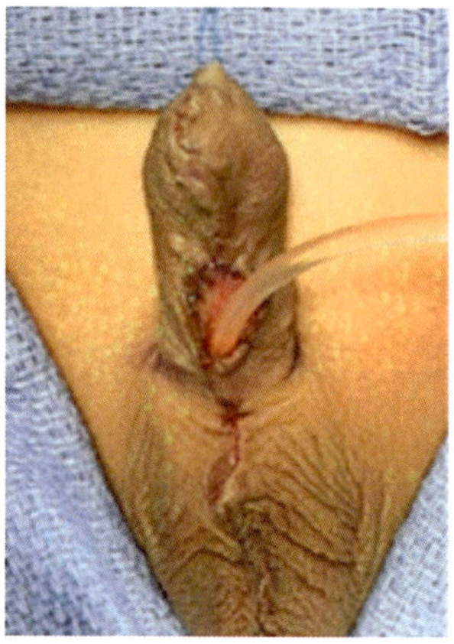

Figure 10. Appearance after STAC 1.
The proximal urethrostomy was made, and the ventral shaft covered with penile skin equal in length to the dorsal shaft skin. Prepucioplasty gives the penis a natural appearance, while scrotoplasty removed the cleft and any shiny skin in the median raphe.

Prepucioplasty

Another important maneuver to ensure there is adequate skin for both shaft coverage and urethroplasty grafting during STAC 2 is prepucioplasty. We emphasize again that the dorsal foreskin hood is *not* split into flaps to provide ventral shaft coverage. Instead, the initial ventral skin incisions are now extended towards the corners of the foreskin on each side to begin the prepucioplasty. The inner prepucial layer is first approximated together using interrupted subepithelial 7-0 Vicryl stitches, and then the outer skin is similarly closed (Figure 9). The goal is to preserve the foreskin and, by creating a phimotic ring distal to the glans, to help it stretch during natural postoperative erections. Therefore, the skin closure extends up and past the tip of the glans without worry about creating phimosis, but avoiding transverse tension that might cause the foreskin to dehisce.

Most dorsal skin humps are bilateral and located on the foreskin or distal shaft. The medial edges of those on the distal shaft can be entered to help lengthen the ventral shaft skin as shown above. Less often, single midline humps are found in the dorsal shaft, usually in the midshaft - and these are *not* disturbed during STAC 1. We have learned that trying to flatten them for aesthetic reasons can devascularize the foreskin distally and cause it to slough. These humps are managed during STAC 2 when the penis is fully degloved.

The ventral shaft skin is closed with interrupted subepithelial stitches. Skin edges near the meatus are sewn to urethral mucosa, using 7-0 Vicryl stitches through the epithelium. Leaving the meatus tapered towards a distal point facilitates smooth skin closure around it to complete the proximal urethrostomy.

Abnormal shiny skin in the scrotal raphe is excised, as is any cleft. Then the scrotal skin edges are approximated using a continuous subepithelial 6-0 PDS.

The final intraoperative appearance is seen in Figure 10.

By tacking the ventral shaft skin to the corpora at the penoscrotal junction and performing prepucioplasy, we have consistently found there is enough skin for both normal, symmetric, penile shaft coverage and the urethroplasty graft during STAC 2.

Following these steps leaves no need for Byars foreskin or scrotal flaps to cover the ventral shaft. Furthermore, oral mucosa is almost never needed to make the urethroplasty graft at STAC 2 in primary repairs.

Catheter and Bandage

An 8Fr foley is inserted into the bladder and the balloon inflated.

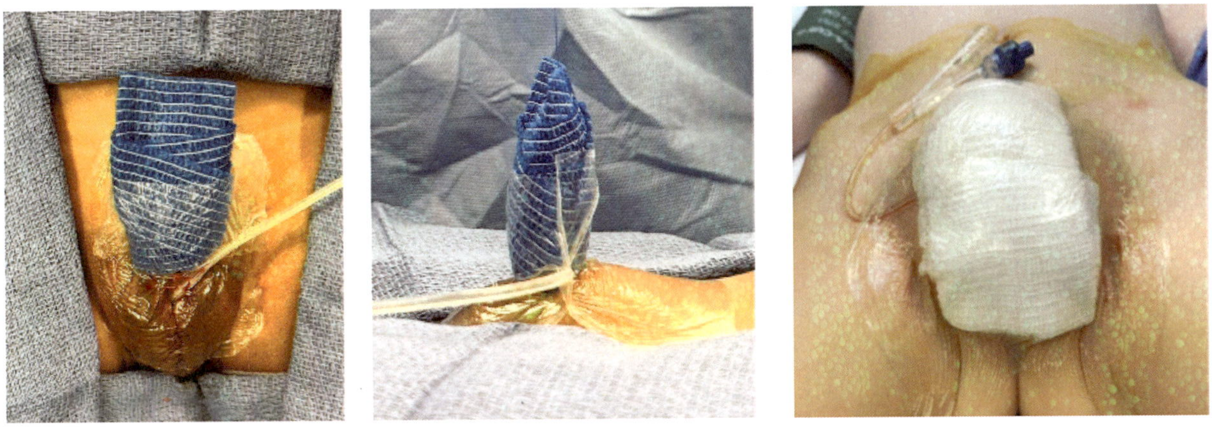

Figure 11. Bandage after STAC.
A,B, An elastic self-adherent bandage, similar to 3M's Coban™ dressing, is gently wrapped around the penis, ensuring it is not too tight. Then, to avoid the child being able to accidentally pull off the bandage in the early postoperative hours, Tegaderm dressing is used to further secure the bandage as shown. C. Additional gauze and Tegaderm are applied over this.

We initially experimented with a rolled vaseline gauze over the closed penis to compress the corporotomies, but the tie-over Prolene stays pulled too much on the shaft skin. Instead, we now wrap the penis with Adaptic followed by Coban™ or similar elastic self-adherent wrap to provide gentle compression, shown in Figure 11. Gauzes are then placed over the ventral penis, which is immobilized against the abdomen with large Tegaderms the same as previously demonstrated bandages. The patient is asked to sponge bathe for 4-5 days. The inner and outer bandages usually come off spontaneously in the days after they start bathing.

Postoperative Care

Urinary Diversion

The catheter drains into diapers for 1 week. If the catheter stops draining before that time it can safely be removed and does not need to be replaced.

Medications

Discomfort in boys less than 1 year of age can most often be relieved with acetominophen alternating with ibuprofen every 4 hours for approximately 36 hours, and then as needed. Patients 1 year and older are provided acetominophen with hydrocodone to use as needed instead of plain acetominophen.

Oxybutynin 0.2mg/kg is given twice daily to boys ages 1 to 3 years, increasing to three times daily for those older, or a daily extended release pill.

Trimethoprim / sulfamethoxazole is given once daily during urinary diversion.

Emollients and Creams

The bandage falls off spontaneously, and is not replaced. Then the parents begin applying Aquaphor (petroleum with lanolin) over the incisions and adjacent skin with each diaper change.

Beginning 1 month postoperatively they add betamethasone 0.1% cream twice a day continuing for 12 weeks.

We also advise parents to gently stretch the penis when applying emollients beginning approximately 1 month after surgery.

Despite these measures, the penis may appear slightly bent postoperatively. This nearly always results from mild ventral skin contracture which is easy to correct during STAC 2.

STAC 1 Results

STAC 1 reliably makes a straight penis with symmetric penile skin circumferentially. In other words, it makes a penis which is normal except for the lower

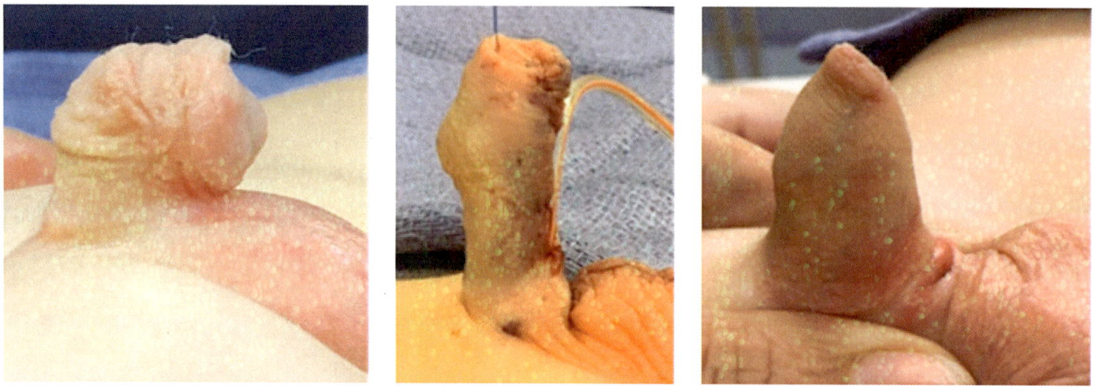

Figure 12. Typical appearance after STAC.
A, the penis is bent and there is essentially no ventral penile skin. B, intraoperative appearance at the conclusion of the STAC repair. The dorsal midline hump was not smoothed because dissection under or into it can disturb vascularity to the distal foreskin. C, appearance 6 months later. Note the penile skin is symmetric circumferentially. The foreskin is also intact after prepucioplasty and circumcision will provide the needed urethroplasty graft to extend from the penoscrotal meatus to the tip of the glans.

meatus. A typical result is seen in Figure 12. Once this is achieved, typical 2-stage graft urethroplasty is most often successful.

Penile Straightening

We verified that 3 corporotomies successfully straightens VC averaging 70° and ranging to 130° as reviewed in Chapter 2. 85% had a straight penis at STAC 2, while 15% had residual curvature averaging 23° corrected by a Heineke-Mikulicz dorsal plication. 99% had no VC at stage 3.

Penile skin reallocation

We measure and record the dorsal and ventral skin lengths from the penopubic and penoscrotal junctions to the distal-most aspect of dorsal and ventral skin, respectively, at the beginning of STAC 1, and again at its conclusion. Typical measurements would be approximately 40mm dorsally, and only 6-10mm ventrally. These measurements confirm the increase in ventral shaft skin length and prove coverage is circumferentially symmetric. Similar measurements at STAC 2 and 3 demonstrate this increase in length is durable, although some ventral skin flap contraction (approx 25%, for instance from 40mm at completion of STAC 1 to 30mm at onset of STAC 2) is quite common.

Complications After STAC 1

Although nearly all patients return for STAC 2 with a completely straight penis, a few have ventral curvature less than 30°. As mentioned above, 15% have residual corporal curvature straightened by dorsal plication. Other reasons for VC include slight contraction of the relocated ventral skin flaps, usually associated with tethering from the urethrostomy. A few had more extensive skin scarring requiring another skin revision.

Minor skin contraction and urethrostomy tethering

Slight skin contracture, usually associated with tethering from the urethrostomy, is the most common reason for penile curvature after STAC 1. That skin shrinkage is easily verified by comparing the ventral skin length at the beginning of STAC 2 to its measurement at the conclusion of STAC 1. Ventral degloving at STAC 2, plus small cuts along or obliquely into the skin edges as needed, resolve bending from short skin. Similarly, releasing the meatus and dissecting it proximally 1-2cm until it is freed from tethering scar tissue, helps with straightening. Repeat artificial erection should then confirm the penis is straight (Figure 13).

We inform all caregivers that mild recurrent curvature can develop after STAC 1 from skin contraction. This is not surprising, since the short ventral skin

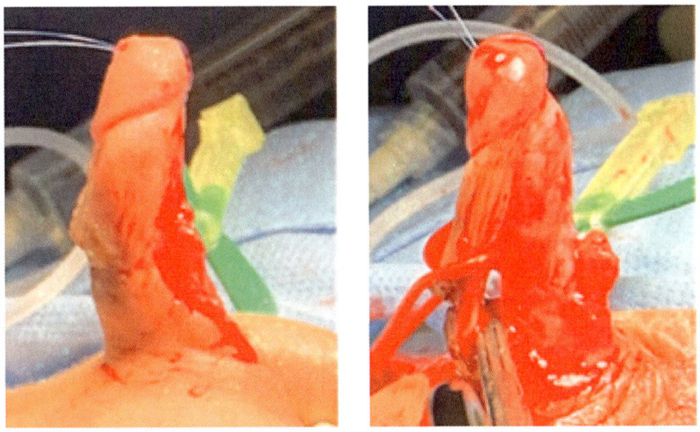

Figure 13. Recurrent ventral curvature after STAC. A, apparent recurrent ventral curvature after STAC 1. B, artificial erection after ventral degloving and short incisions into the skin edges to lengthen them still demonstrates slight bending. C, the meatus was dissected proximally 1cm, releasing it from scar to the coropora, and repeat erection confirms the penis is straight.

found in most hypospadias has abnormal vascularity that is further impacted by degloving and incisions made to lengthen the skin. This can result in ischemic necrosis of the ventral skin which usually manifests at 10-14 days postoperatively (Chapter 21, Figure 16). Accordingly, we request photographs of the ventral penis 2 weeks after STAC 1 specifically to identify this reaction, and recommend Manuka honey be applied with each diaper change until the skin heals, to provide debridement and antimicrobial protection.

Similar postoperative skin reaction can develop after distal repairs or surgery to correct congenital penile curvature or penile torsion but is rarely encountered after circumcision in typical boys, again indicating the penile skin in these anomalies has altered vascularity.

Extensive skin necrosis with scarring

We observed that 7% of patients developed more extensive ventral skin contracture after STAC 1, nearly all associated with either a single midline dorsal skin hump or penile torsion (Figure 14) as further discussed in Chapter 21. These associated skin anomalies likely made their vascularity tenuous. All those patients had sufficient skin contraction that the second operation was devoted to skin revision followed by postoperative HBOT to lengthen and revitalize the shaft skin before urethroplasty grafting was done.

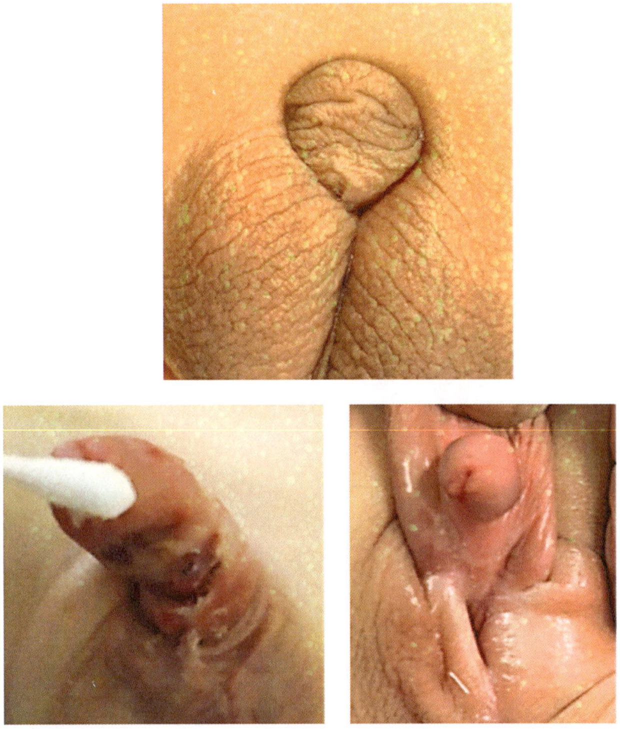

Figure 14. Skin necrosis after STAC 1 with scarring. A, preoperative photo showing a single skin hump on the midshaft which has increased risk for postoperative skin ischemia. B, 2-week postoperative picture send by the caregivers demonstrating ventral shaft skin necrosis. C, Visible skin scarring with loss of length on the right side best managed by skin revision without proceeding to STAC 2 urethroplasty grafting.

Currently we advise preemptive HBOT with STAC 1 when these skin anomalies are found, trying to avoid or minimize these ischemic reactions.

This specific skin reaction was not previously recognized after STAG repairs because it was accompanied by graft contracture. Contraction of either the urethroplasty graft or adjacent shaft skin causes the other to contract, too. Therefore, an advantage of STAC is that poorly vascularized skin is identified and managed before graft placement, increasing the likelihood for successful graft take.

Recurrent corporal curvature

Persisting VC after releasing the ventral shaft skin and meatus indicates recurrent corporal bending. This is uncommon when 3 corporotomy incisions were used and nearly always measures less than 30°. In those cases we complete degloving dorsally and then mimic straightening by plication using Adson forceps with the penis firmly erect. There is usually little resistance to pulling the erect penis straight, indicating that a Heinike-Mikulicz plication should provide durable correction.

We have not encountered persistent or recurrent VC after STAC 1 that required repeating 1 or more corporotomies. Should that happen, those corporotomies would be left to heal after a repeat STAC 1, delaying the urethroplasty grafting until straightening was confirmed.

Foreskin dehiscence or loss

Occasionally the foreskin dehisces after STAC, even though prepucioplasty was done without tension. We have found there is nearly always sufficient foreskin remaining for the urethroplasty graft at STAC 2 despite this occurrence.

Rarely, the foreskin is lost after STAC 1. This is most likely when there are skin anomalies in addition to the ventral skin deficiency – such as midline humps or penile torsion. This also supports preemptive HBOT for patients with these anomalies.

STAC 2

After STAC 1 corrects VC and reallocates penile skin to measure the same length dorsally and ventrally (from the penopubic junction and penoscrotal junction to tip of prepuce dorsally and ventrally, respectively), only urethroplasty remains to complete the repair. That is accomplished using a 2-stage graft technique, comprising STAC 2 and STAC 3.

We wait 6 months after the first stage before continuing the repair. The interval can be longer, but there is

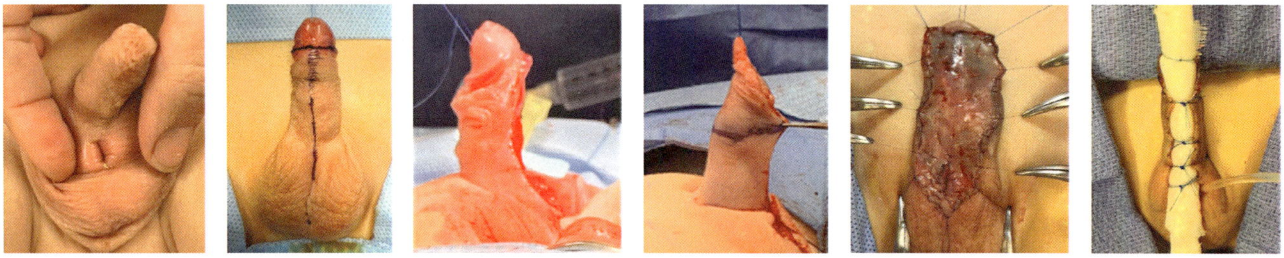

Figure 15. 2nd stage foreskin urethroplasty grafting.

A, healing after 1st stage STAC with urethrostomy in the distal scrotum. Note the otherwise normal appearance of the penis and reconstructed foreskin.

B, the foreskin is retracted and a ventral incision marked down the shaft and around the urethrostomy. The line for circumcision is also marked along the inner prepuce, and will be incised after repeat artificial erection confirms the penis is straight. The circumcision will be made 3mm below the corona to preserve as much foreskin as possible for the graft.

C, artificial erection confirms the prior corporotomies successfully straightened the penis.

D, the circumcision line for graft harvest is marked around the outer skin along the corona with the penis held taut. Note that the skin at the penoscrotal junction has been temporarily approximated to prevent inadvertant shortening of ventral shaft skin during graft harvest.

E, the glans is opened flat and the graft quilted into the space from its tip down to the meatus, with the graft buttonholed to surround it. This adds penile skin to this area which sometimes has troublesome skin deficiency and helps avoid getting scrotal hair into the neourethra and the next stage. When the meatus is deep within the scrotum, we spatulate the dorsal side approximately 4mm and then advance a V of graft within it instead of buttonholing around it. After sewing the perimeter of the graft, it is next quilted to the corpora in 3 rows – the first down the center and then one row to each side. Quilting stitches are *not* placed farther lateral than the edge of the corpora, which would result in quilting the graft to the dorsal shaft skin.

F, tie-over Vaseline gauze bandage and 8Fr foley catheter.

There is no reason to attempt to restrict activities in infants and toddlers after urethroplasty grafting, since they are likely to kick and scream if their parents try. Quilting the graft and using the tie-over bandage provides the immobilization the graft needs to revascularize. Older children are easier to distract so that they are less mobile, but the same reasoning applies to them that their indoor activity does not impact graft healing.

Certainly, there is no medical indication to admit children to the hospital for bedrest after grafting. We place grafts in all ages of boys and men as outpatient procedures.

The Tegaderm bandages fall off spontaneously and are not replaced. The catheter and tie-over bandage are removed at 1 week. Occasionally, the tie-over bandage comes off earlier, but is not replaced. There is no need or benefit to leave bandages on longer than a week.

Emollients and Graft Massage

Parents are instructed to apply Aquaphor (petroleum jelly with lanolin) generously over the graft and suture lines with each diaper change for at least 4 months, although they can continue using it until the next operation. Emollients keep the graft and skin moist, which is beneficial during healing.

Beginning 1 month postoperatively, they are told to substitute betamethasone 0.1% ointment and apply that to the graft and adjacent skin morning and evening, while continuing Aquaphor at other diaper changes. Steroid applications continue for 3 months. Wounds have a tendency to contract, which topical steroids help reduce. This treatment was also recommended by others for graft care (Ferro et al, 2002).

In addition, we advise parents to massage and stretch the graft while bathing to further counteract a tendency to contract beginning at approximately 1 month postoperatively.

STAC 2 Results

An important goal of staged graft repairs is achieving good graft take resulting in a supple, elastic neo-urethral plate to tubularize at the final stage. Even though focal scars or contractures in grafts can often be managed during tubularization, it is far better for the graft to require little or no manipulation.

Our primary prepucial graft success is nearly 95%. This is consistent with most reports on non-urethroplasty full-thickness grafts, finding that most take but a small percentage contract for unclear reasons. As discussed below, we changed from 2-stage STAG to 3-stage STAC in large part to improve graft health, having realized that grafts placed onto corporotomies take less well, and that the penile skin transferred to the ventral shaft during proximal repairs cannot reliably help revascularize the junction to the graft, which then scars and contracts. These problems are nearly eliminated by STAC repair.

Caregivers, and sometimes surgeons, naturally worry if the graft appears healthy. We tell them when the graft is placed that its appearance is unreliable, and that the final determination of graft suitability for tubularization is made during the final stage when it can be carefully inspected for scars and contractures and grasped and stretched with forceps. Furthermore, prepucial grafts often appear poorly vascularized when the bandages are removed yet nearly always heal as desired. We reassure caregivers that if we surgeons cannot accurately determine the health of the graft until the next operation is underway, they should not worry about its appearance beforehand, either.

STAC 3

Tubularization of the graft neo-urethral plate is done 6 or more months later. Some surgeons wait as long as a year after grafting believing that improves the quality of the graft. However, a graft which has healed with scars and/or contractures from poor revascularization evident at 6 months is not likely to significantly improve by waiting another 6 months. Similarly, we have not found grafts tubularized more than 6 months after placement to be noticeably better than those tubularized sooner.

At this stage the graft is now a revascularized neo-urethral plate. However, for simplicity and clarity we will continue to refer to it as a graft in this section.

Key steps in STAC 3 are show in Figure 24.

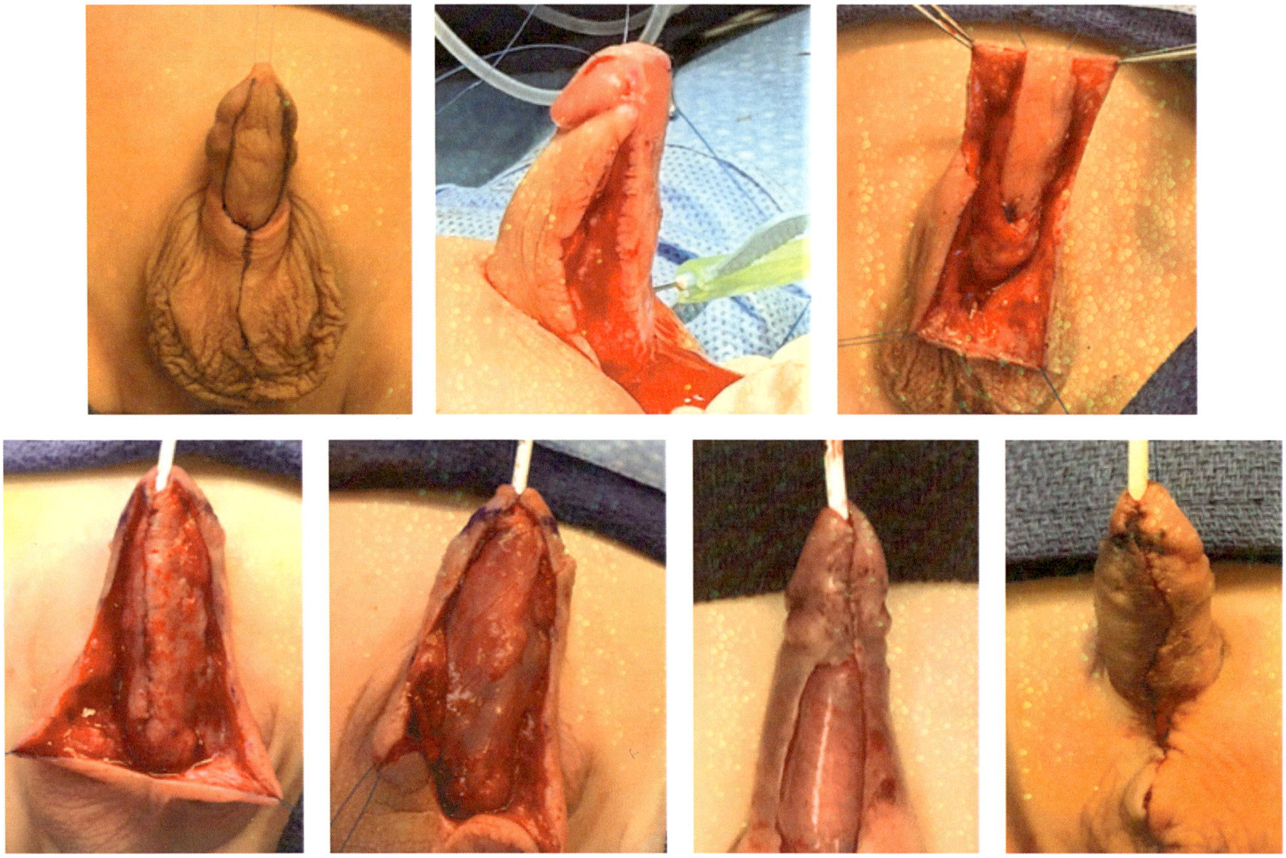

Figure 24. STAC 3, tubularization of the prepucial graft neoplate.
A, the graft appears healthy without visible scars, and measured nearly the same dimensions as when it was placed. Lines for incision are marked alongside the neo-plate at its junction to the skin, then into the meatus to exclude hair follicles, and down the midline of the scrotum to later give access to a testicle to harvest a tunica vaginalis flap. B, after ventral degloving, artificial erection is done to verify again that the penis is straight before proceding with urethroplasty. There is no need to completely deglove the penis during STAC 3. C, next glans wings are created and dissected open widely for later tension-free approximation over the neourethra. D, the neo-urethral plate is tubularized in 2 layers. The first layer, shown here, begins distally and is sewn using interrupted subepithelial 7-0 Vicryl. Then a continuous subepithelial 6-0 or 7-0 PDS is run proximally to distally for a second layer. This is the same tubularization done in proximal TIP repair. E, the neourethra is then covered by a tunica vaginalis flap, as in proximal TIP. F, glansplasty is completed with 3 interrupted subepithelial 6-0 Vicryl stitches, the first placed at approximately the midglans, and the 3rd at the corona. The 2nd includes a bite of tunica vaginalis to hold it up as the glans is closed. Glans wings are not sewn to the urethral opening, and no stitches are placed through the epithelium. This is the same glansplasty done in TIP repair. Note the mucosal collar has also been approximated. G, the skin at the penoscrotal junction is tacked to the coropora using 5-0 PDS and then the remaining shaft skin is closed into a median raphe using interrupted subepithelial 7-0 Vicryl.

Graft Inspection and Measurement Before Skin Incision

A 5-0 Prolene stay stitch is placed horizontally across the glans just beyond the future neomeatus. Then the penis is stretched and the length and widths of the graft are measured while forceps hold it fully expanded. The graft is also carefully inspected for obvious scars that might influence the skin incision.

Skin Incision

Most often the incision extends along the visible junction of the graft to adjacent shaft skin, just within the meatus to exclude any hair-bearing skin, and then down into the midscrotum as shown in Figure 25. We mark the glans wings and inject with 1:100,000 epinephrine, but do not incise along them until the penis is confirmed straight and the graft healthy for tubularization. Most graft contracture occurs below the glans near the urethrostomy, and repairs to the graft can usually be made preserving the healed portion within the glans intact and undisturbed in the small percentage of boys who need a partial patch graft.

Sometimes there is a visible and /or palpably indurated scar somewhere along the graft margin. If adjacent shaft skin is adequate to close easily over the neourethra, the incision is moved laterally just beyond the scar so that the neourethra tubularizes more readily.

At other times the graft may be wider than needed in a region with deficient shaft skin. In this case the incision is moved medial to the skin junction, leaving some of the graft to be used in the skin closure.

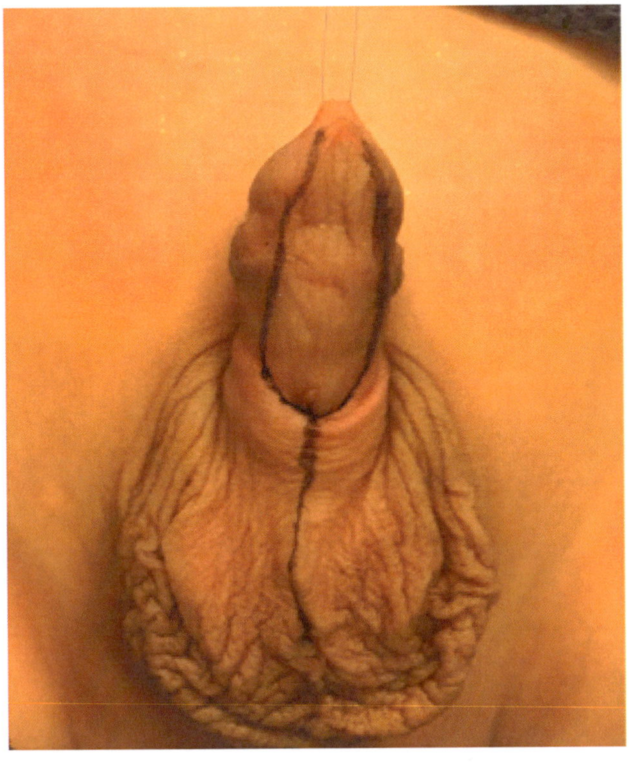

Figure 25. Marks showing the initial skin incision. The junctions of glans wings to the neo-urethral plate are marked, as are the junctions of the skin to the graft neo-plate. The incision goes into the meatus proximally to exclude hair-bearing skin, and continues a short distance down into the scrotum to later access the tunica vaginalis.

The incision continues down into the scrotum to later access a testicle for a tunica vaginalis coverage flap.

Dissecting Skin and Graft

Dissection is then done along the corporal margins to free the skin laterally from the urethrostomy up to the corona sufficiently for later closure.

Next, the graft is lifted and stretched with forceps along its course searching for any lines of tension. Even though a graft maintains its original dimensions and appears supple, contracted dartos along its edge can exert tension and hinder tubularization. We excise the dartos, or incise it longitudinally to release tension, which also slightly lengthens the graft. This process continues until the graft feels elastic along its entire length.

There may be a transverse scar at the junction of the graft to the meatus making it less pliable. This can safely be released and the graft widened at this point using a TIP incision. This incision normally is < 5mm long and heals without stricture, so inlay grafting is not necessary. Should a longer incision be needed at the urethrostomy or elsewhere along the neoplate, inlay grafting is done and then the neo-urethral plate is tubularized.

Management of graft healing problems is discussed in Chapter 11.

Artificial Erection

At this point artificial erection is done to confirm the penis is straight.

Creating Glans Wings

Once it is verified that the penis is straight and the graft is healthy for tubularization, glans wings are created. As in TIP repair, incision into the epithelium is done superficially using a Beaver 69 blade. Then it is deepened with tenotomy scissors dissecting along the surface of the corpora laterally to 3 and 9 o'clock. The wings are then checked for tension, and further dissection is done superiorly off the corpora as needed. It is important that the glans wings be mobile without tension to reduce likelihood for glans dehiscence, as shown in Figure 26 (Snodgrass and Bush, 2016).

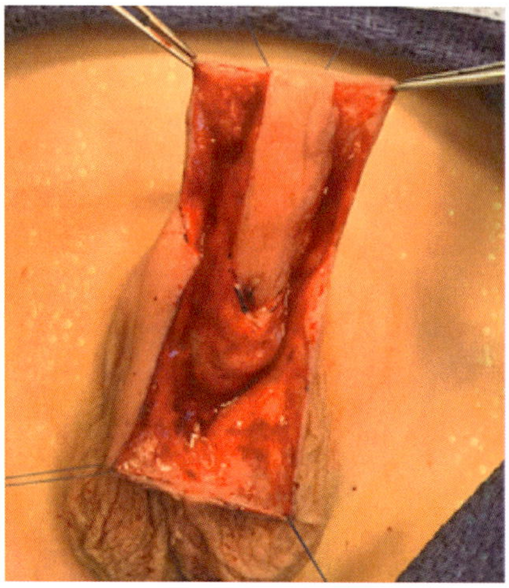

Figure 26. Appearance after glans wing mobilization. The glans wings are dissected laterally and also superiorly, as needed, for later tension-free closure over the neourethra. This is a key maneuver to reduce likelihood for glans dehiscence.

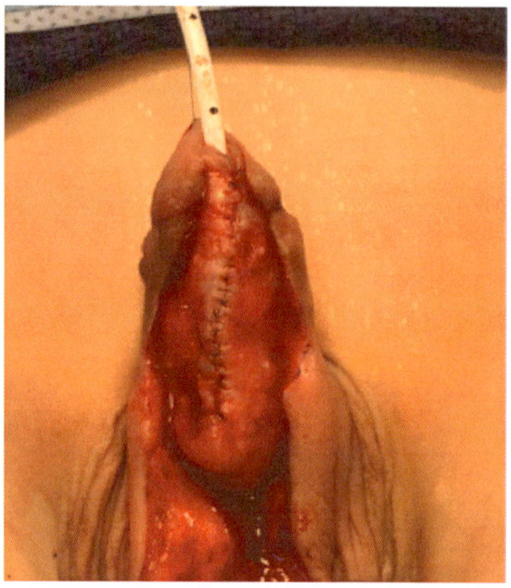

Figure 27. 1st layer tubularization of the neo-urethral plate.
The distal stitch is placed first to create an oval opening. We stress that the first layer of a proximal urethroplasty should be done with *interrupted* subepithelial stitches as shown. A second, continuous, layer will reinforce and bury these, helping to ensure the tubularization is watertight.

Neo-plate Tubularization

A 6Fr stent, or 5Fr feeding tube when the glans width is 13mm or smaller, is passed into the bladder and tied to the glans stay stitch. As we mentioned in Chapter 6, the neourethra is *not* sized to the stent. The stent only provides urinary diversion during the time of greatest postoperative edema within the neourethra.

Then, as with TIP repair, tubularization begins distally at the midglans level, which should be no closer than 3mm to the junction of the end of the neo-plate to the glans. The opening should be oval, and not rounded. Like in proximal TIP, a 2-layer subepithelial closure is done, the 1st with interrupted stitches. This is important to properly align the edges which may not heal entirely symmetrical, and to keep even tension on the sutures (Figure 27). We use 7-0 Vicryl on a TG 140-8 needle for prepucial graft tubularization.

After the first layer is completed, an angiocatheter is inserted into the opening and the neo-urethra distended with fluid to check for leaks. Those are stitched closed. Then a 2nd layer reinforces the closure using 6-0 or 7-0 PDS running from proximally to distally.

These technical details are important. Two-layer closures have fewer fistulas than single layer tubularizations. Interrupting the first layer and running the second results in 50% fewer fistulas than when the first layer is sewn with a continuous suture and the second is interrupted.

Tunica Vaginalis Flap

As in proximal TIP, a hemiscrotal compartment is entered and a testicle delivered to create a tunica vaginalis flap. That flap extends from the testicle to the external ring to avoid creating tension on the penis that would pull it to the side. Then the testicle is suture pexed back to the scrotum and a scrotal flap sewn over it to keep it from migrating medially.

The tunica vaginalis flap covers the entire neourethra (Figure 28). If bands of dartos muscle are seen in the flap, these are incised transversely to prevent intermitent penile torsion, taking care not to injure the flap vascular pedicle. We explained in Chapter 6 that these flaps significantly reduce fistulas in proximal repairs compared to dartos coverage flaps.

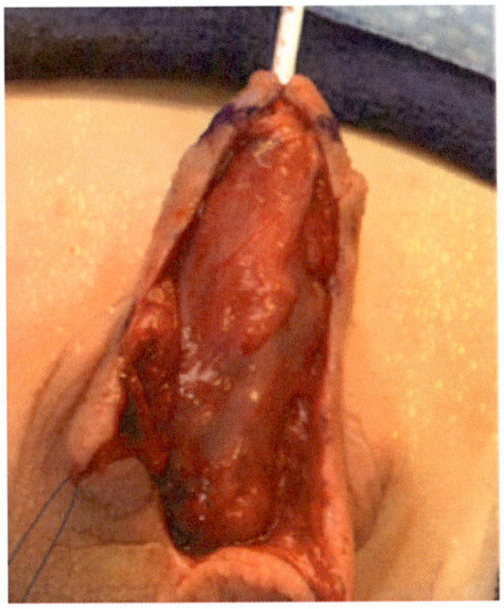

Figure 28. Tunica vaginalis flap covers the neourethra. Tunica vaginalis provides greater protection against fistulas than does dartos in proximal repairs. The flap should be dissected to the external ring and then moved medially and sewn without tension over the entire suture line. The testicle should be suture pexed back into its normal position and the hemiscrotal compartment closed to keep it from migrating medially.

Glansplasty

Glansplasty is also the same as in TIP repair, described in Chapter 6. Before approximating the glans wings over the neourethra they are again stretched and checked for residual tension, which is released before proceeding. Typically, 3 subepithelial interrupted stitches of 6-0 Vicryl create normal glans fusion below the meatus (Figure 29). The first approximates the midpoint of the glans wings and the third joins the corona. The 2nd stitch includes a bite of tunica vaginalis to hold it in place over the distal neourethra suture line.

The glans wings are not sewn to the opening in the tubularized neourethral plate. No epithelial stitches should be used during glansplasty. When the glans wings have been sufficiently dissected, single layer supepithelial closure effectively completes glansplasty with minimal risk for dehiscence and does not make visible scars that epithelial stitching often creates.

Creating the Mucosal Collar

The inner prepuce is carefully maintained during the earlier 2 stages so that it can be approximated at this point. This is not only important aesthetically, but it

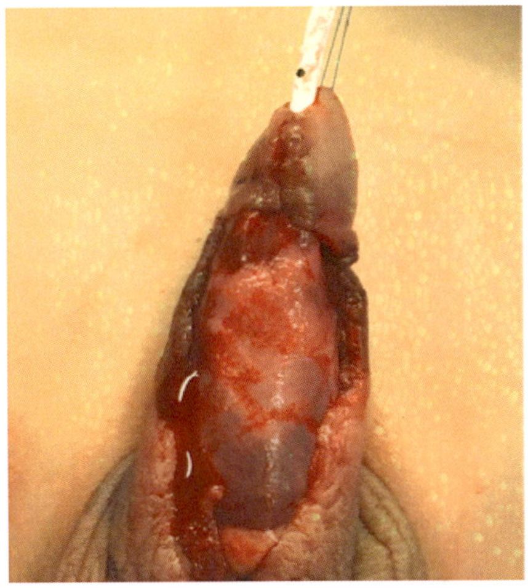

Figure 29. Completed glansplasty.
As in TIP repair, the glans wings are sewn together over, and not to, the neourethra. The first glans stitch is in the midglans. The 3rd aligns the corona. The 2nd, between those two, includes a bite of tunica vaginalis to hold it in place under the glans. We close the glans with only this single layer of subepithelial stitches. A second layer through the epithelium is not necessary, and is commonly harmful – creating visible scars and even gashes into the glans.

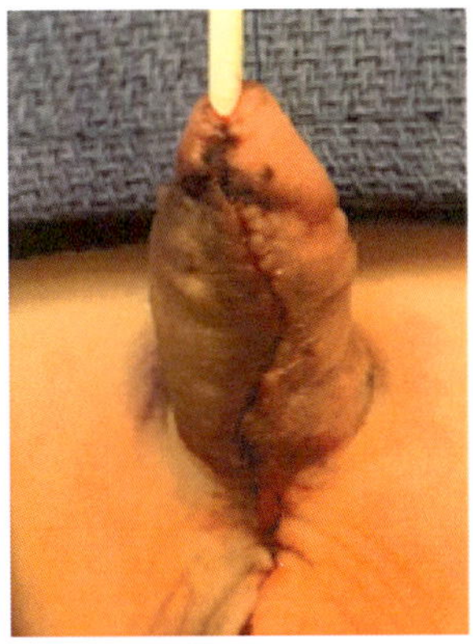

Figure 30. Final appearance after skin and scrotal closures. As in TIP repair, skin edges are all closed using subepithelial stitches.

also reduces fistulas and glans dehiscence. The mucosal collar buffers against tension that the ventral skin might exert on the glans. This step is the same as in TIP repair (Chapter 6).

Creating the Penoscrotal Junction

The proper location for the penoscrotal junction is determined, and then the proximal shaft skin is stitched to the corpora on each side lateral to the neourethra using 5-0 PDS. If there is ventral skin deficiency the junction can be moved up to 5mm distally to make skin closure easier.

Shaft Skin and Scrotal Closure

These steps are also done in the same way as described for proximal TIP repair. The scrotum is closed with a continuous subepithelial 6-0 PDS, while the shaft skin is approximated using interrupted subepithelial 7-0 Vicryl to make a median raphe, as shown in Figure 30

A clear advantage to the surgical algorithm of this textbook is that so many key steps in proximal TIP and the final stage of STAC are the same. Given that most urologists do few proximal repairs, it is easier to perform those steps optimally when they are the same in different situations.

Postoperative care

Urinary Diversion

The stent drains into diapers for 2 weeks. Occasionally it stops draining or is dislodged earlier. When that occurs within a few days of repair we replace the stent under sedation. If it happens a week or more after surgery we leave it out unless extravasation or retention develop, which are both unusual following a 2-layer urethroplasty that is confirmed intraoperatively to be watertight.

Medications

Hydrocodone with acetominophen is given alternating with ibuprofen on a regular schedule for 48 hours, and then as needed.

Oxybutynin suspension 0.2mg/kg is given twice daily to boys less than 3 years, increasing to three times daily for those older, or a single extended release tablet daily for patients old enough to swallow pills.

Trimethoprim / sulfamethoxazole is given twice daily during urinary diversion.

Emollients

Once the bandages fall off, parents are instructed to apply a coating of Aquaphor (petroleum with lanolin) over the incisions and adjacent skin with each diaper change.

If there was concern intraoperatively about snug penile skin, or the median raphe appears to be contracting postoperatively, bethamethasone 0.1% cream is

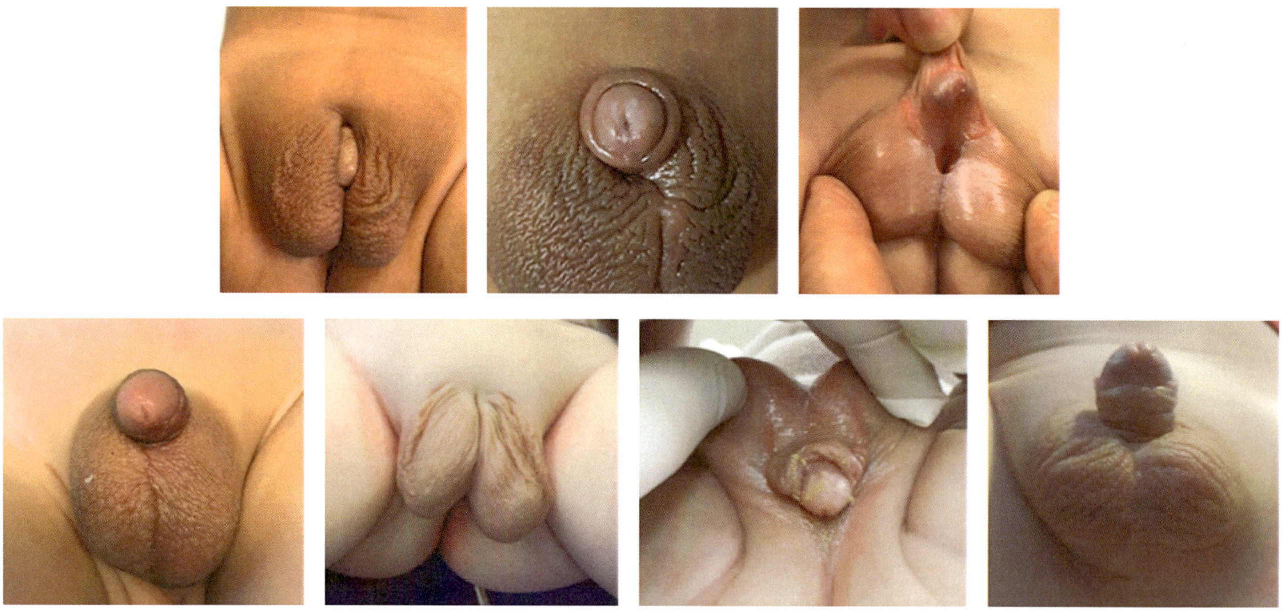

Figure 31. STAC repair in 3 patients with perineoscrotal hypospadias.
3-stage STAC repair routinely achieves the goal of changing the abnormal anatomy of even the most severe hypospadias into a normal penis. No other technique so reliably achieves these results, and many “2-stage” repairs actually involve 3 or more operations.

applied to the incision beginning 1 month postoperatively and used twice daily for 6-12 weeks.

Results

The final stage tubularization is successful without complication in 87% of cases (Snodgrass and Bush, 2024), which is the same as with proximal TIP. The most common urethroplasty complications are fistulas and glans dehiscences, occuring in similar numbers of patients. These are almost always corrected with 1 additional reoperation.

Therefore, the goal of making a penis with normal anatomy is achieved using STAC in over 98% of patients. Pre- and postoperative pictures of example cases are shown in Figure 31.

We are not aware of another procedure which can reliably achieve similar results.

Why we stopped doing 2-stage repairs

WS quickly abandoned the 1-stage transverse island flap repair he was taught during training when every patient in a small series developed postoperative complications. He next tried 2-stage Byars flaps combined with a distal TIP in the glans, which also resulted in 100% complications. These results are similar to those more recently reported by Stanasel et al, 2015, McNamara et al, 2015 and Long et al, 2017, as recounted in Chapter 1.

Influenced by Bracka, he eventually moved to 2-stage graft repairs. However, he realized the chordee excision Bracka used to straighten curvature would not work for the bending commonly encountered in boys with proximal hypospadias. He instead developed the 3 corporotomies to straighten the penis and allow simultaneous urethroplasty grafting during the first stage.

Initially he believed grafts took reliably when placed over corporotomies, until he and Bush started measuring graft dimensions when they were placed and again at the next stage. It was soon apparent that grafts heal best when they are placed onto intact corpora. Consequently, we stopped doing 2-stage STAG repairs when the mobilized urethra did not reach beyond the most distal corporotomy incision.

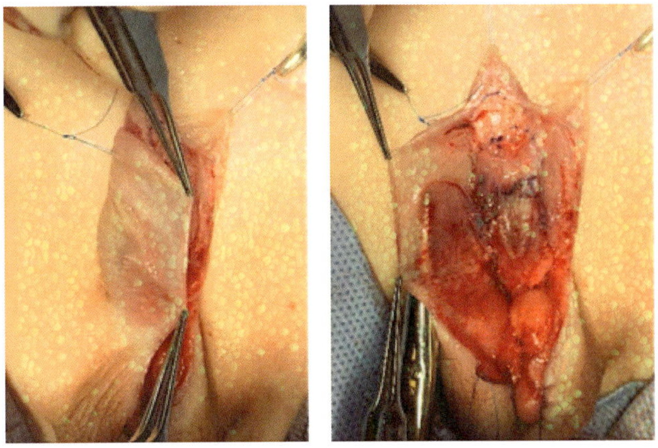

Figure 32. Thin ventral skin cannot reliably support a urethroplasty graft.
A, assessing skin to cover the ventral shaft. B, the ventro-lateral skin in proximal hypospadias lacks the robust dartos layer underlying normal penile skin. That results in this “thin” appearance in which the scissors can be seen through the skin. This skin needs time to heal before urethroplasty grafting, as it would be unlikely to sufficiently support revascularization along the edges of a graft sewn to it.

Nevertheless, some grafts still contracted, and a review of photographs taken of those cases revealed this happened when there was little ventral shaft skin. We learned that skin transposed to cover the ventral penile shaft deficiency needs time to recover before facing the additional stress a skin graft causes (Figure 32). That realization led to routine STAC repair for proximal hypospadias, since nearly all these patients have little or no ventral shaft skin.

STAC vs STAG

We reported a comparison between 220 consecutive STAG repairs done from 2014 to mid 2020 and 148 consecutive STAC from mid 2020 to 2022. All had 3 corporotomies for straightening, all had the meatus repaired to the tip of the glans, and none received testosterone. We found STAC grafts were healthier, having an average of 6% contracture versus 23% in STAG, p=0.001. The skin in STAC was also healthier as determined by problems at closure of the final operation. Nearly 1 of every 10 STAG patients needed a scrotal skin flap, Cecil maneuver, or external penile skin graft versus 0 in STAC, p=0.005. Finally, urethroplasty complications were fewer after STAC, 13% versus 23%, p=0.037.

STAG patients underwent an average of 2.8 operations to complete their planned 2-stage repair, and 4 could never tubularized due to inability to achieve a sufficiently healthy graft. STAC patients underwent an average of 3.2 operations to complete their planned 3-stage repair and all were tubularized (Snodgrass and Bush, 2024).

These data should be convincing to adopt routine STAC repair for proximal hypospadias.

Modified STAC

Chapter 9 presents a "simplified" STAC repair for surgeons to use during a transition from flap or 2-stage flap repairs. Chapter 10 discusses 1 and 2-stage variations on STAC when repairing chordee without hypospadias or distal hypospadias with ≥ 30° VC, respectively. These show the versatility of 3 corporotomies for straightening and STAC repair for varying circumstances.

Helpful information for parents

The neo-urethra created by STAC has similar characteristics to the neo-urethra made from the urethral plate in proximal TIP. The same explanations of what to expect postoperatively discussed in Chapter 6 are given to parents before STAC 3, and copied here.

The longer neourethra created by proximal hypospadias repairs behaves in ways that are noticeable, and sometimes worrying, to parents. For example, postoperative edema temporarily alters the lumen of the neourethra following STAC 3. After the stent is removed parents may notice the stream is thin and/or deflected. This does not indicate meatal stenosis, and neither calibration nor dilation should be done.

During this phase of postoperative edema and turbulent urine flow, urine infection may occur, which almost never happens after distal repairs. In the few who develop an infection, the first typically happens a few weeks after the stent is removed and is often febrile. We simply treat with a 1-week course of oral antibiotic, and do not pursue any other diagnostic tests such as renal sonography or VCUG. These few boys sometimes go on to experience additional episodes of cystitis, which we treat with 3 days of antibiotic. We cannot recall a patient who continued this pattern beyond 1 year following surgery. In contrast, UTIs that occur well after healing and resolution of edema may indicate a complication.

The steam gains force and straightens over the first several postoperative months. But even after healing it remains prolonged compared to typical boys. Parents notice this when they watch their son who had hypospadias repair urinate at the same time as his brother or a friend. Uroflowmetry also commonly demonstrates a decreased Qmax and flattened curve. Interestingly, this difference in voiding is rarely noticed by patients, either as children or adults, or their friends. We routinely ask older boys if their friends ever comment that they take longer to urinate and the answer is invariably no.

The neourethra is not a natural urethra, regardless of the technique used to create it. It has less elasticity, which likely accounts for the slower flow rate and flattened curve. In addition, this explains the post-void dribbling probably all patients experience after proximal repair. Like a garden hose dribbles when the faucet is closed because it is stiff, the neourethra does not collapse like the normal urethra as bladder emptying finishes, leaving a few drops to expel when urination is otherwise complete. Usually the leakage is small, and older boys and men learn to manage it.

Key Points

Even the most severely abnormal hypospadias anatomy can be repaired into normal penile anatomy by STAC. To achieve this requires surgeons to re-think traditional teachings. First, the decision if a repair should be done by TIP tubularizing the urethral plate in 1 stage, or by STAC transecting the urethral plate and creating a graft neo-plate is determined by the extent of VC, and not by whether the meatus is nearer the glans or the scrotum.

Second, initial degloving should be done ventrally, rather than circumferentially. Even when the hypospadias meatus is distal, 15% of patients will have ventral curvature that measures 30° or more but is not always apparent preoperatively. Consequently, we rarely begin hypospadias repair with a traditional circumferential degloving incision anymore so that the prepuce can be saved for urethroplasty grafting.

Third, *when VC measuring 30° or more is found, the single most important step in the entire repair is making the penis durably straight.* This is most reliably done using 3 ventral corporotomies, and not by any method of dorsal plication.

Fourth, attention must be paid to the penile skin from the outset to ensure the penis will be covered by symmetric, healthy penile skin when the repair is finished.

Fifth, graft neourethras are superior to those made from flaps, which means that surgeons repairing proximal hypospadias have to become adept at grafting. These are best placed at a 2nd stage after the penis has been straightened and skin transposed ventrally has healed.

Once there is a healthy graft neoplate on a straight penis with symmetric, healthy penile skin, final stage tubularization creates a durable neourethra ending in a neomeatus at the tip of the glans.

Surgeons can make proximal hypospadias into a normal penis – if they use the best technique, STAC, and do each step the best way.

References

Badawy H: Reported to the Hypospadiology email group, 2019

Bush NC, Villaneuva C, and Snodgrass W: Glans size is an independent risk factor for complications after hypospadias repair. *J Pediatr Urol* 9:1118, 2013

Duckett JW, Jr: Transverse prepucial island flap technique for repair of severe hypospadias. *Urol Clin North Am* 7: 423, 1980

Ferro F, Zaccara A, Spagnoli A, Lucchetti MC, Capitanucci L, Villa M: Skin graft for 2-stage treatment of severe hypospadias: back to the future? *J Urol* 168: 1730, 2002

Long CJ, Chu DI, Tenny RW, Morris Ar, Weiss DA,Shukla AR, Srinivasan AK, Zderic SA, Kolon TF, Canning DA: Intermediate-term followup of proximal hypospadias repair reveals high complication rate. *J Urol* 197: 852-858, 2017

McNamara ER, Schaeffer AJ, Logvinenko T, Seager C, Rosokliga I, Nelson CP, Retik AB, Diamond DA, and Cendron M: Management of proximal hypospadias with 2-stage repair: 20-year experience. *J Urol* 194: 1080, 2015

Snodgrass W and Bush N: TIP hypospadias repair: a pediatric urology indicator operation. *J Pediatr Urol* 12:11, 2016

Snodgrass W and Bush N: Staged tubularized autograft repair for primary proximal hypospadias with 30-degree or greater ventral curvature. *J Urol* 198: 680, 2017

Snodgrass W and Bush NC: Persistent or recurrent ventral curvature after failed proximal hypospadias repair. *J Pediatr Urol* 15: 344, 2019

Snodgrass W and Bush NC: Graft and skin complications in 342 primary proximal hypospadias repairs: STAG versus STAC. ESPU abstract, 2024

Stanasel I, Le HK, Bilgutay A, Roth DA, Gonzales ET, JR, Janzen N, Koh CJ, Gargollo P and Seth A: Complications following staged hypospadias repair using transposed prepucial skin flaps. *J Urol* 194: 512, 2015

Chapter 9

Transitioning From Byars Flaps To (Simple) STAC

Probably the least technically demanding operation for proximal hypospadias is the Byars flap repair. That relative simplicity most likely accounts for its widespread use today, since most hypospadias surgeons do fewer than 5 proximal repairs a year. For many, like WS, it replaced the Duckett tubed flaps they learned in training because those were more complex and had too many complications.

Unfortunately, Byars flap repairs also have many complications (Stansel et al, 2015; McNamara et al, 2015; Long et al, 2017). WS connected the Byars flaps to the urethral plate preserved in the glans, and then did a combined glanular TIP- second stage flap tubularization. However, 54% of his patients developed diverticulum. Thinking that he might be making the urethroplasty incisions too wide at the 2nd stage, he intentionally made the next one more narrow and instead created a urethral stricture. In his series, 100% of patients needed at least 1 more than the planned 2 procedures.

Others also report that patients repaired with Byars flaps usually need more than 2 procedures. For example, Stanasel et al found that 7% of 1st stages required revision before tubularization could be done, and that 66% of all their patients required more than the planned 2 stages. Similarly, Shukla et al (2004) reported that 70% of their patients undergoing Byars flaps required 3 or more operations.

Because of disappointing results many surgeons today have given up trying to repairing proximal hypospadias into a normal penis, and instead convert it to distal hypospadias hoping to reduce surgical complications. One problem with that approach is that a coronal meatus risks a lifetime of urine spraying. Another is that chordee excision and dorsal plications that many use to straighten curvature usually leave the penis bent to cause urethroplasty complications and future sexual dysfunction.

A better option is to transition to STAC repair. However, many hypospadias surgeons were not trained to harvest and place grafts, and few have straightened curvature with corporotomies or done prepucioplasties needed to save foreskin. Considering those now when they operate on no more than a handful of proximal hypospadias each year may deter them from performing the STAC we described in the preceding chapter.

For these reasons we propose a "Simple" STAC in this chapter – an easier graft repair that surgeons using Byars flaps can quickly master, and which corrects proximal hypospadias to a normal penis. Using this method should immediately improve results, and give surgeons the confidence to learn the few additional steps to do a regular STAC repair

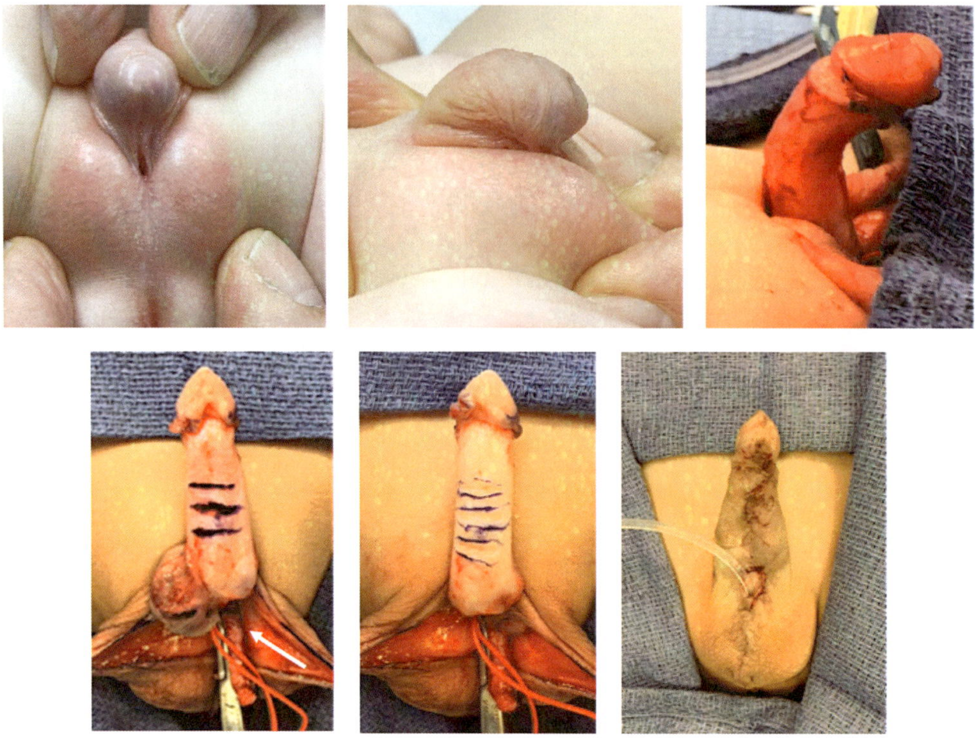

Figure 1. 'Simple' STAC repair.
A, B, scrotal hypospadias with VC and near-absent ventral penile shaft skin. C, the penis is completely degloved and artificial erection confirms VC > 30°. D, the urethral plate has been transected and dissected with the urethra into the distal scrotum (arrow). Repeat artificial erection was done and then lines for 3 corporotomies marked. E, the corporotomy incisions are made through the tunica albuginea from 3 to 9 o'clock. These are covered with a dartos flap from relocated penile skin, or from a scrotal dartos flap. F, in contrast to a normal STAC repair, the dorsal foreskin was split into Byars flaps, which were rotated ventrally to cover the penile shaft and approximated into a median raphe. This relocated shaft skin was also sewn to the urethral mucosa to create a proximal urethrostomy. Excess skin was then removed for circumcision, rather than preserved by prepucioplasty.

1st Stage

The simplified STAC 1 as shown in Figure 1 is quite similar to a Byars flap first stage. The penis is completely degloved and artificial erection done. When curvature ≥ 30° is measured, the urethral plate is transected at the corona and dissected off the corpora in continuity with the urethra past the penoscrotal junction into the upper scrotum. This is sufficient dissection to identify the area of curvature, incise the 3 corporotomies, and make the proximal urethrostomy.

Surgeons already experienced in making a single corporotomy with corporal grafting will find it easier to instead incise 3 corporotomies without grafting the defects. As discussed in Chapter 2, VC in proximal hypospadias *averages* 70°, which a single incision with corporal grafting may not completely straighten. Others who have not done ventral lengthening can readily learn this straightening maneuver. *This change is extremely important.* Successful hypospadias repair requires the penis to be straight, and no other straightening procedure is as reliably successful and durable as 3 corporotomies (Snodgrass and Bush, 2017).

WS has used this straightening technique for 20 years, and, as explained in Chapter 2, 3 corporotomies without corporal grafting do not bleed excessively intraoperatively or postoperatively, nearly always heal without scarring or recurrent VC, and do not cause erectile dysfunction.

When the 3 incisions have been made, a dartos flap is next created from under the penile shaft skin on one side, or dorsally and brought around one side. This is freed sufficiently to not torque the penis when it is advanced over the corporotomies. Then it is sutured to the corpora around the perimeter of the incisions and to the isthmuses between them to contain any bleeding.

The urethra is advanced back distally and secured at intervals to the corpora cavernosa in the midline. A proximal urethrostomy is made wherever the urethra reaches without tension. That might be below the corporotomies, on an isthmus, or, occasionally, distal to the incisions.

Then the skin at the penoscrotal junction is tacked to the corpora on either side of the urethra with a 5-0 PDS, a maneuver which most surgeons already use to prevent the penis from telescoping after the final operation. This stitch provides a fixed point for postoperative erections to stretch the skin on the penile shaft.

Finally, the dorsal foreskin is split down the midline, creating Byars flaps that are moved ventrally to fill the skin deficit. This is done *without* making glans wings or advancing the flaps into the glans.

Finally, adjacent shaft skin is sewn to the urethral mucosa at the meatus to complete the proximal urethrostomy. Remaining excess skin is removed to finish the circumcision.

2nd Stage

This operation begins with a *ventral* midline incision from the corona to the urethrostomy, continuing around it for a short distance. Complete degloving is not necessary. The skin is opened down to the corpora. Visible dartos on the surface of the corpora is excised, being careful not to make small corporotomies. Then artificial erection is done to verify that the penis is straight.

Glans wings are next opened laterally to 3 and 9 o'clock until that they are flat like a book opened to the middle. 6-0 Prolene stays are placed in the corona on either side to hold the wings open, and later to tie over the Vaseline gauze covering the graft.

Then oral mucosa is harvested from the lower lip when the meatus is on the proximal shaft or lower. An upper lip graft suffices when the meatus is mid- or distal shaft. Graft harvest is described in Chapter 11. Cheek should not be used, since it heals thicker than lip, leading to more glans dehiscence (Snodgrass and Elmore, 2004).

After defatting, the graft is laid into the defect and then stitched around the perimeter and quilted to the corpora as shown in Figure 2 and described in Chapter 11. The proximal end is button-holed to encompass a meatus on the penile shaft or at the penoscrotal junction. When the meatus is within the scrotum, it is spatulated dorsally a distance of 4mm and graft is advanced within it and sewn to the urethra mucosa. 5-0 Prolene stays are placed at 1.5cm intervals bilaterally along the graft. An 8Fr foley catheter is inserted and then the stays are tied over a tightly rolled Vaseline gauze to provide gentle compression to the graft.

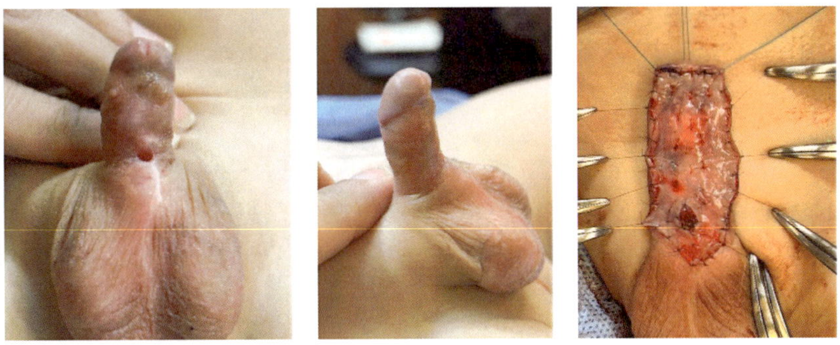

Figure 2. 2nd stage simple STAC repair, urethroplasty grafting.
A, B, appearance after simple STAC at the start of STAC 2. C, Once artificial erection shows the penis to be straight, glans wings will be opened widely. Lower lip graft, not cheek, has been harvested and sewn into the defect from the urethrostomy to the tip of the glans. The lip graft is buttonholed around the proximal urethrostomy to ensure no hair-bearing scrotal skin is inadvertently incorporated into the neourethral at the final STAC 3.

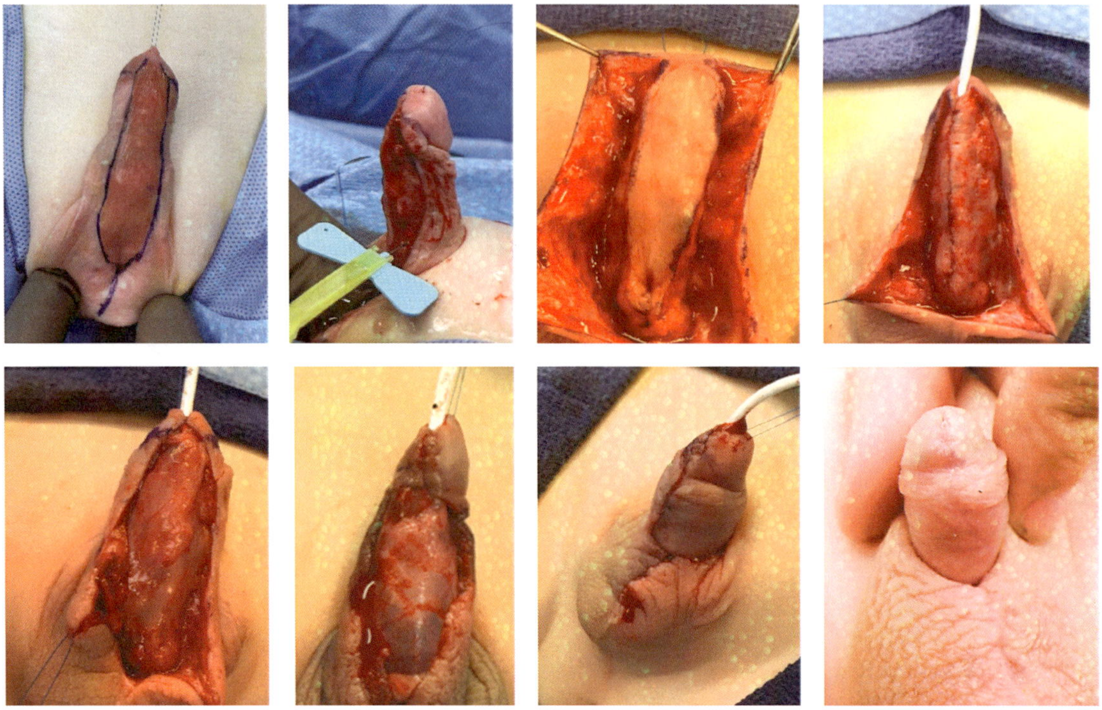

Figure 3. Tubularization of the oral graft neo-plate.
A, the graft appears healthy, without visible scars, and measured essentially the same dimensions as when it was placed. Lines for incision are marked alongside the neo-plate at its junction to the skin, then into the meatus, and down the midline of the scrotum. B, after ventral degloving, artificial erection is done to verify again that the penis is straight before proceding with urethroplasty. C, next glans wings are created and dissected open widely for later tension-free approximation over the neourethra. D, the neo-urethral plate is tubularized in 2 layers. The first layer begins distally and is sewn using interrupted subepithelial 6-0 Vicryl. Then a continuous subepithelial 6-0 PDS is run proximally to distally for a second layer. Except for the larger sutures used in oral grafts, this is the same urethroplasty done for regular STAC repairs. E, the neourethra is then covered by a tunica vaginalis, not dartos, flap. F, glansplasty is completed with 3 interrupted subepithelial 6-0 Vicryl stitches, the first placed at approximately the midglans, and the 3rd at the corona. The 2nd includes a bite of tunica vaginalis to hold it up as the glans is closed. Glans wings are not sewn to the urethral opening, and no epithelial stitches are placed. This is the same glansplasty done in regular STAC repairs. G, the skin at the penoscrotal junction is tacked to the coropora using 5-0 PDS and then the remaining shaft skin is closed into a median raphe using interrupted subepithelial 7-0 Vicryl. H, final, normal appearance 6 months later.

3rd Stage

Key steps of the final stage are shown in Figure 3.

This procedure is quite similar to the 2nd stage of a Byars flap repair, with a U-shaped incision made around the graft and into the proximal urethrostomy to exclude any skin previously sewn to it which might grow hair during puberty. Artificial erection is performed again before the graft is tubularized to confirm a final time that the penis is straight.

Tubularization is the same as described in Chapter 8 for regular STAC repairs, except the suture used for oral grafts is 6-0 Vicryl instead of the 7-0 which we use for prepucial grafts, since oral grafts are slightly thicker than prepucial grafts. The first layer uses interrupted subepithelial 6-0 Vicryl to align the edges precisely, followed by a 2nd continuous subepithelial layer of 6-0 PDS.

As in all proximal repairs, the neourethra is then covered by a tunica vaginalis, rather than dartos, flap.

Glansplasty is the same as in TIP repair, approximating the glans wings over the neourethra, but not to it, using 3 interrupted subepithelial 6-0 Vicryl stitches. The neomeatus is in the anatomically correct location with normal glans fusion below it.

Shaft skin closure includes tacking the penoscrotal junction to the corpora on each side again using 5-0 PDS. Skin edges are closed with subepithelial stitches into a median raphe.

The pictures tell the story, that simple STAC repair can easily be done by surgeons currently using Byars flaps, and that the final results are better than achieved by flap operations. The simple STAC makes a normal penis in the same number of operations actually done for most Byars flap repairs. WS was not able to make a normal penis using Byars flaps, and the published experience of other centers indicate this is a problem with the operation, and not the surgeon or the severity of the hypospadias.

Moving From Simple Stac to Full Stac

After learning Simple STAC, converting to a full STAC only involves a few changes in skin management during the first operation. Specifically, rather than completely degloving the penis, the skin incision is made ventrally so that prepucioplasty can be done. Then artificial erection, transection of the urethral plate and its mobilization along with the urethra into the scrotum, 3 transverse corporotomies, a dartos flap covering those incisions, and a proximal urethrostomy are done as described above and in the preceding chapter. The shaft skin is lengthened to fill the ventral defect without using Byars flaps from the foreskin. Finally, prepucioplasty is done so that the preserved foreskin will stretch during natural postoperative erections before STAC 2.

STAC 2 is now done using prepucial graft harvested by circumcision, rather than oral mucosa. STAC 3 involves the same steps to tubularize the neourethra, cover it with tunica vaginalis, and then close the glans with the neomeatus at the tip.

Key Points

It should not be a difficult transition for surgeons using Byars flap repairs for proximal hypospadias to start doing the simple STAC. Traditional degloving is done. Once VC ≥ 30° is confirmed, the urethral plate and urethra are dissected from the corpora into the distal scrotum, which is a maneuver most urologists are familiar with. 3 corporotomies across the area of bending are easy to perform and reliably straighten the curvature, without need to graft the corporal defects. Every hypospadias surgeon can develop a dartos flap from the skin to cover those incisions, and then bring the urethra back distally and make a proximal urethrostomy. Finally, skin closure splits the foreskin to fill the ventral deficiency, in a manner similar to completing a Byars flap repair except that the glans is not opened.

All hypospadias surgeons should be able to harvest lip mucosa at the second stage and then secure it from the end of the opened glans to around the urethrostomy. Final stage tubularization resembles the 2nd stage of a Byars flap repair or a proximal TIP. Urologists are familiar with surgery on the tunica vaginalis from hernia repairs and orchiopexies and can easily adapt that experience to making it into a coverage flap over the neourethra. Glansplasty is the same as done in a distal TIP, and there should be sufficient ventral shaft skin for symmetric closure around the shaft.

Surgeons whose volume of proximal repairs is so low that they are uncomfortable making these adjustments should refer those few patients to others, rather than persist in using the Byars flap repair which has unacceptably high complication rates regardless of who does the surgery according to the published literature. Surgeons who continue performing Byars flap repairs should objectively measure glans fusion, and if they are achieving normal glans fusion without diverticula or stricture, then the technical modifications which have enabled them to achieve this should be published for others to learn from. Glans fusion can easily be measured in the office with a ruler in those patients returning for postoperative visits. Monitoring for a splayed/deflected urine stream is more difficult, as it typically does not become symptomatic until around age 8 years as mentioned in previous chapters, and may only occur intermittently.

Nonetheless, older patients who have undergone Byars flap repairs can be assessed for this with direct questioning and patient/parental observation while voiding. For those who do transition to STAC, the ability to make even the most severe hypospadias into a normal penis is reward for the surgeon and life-changing for the patient.

References

Long CJ, Chu DI, Tenny RW, Morris Ar, Weiss DA,Shukla AR, Srinivasan AK, Zderic SA, Kolon TF, Canning DA: Intermediate-term followup of proximal hypospadias repair reveals high complication rate. *J Urol* 197: 852-858, 2017

McNamara ER, Schaeffer AJ, Logvinenko T, Seager C, Rosokliga I, Nelson CP, Retik AB, Diamond DA, and Cendron M: Management of proximal hypospadias with 2-stage repair: 20-year experience. *J Urol* 194: 1080, 2015

Shukla AR, Patel RP and Canning DA: The 2-stage hypospadias repair: is it a misnomer? *J Urol* 172: 1714, 2004

Snodgrass W and Elmore J: Initial experience with staged buccal graft (Bracka) hypospadias reoperations. *J Urol* 172:1720, 2004

Snodgrass W and Bush N: Staged tubularized autograft repair for primary proximal hypospadias with 30-degree or greater ventral curvature. *J Urol* 198: 680, 2017

Stanasel I, Le HK, Bilgutay A, Roth DA, Gonzales ET, JR, Janzen N, Koh CJ, Gargollo P and Seth A: Complications following staged hypospadias repair using transposed preputial skin flaps. *J Urol* 194: 512, 2015

Chapter 10

STAC Variations

STAC for proximal hypospadias is a 3-stage repair. But there are 2 circumstances in which the operation sometimes can be adapted to make the penis normal in 1 or 2-stages: congenital penile curvature ("chordee without hypospadias") and distal hypospadias with VC ≥ 30°. This chapter describes those.

In both, the urethra is dissected off the corpora from near the corona down into the scrotum without transecting it, taking advantage of its natural elasticity to gain length and avoid need to create a graft neourethra. 3 corporotomies are done with the urethra retracted to the side. Then, with the penis kept taut, the urethra is assessed to be certain it does not exert downward tension on the now straightened, longer penis.

Mobilizing the urethra without transecting in this way is similar to urethral mobilization for stricture repairs, which does not devascularize it. We have successfully straightened VC between 30° and 60° using this maneuver, which corrects congenital penile curvature in 1 operation, and distal hypospadias with 30° or more VC in 2 operations, the second being a distal TIP repair. If the urethra remains taut, further dissection can be done mobilizing it to near the sphincter. If tension remains, the urethra is transected and Johansen STAC or 3-stage STAC is done, for congenital penile curvature or distal hypospadias, respectively.

Congenital Penile Curvature

Because the anatomy of the glans and meatus are, by definition, normal in this condition, they should be maintained. Single stage repair can be done if the urethra mobilized off the corpora is sufficiently elastic to stretch without tension when the curvature is straightened.

Key steps are shown in Figure 1. The penis is degloved ventrally. After artificial erection confirms VC is 30° or more, the urethra is dissected off the corpora from near the corona to within the scrotum. This dissection can continue as needed to the membranous segment until it is established that the urethra is sufficiently elastic to allow 3 corporotomies beneath it without tension. Those incisions are made and then covered with a dartos flap to contain any bleeding. Then the repair is completed by anchoring the urethra, gently stretched distally, back to the corpora. When desired, circumcision is done.

If the urethra does not stretch without tension, a Johansen – modified STAC 1 is done, maintaining the foreskin for the next operation. This is shown in Figure 2.

Despite similar dissection, sometimes tension remains within the mobilized urethra, which does not raise far away from the corpora (compare the photos in Figure 1B and Figure 2B). When this is found, additional length will need to be added to the urethra. Since the glans and meatus are normally formed, they are left intact and the urethra is transected lower, on the penile shaft. The cut ends separate from each other naturally, revealing the distance that will have to be bridged.

A distal and a proximal urethrostomy are created. While a graft potentially could be placed at this time, assuming it would not rest on any of the corporal incisions, we advise delaying that until the second procedure since the ventral skin is also short and requires

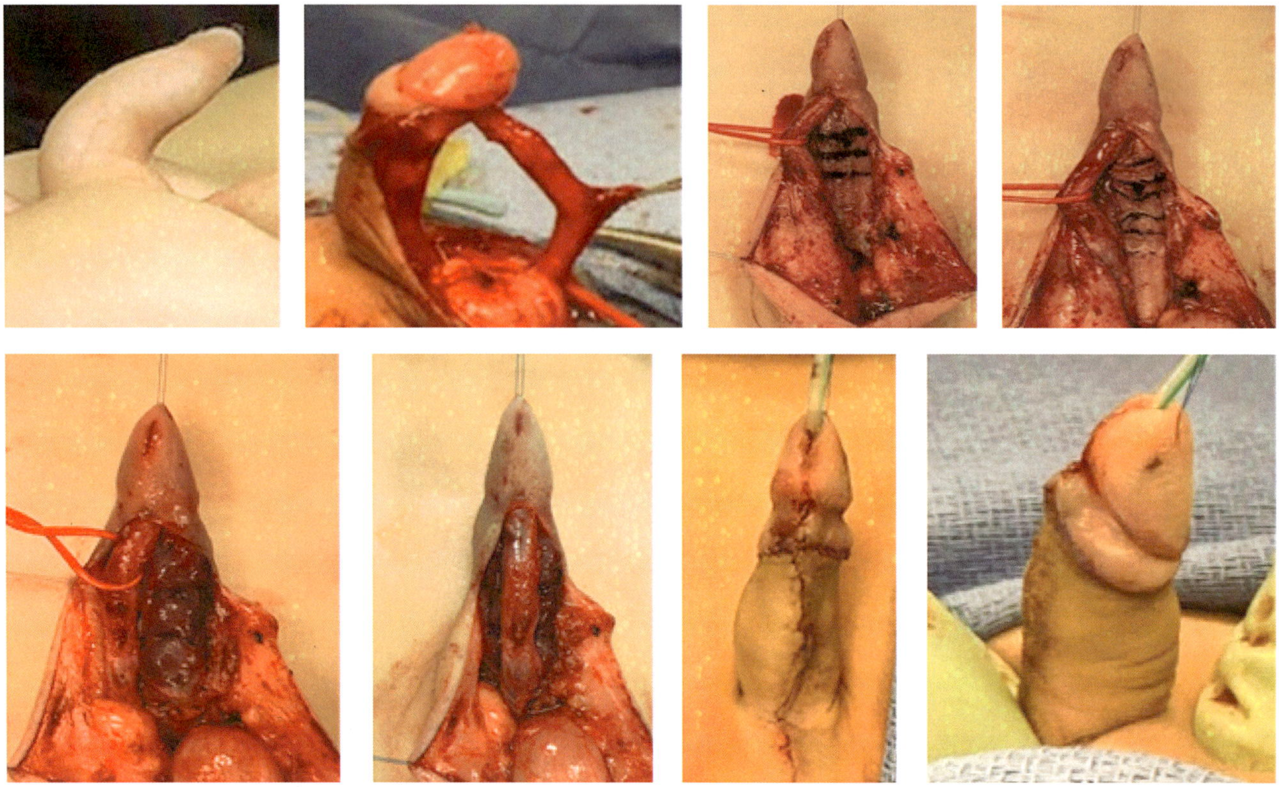

Figure 1. 1-stage correction of congenital penile curvature.
A, congenital penile curvature. B, after ventral degloving, VC measured 50°. The urethra was next dissected off the corpora from the corona into the distal scrotum as shown. There was sufficient length gained to straighten the corpora without transecting the urethra. C, with the urethra retracted laterally, lines for 3 corporotomies are marked across the arc of the bending. D, incisions have been made for straightening, which also lengthen the penis. Note the urethra remains lax. E, a dartos flap placed under the urethra now covers the incisions and has been sutured to the corpora to make the area watertight. F, the urethra has been stitched back to the corpora. G,H, final appearance after circumcision.

lengthening. As discussed in Chapter 8, the need for lengthened ventral skin to recover before it is additionally stressed by the demands of a graft is a major the reason we stopped using STAG and developed STAC.

Steps of this Johansen-modified STAC are shown in Figure 2.

We first applied STAC modifications to patients having congenital penile curvature, reasoning there was no benefit to reconstructing the glans and meatus since they were already normal. In most cases urethra mobilization effectively lengthens it so that an additional neourethra segment, shown in Figure 2, is typically not needed except for the most severe degrees of congenital penile curvature.

Distal Hypospadias with VC ≥ 30°

Success with this approach for congenital penile curvature then led us to consider similarly correcting VC exceeding 30° in boys with distal hypospadias. The goal was to use TIP rather than a staged graft repair for the urethroplasty after first straightening curvature using 3 corporotomies under a mobilized urethra. An example is shown in Figure 3.

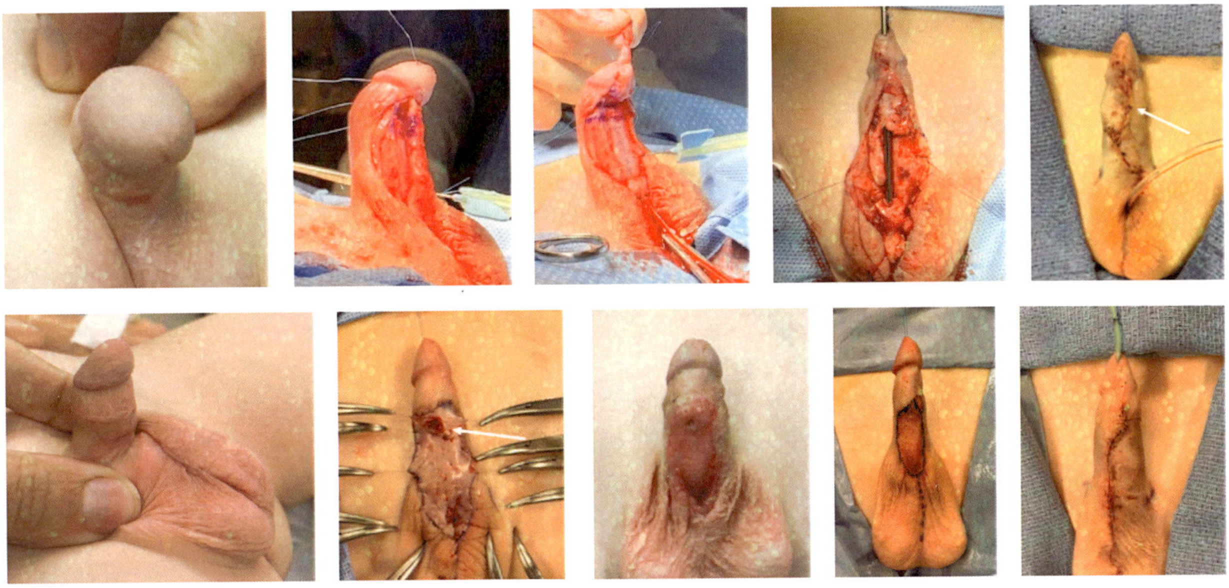

Figure 2. 3-stage STAC with Johansen modification.
A, congenital penile curvature diagnosed after circumcision, with very distal curvature that measured 60° after ventral degloving. B, the urethra exerted tension despite mobilizing it well down into the scrotum to near the sphincter. C, the urethra was transected in the midshaft and the distal end is being held upwards. The marks for corporotomies can be seen distally. Only 2 incisions could be made across the arc of curvature, avoiding an incision at or above the corona. D, after covering the corporotomies with dartos, the urethra was laid back down and sutured to the corpora. The sound indicates the 2 stomas and shows the length of neourethra that will be needed to restore urethral continuity. E, shaft skin has been closed between the distal (arrow) and proximal urethrostomies. F, the penis appears straight with healthy skin 6 months later. G, incision was made between the stomas and lower lip graft inserted between them, encircling both. The arrow points to the distal urethrostomy. H, healthy, well-healed graft at STAC 3. I, incision marked along the graft edges and into the scrotum to harvest a tunica vaginalis coverage flap. J, artificial erection confirms the ventral curvature remains corrected, the graft is tubularized, then the neourethra is covered with tunica vaginalis, and the skin is closed.

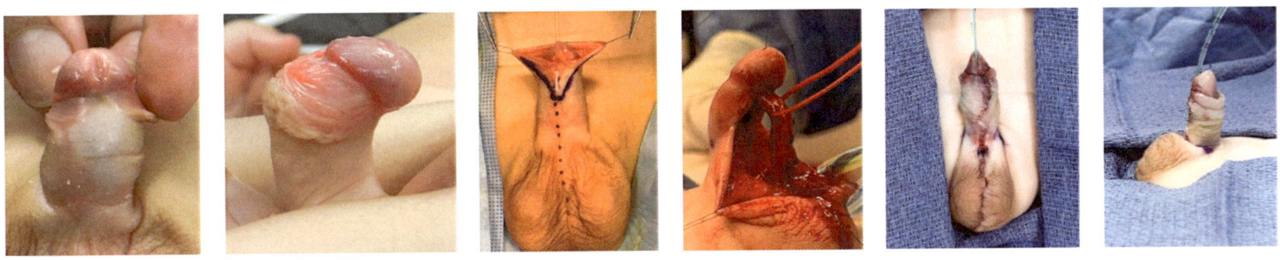

Figure 3. STAC-TIP.
A, glanular hypospadias with insufficient glans fusion measuring 1mm. B, ventral curvature that could be due to short skin or a short ventral corporal sheath. C, because the etiology of VC cannot be determined until the skin is released, a ventral skin incision was made, preserving the option for 3-stage STAC if the urethra was found to not be sufficiently elastic. D, VC meaured 45°. Leaving the distal hypospadias intact, the urethra was mobilized from the corpora to facilitate straightening with 3 corporotomies. The urethra was sufficiently and elastic to avoid transection. E, after straightening, the skin was closed with partial prepucioplasty, preserving the foreskin in case there was postoperative contraction of either the urethra or the shaft skin, but not closing it over the glans. If circumcision is desired it will be done along with distal TIP at a second operation.

Results

Our experience indicates that the urethra in boys with chordee without hypospadias and distal hypospadias with VC of 30° most often can be maintained intact while straightening the curvature by 3 corporotomies. Dissecting the urethra off the corpora from near the corona into the scrotum provides access to the ventral corporal surface to make the incisions, and allows the urethra to gently stretch longer to accommodate the increased penile shaft length after straightening. It has not been difficult to recognize the few whose urethra remains taut despite mobilization, who then have it transected for either a Johansen-modified STAC when the meatus is normal, or a traditional STAC when there is hypospadias. In those undergoing a staged repair, we preserve the foreskin to the second operation to use should there be skin complications or contraction of the mobilized urethra. To date, only one patient had enough tension on the native subcoronal urethra at the time of his second surgery that TIP was not felt to be possible, and the patient underwent grafting in a typical STAC 2 instead. Because the needed graft is short, and because fully reconstructing the foreskin around the hypospadiac distal meatus can cause some scarring in the area where TIP is performed, after initially performing a full prepucioplasty as we do for 3-stage STAC, we no longer manipulate the foreskin during the STAC portion of a STAC-TIP repair, and instead leave the hooded prepuce.

Key Points

As STAC is mastered, variations in the procedure can be used in special circumstances, including chordee without hypospadias and distal hypospadias with 30° or more VC. These arise from the principle that the goal of penile surgery is to make abnormal anatomy normal, and so when the glans and meatus are normally formed, as in chordee without hypospadias, there is no need to disturb them. A one-stage repair that lengthens the penis using 3 corporotomies, rather than shorten it with less reliable plications, is an obvious advantage.

Similarly, if VC can be straightened with 3 corporotomies without transecting the urethra in the 15% of boys who have distal hypospadias with VC ≥ 30°, then distal TIP can complete the repair in a second operation – avoiding need for urethroplasty grafting.

Chapter 11

Urethroplasty Grafts

Urologists have taught themselves that flaps are better than grafts for hypospadias urethroplasty. It seems intuitively true, moving the foreskin ventrally still connected to its blood supply must be more reliable than removing the foreskin, sewing it back on ventrally, and then relying on re-vascularization to keep it alive.

However, multiple observations suggest the opposite is true. First, there is the clinical evidence showing that flap urethroplasties consistently have at least double the complication rate of grafts in proximal hypospadias repairs (Snodgrass and Bush, 2017). In addition, those flap complications include more meatal stenosis and urethral strictures than occur with grafts, indicating that the ends of flaps have less reliable vascularity. John Duckett said as much, writing in an editorial comment years ago that inspection after intravenous fluorescein sometimes showed those ends to be "devascularized" and needing to be removed (Duckett, 1981). However, he never wrote how often he performed that test and how often he then needed to excise part of the flaps.

Second, plastic surgeons have known for years that the "random flaps" urologists devise based on a variable vascular pattern are less successful than pedicle flaps with defined blood vessels. Today SPY angiography verifies that fact, demonstrating regions of flaps which may look healthy to the surgeon but which may be compromised.

We have used SPY to inspect grafts when they are healed and ready for tubularization. Prepucial grafts have similar vascularization as the penile skin, while the appearance of oral grafts is similar to their donor sites, as shown in Figure 1. We interpret this to mean that the grafts re-vascularize uniformly, which may explain why meatal stenosis and neourethra strictures are so uncommon after their tubularization.

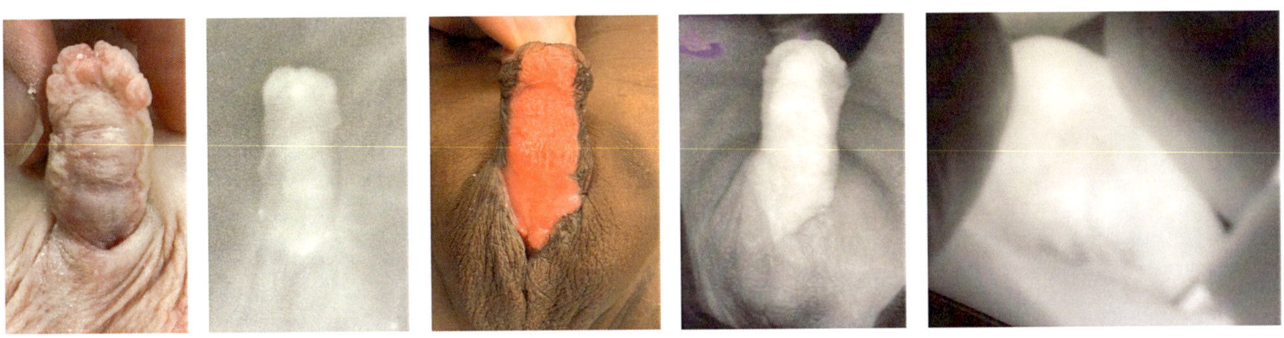

Figure 1. Graft revascularization as seen using SPY angiography.
A, healed prepucial graft, which SPY in B shows similar or increased vascularization compared to adjacent skin. C, healed lip graft. D, vascularization similar to non-operated lip seen in E.

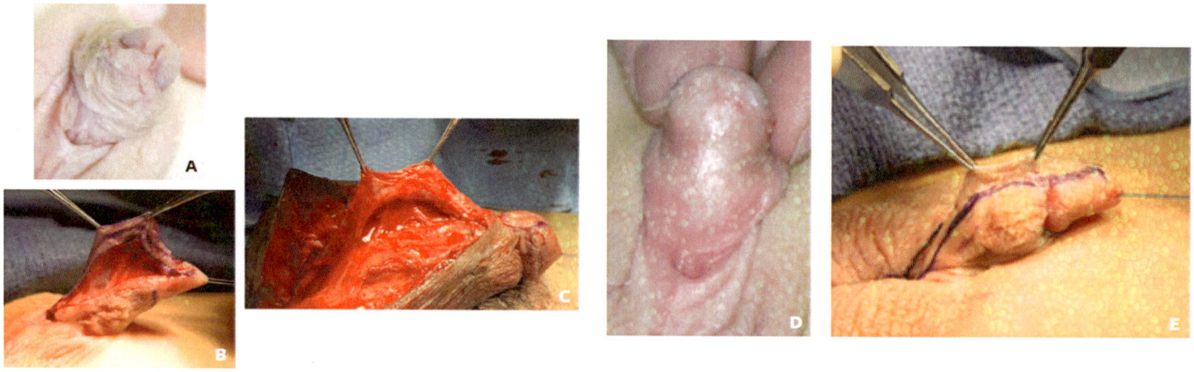

Figure 2. Flaps versus Grafts.
A, irregular, wrinkled appearance of a Byars flap before tubularization. B, the flap is poorly adhered to the corpora because of the underlying dartos. C, tubularized prepucial flap is still not adherent to the corpora 20 years later in another patient. D, smooth appearance of a foreskin graft, which in E is seen well-affixed to the corpora.

Third, grafts are stitched flat to the corpora. That secures them in much the same way as a normal urethra is fixed to the corpora. Rectangular grafts also create a uniform, smooth neourethra. In contrast, flaps do not fix to the corpora and their surface is irregular (Figure 2), making a neourethra which is mobile with a non-smooth lumen. Duckett moved from tubularized flaps to onlay flaps attached to the urethral plate to better stabilize the neourethra and smooth its lumen. Others have tried quilting Byars flaps to the corpora to mimic the fixation of grafts, but the dartos under the epithelium prevents the same attachment that grafts have.

Finally, a graft makes a neourethral plate which tubularizes in much the same way as tubularization of the urethral plate. That includes glansplasty, which for both TIP and graft repairs achieves normal glans fusion. In contrast, surgeons who use flaps stitch the urethral opening circumferentially to the glans wings and therefore achieve less, often subnormal, glans fusion (Figure 3). This abnormal anatomy increases risk for future abnormal urinary function with spraying.

This chapter discusses important technical details to optimize graft take. It also describes various grafting complications and their management. The overriding goal for surgeons is to make healthy grafts which will easily tubularize at the final stage.

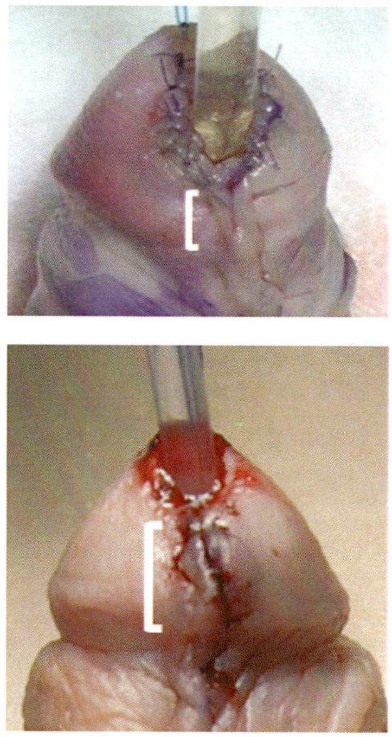

Figure 3. Glans fusion in flaps versus grafts.
A, glans fusion after onlay flap repair in which the flap was stitched to the glans wings. The glans fusion is less than in a glansplasty after staged graft repair as seen in B.

General Considerations

There are a few considerations which apply to grafts used in both primary and reoperative repairs. The first and most important is that grafts derive their neovascularity from the surface of the underlying corpora *and* the adjacent shaft skin sewn to their edges. Therefore, grafts should only be placed onto intact corpora, and health of ventral shaft skin should be optimized before grafting. As explained in Chapter 8, STAC was derived from STAG when we realized that grafts placed onto corporotomy incisions have greater likelihood for scarring and contracture than those placed onto intact corpora. Continued graft scarring subsequently indicated that skin relocated to the ventral surface needs time to replenish its own vascularity before it can reliably nourish the edges of a graft.

When grafting, it is best to create the neo-urethral plate from 1 piece of tissue to avoid junctions, since those add risk for scar contracture. In primary repairs we first size the skin needed to cover the penile shaft and then take all the remaining foreskin for the graft. Similarly, when we take oral mucosa in reoperations we always take all the available graft from within the anatomic region being harvested. That most often ensures there is sufficient tissue to fill from urethrostomy to glans tip and coronal margin to coronal margin without tension. On those unusual occasions when more than 1 piece of graft is needed, the most thin segment harvested should be placed within the glans.

We never re-harvest oral mucosa from a prior donor site. For that reason, surgeons should never take small grafts from the lower lip, preserving that site should a longer graft be needed subsequently. The upper lip supplies sufficient graft to reach from the glans tip to the mid-/ distal shaft, reliably reaching 3-3.5cm, while the lower lip is harvested when a graft longer than 3.5cm is needed to reach the proximal shaft / scrotum.

Hypospadias surgeons must be able to harvest their own grafts. The need to graft cannot always be anticipated preoperatively, and the unexpected finding that one is required but a plastic or oral surgeon is not available to take it results in suboptimal care and complications. Graft harvest is not difficult and is well within the abilities of surgeons who choose to correct hypospadias.

Urethroplasty Graft Sources

Prepuce

The easiest substitute tissue for the urethral plate is the foreskin. There is essentially no donor site morbidity following its harvest. It heals with minimal reaction along its junction to the shaft skin. It remains thin during healing and is therefore easy to both roll into the neourethra and to close the glans wings over. If there is partial dehiscence of the neomeatus the exposed foreskin is not obvious, in contrast to the stark red appearance of oral mucosa. And if shaft skin has healed with any foreshortening, excess prepucial graft can be used to augment the skin closure.

Although it is commonly written that the inner prepuce should be used for urethroplasty grafts, in fact it rarely is large enough to comprise the entire neourethra. In addition, inner prepuce can be so thin that it resembles a split thickness graft, which has a greater risk for contracting. Accordingly, we use the outer skin and discard most or all the inner segment.

Surgeons accustomed to using foreskin flaps might think the available skin will not be large enough to

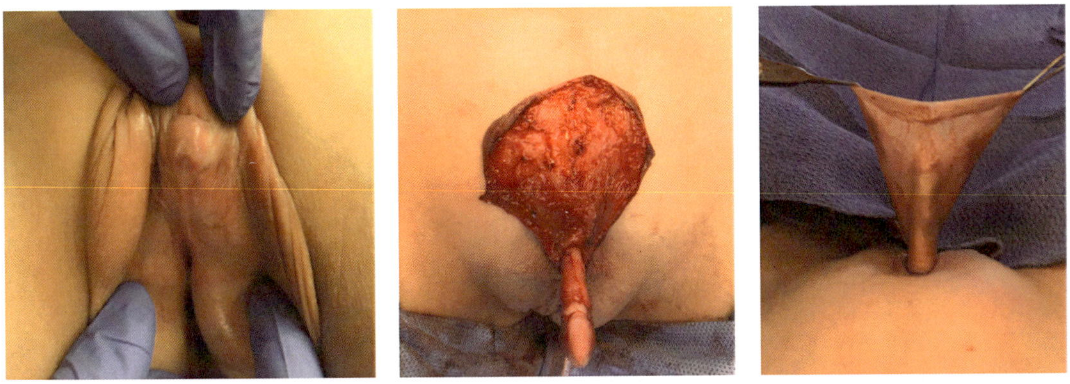

Figure 4. Increased foreskin size from excising its dartos.
A, perineal hypospadias. B, large increase in the size of the foreskin and dorsal penile shaft skin after removing the dartos. C, it is clear there is sufficient skin to cover the penis symmetrically and also make a urethroplasty graft.

reach from a proximal meatus to the glans tip while also providing skin needed for penile shaft closure. However, the skin significantly expands when the underlying dartos is excised (Figure 4). In several hundred primary graft repairs the prepuce has nearly always been sufficient for both purposes. However, we emphasize 2 important caveats:

1. The *first priority* is to use foreskin/penile skin to cover the penile shaft. In the unusual event that the remaining foreskin will not provide an adequate urethroplasty graft, oral mucosa can be used to make part or all of the neourethra.

2. The urethral mobilization we do towards the external sphincter brings the urethrostomy further distally, decreasing the length of graft that is needed. Although we once routinely dissected back to the sphincter to stretch the urethra as far distally as possible, today the most extensive dissection is reserved for those with the most severe hypospadias, i.e. those with a meatus between the perineum and mid-scrotum, so that we can bring the urethrostomy near or to the penoscrotal junction. Otherwise, dissection extends only into the distal scrotum, so that the urethrostomy is on the penile shaft.

Oral Mucosa

Oral mucosa is significantly different than prepuce. The donor site is painful and sometimes contracts, limiting ability to open the mouth and distorting the appearance of the lip. Oral mucosa always heals with variable induration along the junction to adjacent shaft skin, probably because this tissue is foreign to the penis. It also thickens during healing and is always thicker than prepuce, which makes glansplasty more difficult in the smaller-sized glans typically encountered in proximal hypospadias. If the meatus opens with a partial or complete dehiscence, the red oral mucosa is quite obvious and unsightly. Furthermore, any exposed oral mucosa at the meatus dries and forms keratin, resulting in a snakeskin-like film that can deflect or obstruct the urine stream (Figure 5).

For all these reasons, prepuce should be used for urethroplasty grafts in primary repairs. However, when the foreskin has been removed, or the family prefers it to reconstructed to make the penis to look natural, lip grafts are then second choice for urethroplasty.

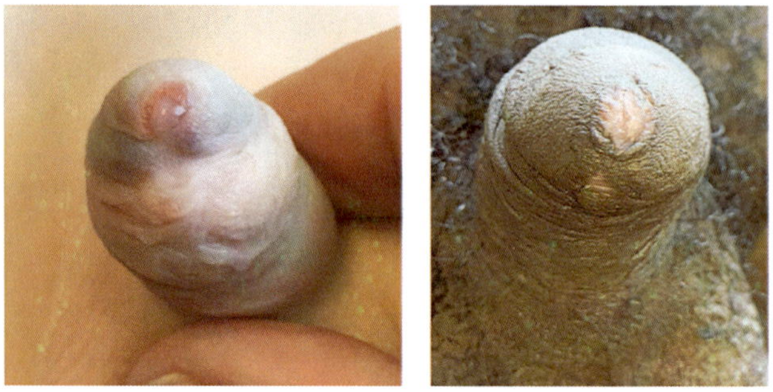

Figure 5. Exposed oral mucosa.
A, unsightly red meatus from partial glans dehiscence.
B, thin film of keratin on exposed oral mucosa in an otherwise satisfactory neomeatus. This film can make it difficult to urinate and/or deflect the stream unless it is wiped away with Aquaphor before urinating.

As mentioned above, we harvest from the upper lip when shorter grafts are needed to extend to the midshaft, and lower lip when grafts reach to the proximal shaft or as far as the perineum. It seems that many urologists consider oral mucosa to mean cheek. Cheek grafts are more thick than those taken from the lips (Figure 6), and significantly increase risk for glans dehiscence (Snodgrass and Bush et al, 2009). They are also shorter and less elastic than lip grafts, increasing likelihood that more than 1 piece will have to be used to make the neo-urethral plate in scroto-perineal hypospadias.

We use cheek most often when a patch re-graft is done on the penile shaft. When oral mucosa is needed for urethroplasty, lip is the first choice. It is a technical error to place cheek graft within the glans.

Lingual

We have very little experience using lingual mucosa. It is thinner that lip, which potentially is an advantage, but it is also much more narrow, increasing need to take more than 1 piece to make into the neo-urethral plate. When used, the donor site is sutured closed along the underside of the tongue. Reported complications include tongue numbness, altered taste, and slurred speech, which 1 study reported could persist a year or longer postoperatively (Xu et al, 2010). For these reasons we have only used lingual grafts on rare occasions when all other donor sites within the mouth have previously been used.

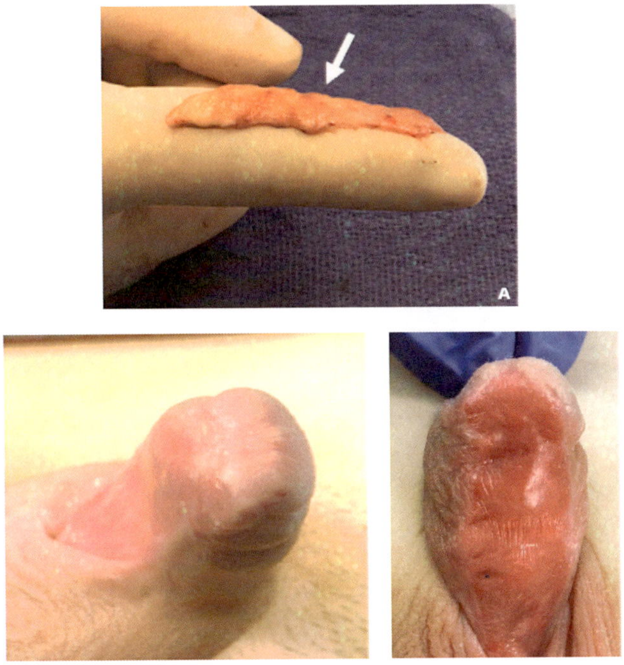

Figure 6. Cheek grafts are thicker than lip grafts. A, arrow indicates the junction of cheek (on the left) to lip (on the right), demonstrating that defatted cheek grafts are more thick than lip grafts. B, cheek graft in the glans is too thick for successful glansplasty, increasing risk for glans dehiscence and visible red tissue at the meatus. C, appearance after lip graft showing the glans wings should easily enclose the neourethra.

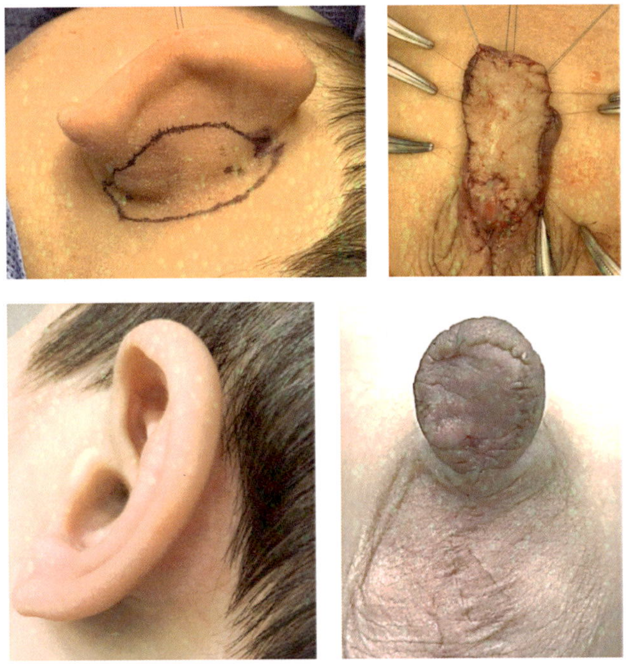

Figure 7. Posterior auricular urethroplasty graft. A, graft donor site. B, graft reaching to the penoscrotal junction, which is the limit for the length one of these grafts provides. C, healed donor site with faint visible scar. D, healed graft. We find these grafts to be less elastic than oral mucosa, and therefore less readily tubularized.

Posterior Auricular

We also have not used these grafts often for urethroplasty, even though they are another option which does not grow hair. The donor site is not visible (Figure 7) and is less uncomfortable during healing than lip and cheek graft harvests. However, the tissue is less elastic, and the grafts that can be obtained are usually smaller than oral grafts. We have also found they will not reliably reach below the penoscrotal junction. A large graft would require harvest from both ears which consumes more time and requires the pieces to be sewn together. Accordingly, we have used posterior auricular urethroplasty grafts in reoperations when oral mucosa was either no longer available or the patient demanded an alternative donor site than the mouth.

Groin

Urethroplasty grafts can be harvested from the adjacent groin crease, providing a strip of skin which is

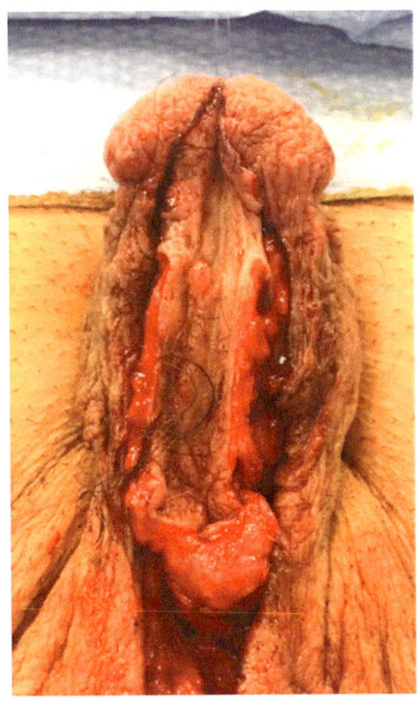

Figure 8. Hair in the neourethra made from scrotum. A scrotal tube comprised the proximal two thirds of this neourethra, and grew hair causing UTIs during puberty. This required a reoperative STAG repair to remove the neourethra and replace it with oral mucosa.

both adequately long and wide. We had a brief experience with these, after being told that defatting would likely remove any hair follicles. However, an adult who wanted to avoid an oral graft and selected this donor site found that hair grew from the graft and required painful, repetitive depilations before it could be tubularized. Skin which might grow hair should *never* be used for urethroplasty.

Scrotum

The shiny skin in a scrotal cleft is tubularized by some surgeons, usually to make the neourethra from a perineo-scrotal meatus reach to the penoscrotal junction to join a tubularized prepucial flap. However, this shiny skin can harbor hair follicles, and so scrotal tubes made from flaps or grafts should be avoided. We have removed many neourethras made with this midline scrotal skin when hair grew within them at puberty and caused symptoms (Figure 8).

Hair grows inside the urethra during puberty, causing UTIs and sometimes, stones. Laser depilation via urethroscopy is difficult and requires several sessions. Most often, these patients need STAG repair, if the penis is straight, to remove the hairy urethra and replace it with one made of oral mucosa.

Graft harvest and donor site management

Prepuce

Harvesting prepuce requires little more than a circumcision. However, dartos on the underside needs to be removed and that is best done while the foreskin is still connected to the penis. We emphasized in Chapter 8 that the skin needed to cover the penile shaft symmetrically should be determined *before* harvesting the foreskin, giving priority to surrounding the penis with healthy, penile skin (Figure 9).

The penis should be held taut when marking the coronal margin along which the foreskin will be cut. We approximate the ventral shaft skin edges between the urethrostomy and the glans with temporary stitches to align the skin and be certain it is the correct length before harvesting the graft. Those stitches are then removed down to the urethrostomy so the graft can be placed.

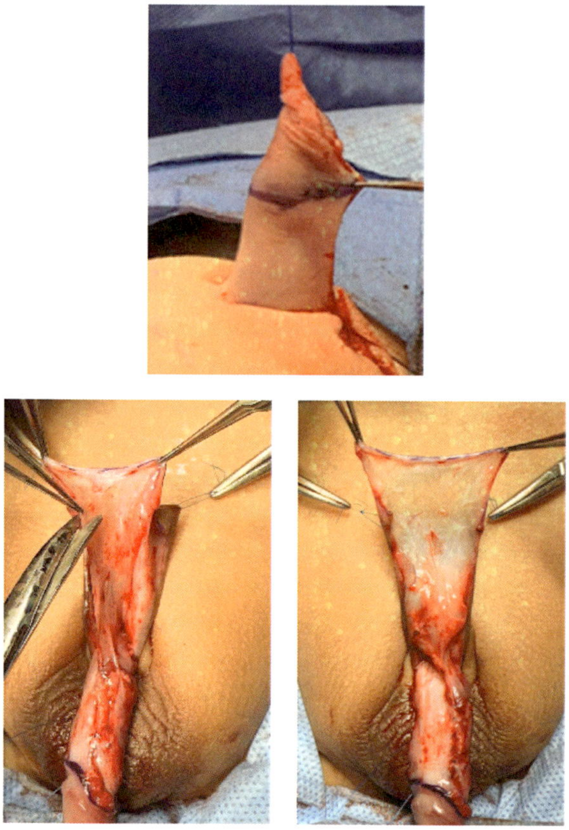

Figure 9. Harvesting prepucial grafts.
After the ventral shaft skin has been sized, the remaining foreskin distally is harvested. The line is marked along the corona as shown in A. Then the dartos is excised from the still-attached foreskin in B, until it resembles C. Note that the dartos is removed from the foreskin which will become the graft, but not the shaft skin.

Oral Mucosa

A first-generation cephalosporin is given intravenously before graft harvest. We do not prep the mouth or change gloves or instruments for graft harvesting.

The visible margin of the lip is marked and 5-0 Prolene stay stitches are placed for retraction to expose the donor site. A damp gauze is packed in the mouth and throat next into the endotracheal tube to limit bleeding down the laryngopharynx.

Then the graft is outlined with a marking pen, also noting the location of Stenson's duct and marking it to avoid injury during any graft harvest in its vicinity. Next, 1:200,000 epinephrine with bupivacaine is injected under the graft.

The incision is made using a 15 blade around the perimeter of the graft. Then the assistant lifts a corner with 0.5 Castroviejo forceps as the surgeon uses tenotomy scissors to develop a plane under the epithelium and above underlying fat and muscle. Dissection continues in this plane until the graft is removed, having a minimum of fat and muscle to then be excised.

The surgeon then completes graft defatting, draping the graft over an index finger, or, when it is too small, stabilizing it on a dampened area of the surgical drape (Figure 10). We never use pin boards when defatting grafts.

"Defatting" actually removes both fat and loose muscle from the graft, leaving a robust subepithelial tissue layer. A yellowish lamina propria with thin streaks of muscle is normal after defatting cheek grafts (Figure 10). Excessive defatting essentially converts a full-thickness graft into a partial-thickness graft which is more likely to contract.

The donor site should *never* be sutured closed after harvesting oral mucosa. There are several reasons for this. First, the intention to close the wound makes it more likely the surgeon will harvest a smaller graft, which might not fill the needed space from urethrostomy to glans tip without tension or requiring an additional graft segment and a junction between the pieces.

Suturing a labial harvest site after taking an adequately sized graft will visibly distort the lip. Suturing the cheek wound *increases* postoperative pain compared to simply leaving the harvest site open to re-epithelialize, as proven in a randomized trial (Rourke et al, 2012).

Immediately after harvest, we pack a gauze soaked with 1:1000 epinephrine against the donor site and then ignore this area until the operation is completed. There is rarely active bleeding at that time which requires cauterization.

No additional care is needed postoperatively. If bleeding develops after discharge from surgery, pressure held on a folded wet washcloth pressed externally over the harvest site will stop the oozing.

However, pain after oral graft harvest often exceeds the discomfort from the genital surgery. Magic Mouth Wash containing lidocaine, Benadryl and Maalox can

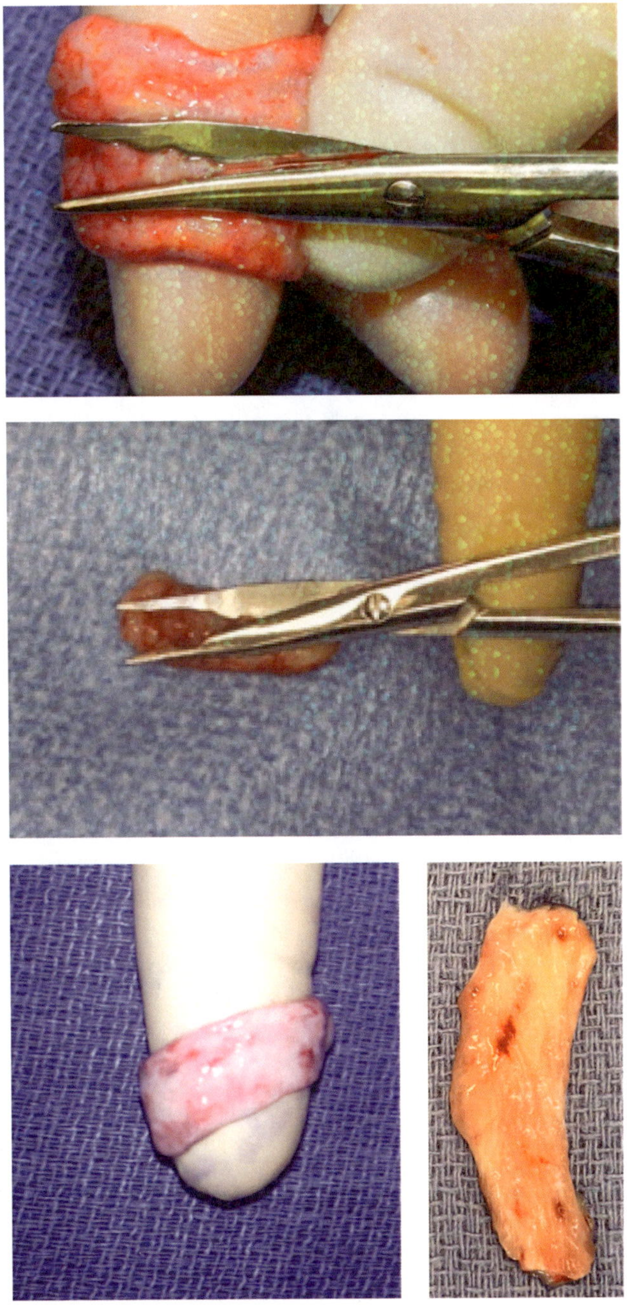

Figure 10. Defatting oral mucosa grafts.
A, it is best to drape the graft over an index finger while defatting, as this way the surgeon can sense the depth of dissection better than if it is placed onto a pin board. Visible fat and muscle are removed. B, small grafts, used for inlays, cannot be stabilized over a finger and so are placed onto a damp spot on the surgical drape to hold them steady while defatting. C, correct appearance of a defatted lip graft, showing no fat or loose muscle but leaving a robust subpeithelium. D, appearance after defatting cheek graft. Note the yellow appearance with streaks of adherent muscle that remain after removing loose fat and muscle.

be compounded and used as needed. It is very helpful in patients who can swish and spit. We do not use it in patients too young to spit out the mouthwash as dabbing it with cotton soaked in the solution, for instance, can increase risk for clots to be inadvertently removed and create bleeding.

It is normal for the patient to experience transient restriction in opening the mouth, and/or distortion of the lip. These usually resolve before the next stage operation. When noticed, the parent or patient can stretch and massage the healing wound beginning approximately 1 month postoperatively to help avoid scar contracture. Betamethasone 0.1% can also be applied by fingertip 2x daily beginning 1 month postoperatively and continuing for 6-12 weeks if contracture appears to be developing. Management of persisting scar contraction in the mouth is discussed below.

Upper Lip

If foreskin is not available, the second-best tissue for urethroplasty grafts is labial mucosa. When the proximal urethrostomy is on the mid to distal penile shaft, upper lip is harvested (Figure 11) to reach from there to the tip of the opened glans. This donor site creates less postoperative discomfort and has less tendency to contract and distort the smile. Furthermore, should there be a need for a longer re-grafting in the future the lower lip, which reaches further proximally, remains undisturbed.

The frenulum limits the length of an upper lip graft, and we do not take this down to make the graft longer.

Lower Lip

When a graft is needed to reach from proximal shaft, scrotum, or perineum to the tip of the glans, lower lip is harvested. We have consistently found that graft taken from within the visible junction to the cheek on each side, and from just inside the visible margin of the lip and along the gum (Figure 12), will reach into the perineum. Small grafts should *never* be harvested from the lower lip.

Grafts from upper and lower lip have similar thickness, which in both is less than the cheek. Lower lip donor sites seem to be more painful to patients than upper lip according to those who have had both sites harvested.

Cheek

A dental retractor opens the mouth wide to visualize the cheek (Figure 13). A damp gauze is packed next to the endotracheal tube and against the tongue to prevent blood from trickling down the throat, and to help retract the tongue medially with a narrow Deaver or ribbon. The head is turned slightly towards the surgeon, who first marks Stenson's duct and then outlines the graft. A horizontal mark is made proximally at the end of the mouth which then extends along the gum line medially and just under the parotid duct laterally before ending near the lip.

The graft is infiltrated with 1:200,000 bupivacaine with epinephrine, and the marked lines are incised using a 15 blade. Then the distal edge is lifted with

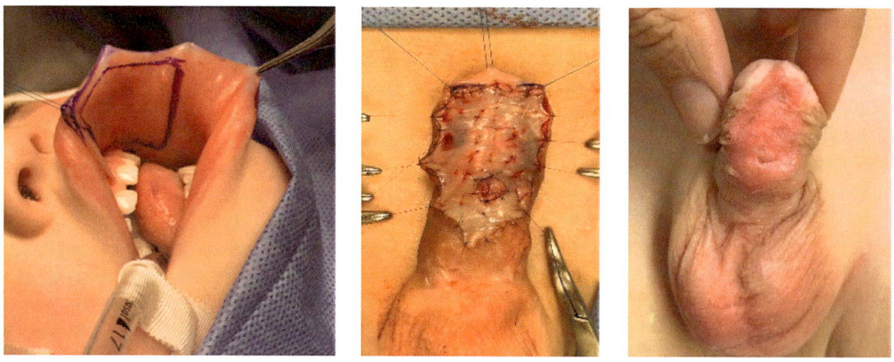

Figure 11. Upper lip graft.
A, the usual anatomic boundaries for an upper lip harvest are the frenulum medially, the gums proximally, a line approximately 2mm within the visible lip margin cephalad, and the cheek laterally. This size graft will provide sufficient tissue to fill between a midshaft meatus and the top of the opened glans as shown in B at the time of STAC 2. C, the upper lip graft in the same patient at the time of STAC 3 6 months later.

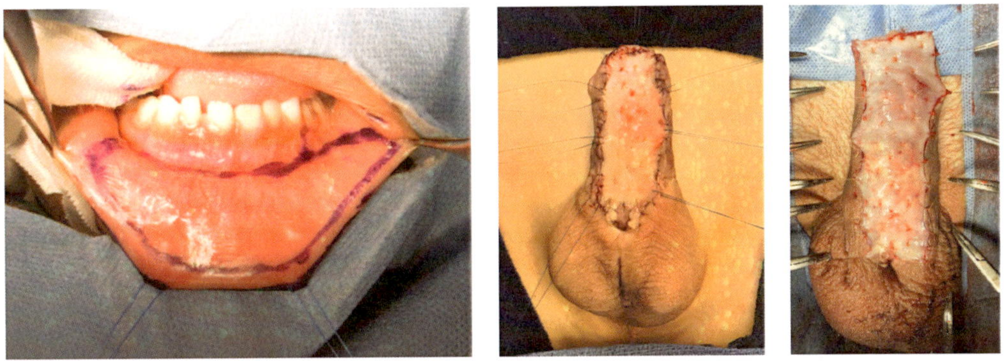

Figure 12. Lower lip graft.
A, the lip is held open with polypropylene stays as shown, and the throat packed with a damp gauze seen exiting to the patient's right side. The graft is outlined running immediately adjacent to the gums and vermillion border and extending on each side to the visible junction to the cheek. B, lower lip graft to the penoscrotal junction in a prepubertal patient. C, similar graft reaching to near the mid-scrotum in an adult.

fine-toothed forceps and the graft dissected above the cheek muscle. This plane is easily established and harvest should leave little muscle or fat to be removed.

The donor site is packed with a gauze soaked in 1:1000 epinephrine and then ignored while hemostasis establishes. The graft is defatted as described above; the donor site is left open to heal.

Placing and securing the graft

The graft is adjusted to best fit the space from the tip of the widely opened glans down to the urethrostomy. It is first sewn to the corona on both sides adjacent to the Prolene stays holding the glans flat. Then it is stitched using 7-0 Vicryl interrupted stitches to the shaft skin. A hemostat is left on every other stitch to maintain the graft width, since otherwise it can be pulled more narrow as stitching continues towards the urethrostomy (Figure 14).

When the meatus is at the penoscrotal junction or more distal, a buttonhole is made in the graft overlying the meatus so that graft will surround it (Figure 15). For a meatus within the scrotum, we spatulate the meatus approximately 4mm on the dorsal side and then advance a V of graft within it. The goal is to create a meatus sufficiently wide for next-stage tubularization into the neourethra without incorporating hair-bearing skin.

An important step for successful graft take is securing it to the underlying corpora. This stabilizes the graft in place and limits the opportunity for hematoma

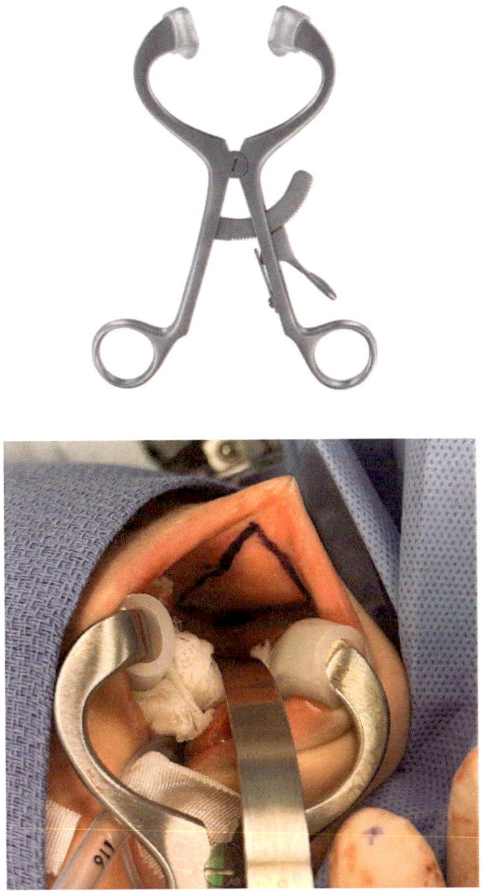

Figure 13. Cheek graft harvest.
A, Molt dental retractor used to expose the cheek. B, outline for left cheek harvest, with exposure gained from the Molt retractor and a narrow Deaver holding the tongue. The margin extends below Stenson's duct (purple dot) towards the junction with the teeth and the lower lip.

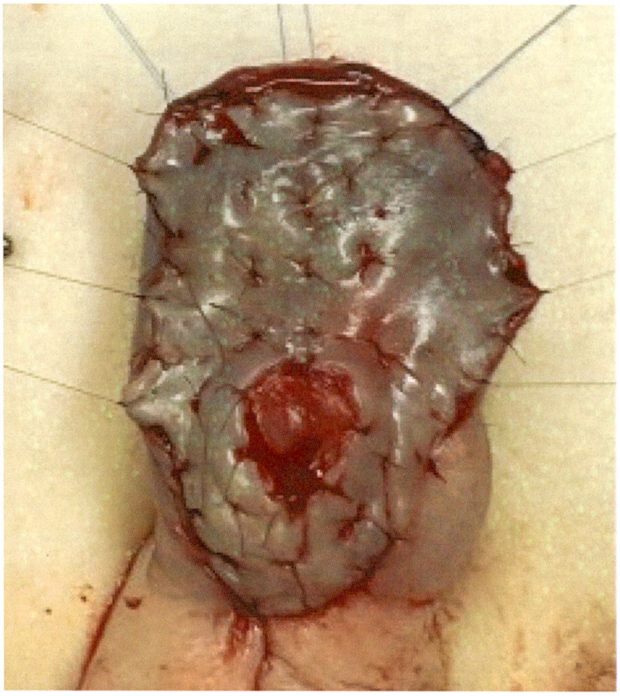

Figure 14. Securing the graft.
The graft has been sewn around the perimeter using 7-0 Vicryl. The stays hold it wide as stitching proceeds from distal to proximal. The distal end of the graft is trimmed to fit and then sewn to the glans. Since this will become the neomeatus at the next operation the stitches to the glans should be placed *subepithelially* to avoid suture marks. Whenever possible, a buttonhole is created in the graft around the proximal urethrostomy.

or seroma to accumulate underneath and impede revascularization.

We emphasize that the graft is quilted to the corpora, and not to the dorsal shaft skin lateral to the corpora. Consequently, quilting is limited to the width of the corpora - which is less than the overall width of the graft placed on the penile shaft in prepubertal boys. We space these quilting stitches approximately 5mm apart, beginning with a row down the center of the graft distally to proximally. Then a second row is placed to one side and a third to the other side. The graft is also quilted to the open glans wings distally on either side (Figure 16).

Graft should not be quilted near the junction to skin, as this could make rolling the graft more difficult.

We find 7-0 Vicryl ideal for stitching the perimeter, and for quilting foreskin grafts. Oral mucosal and posterior auricular grafts are thicker and therefore easier to quilt using 6-0 Vicryl on a RB1 needle.

We always interrupt quilting stitches and have no experience with other sutures for securing the graft.

We are often asked about scoring the graft, making punctures in it to allow fluids underneath to escape. We have never done that, in part from concern that those holes might rapidly fill and not drain. Quilting plus the tie-over bandage accomplish the same purpose of limiting fluid collection underneath the graft.

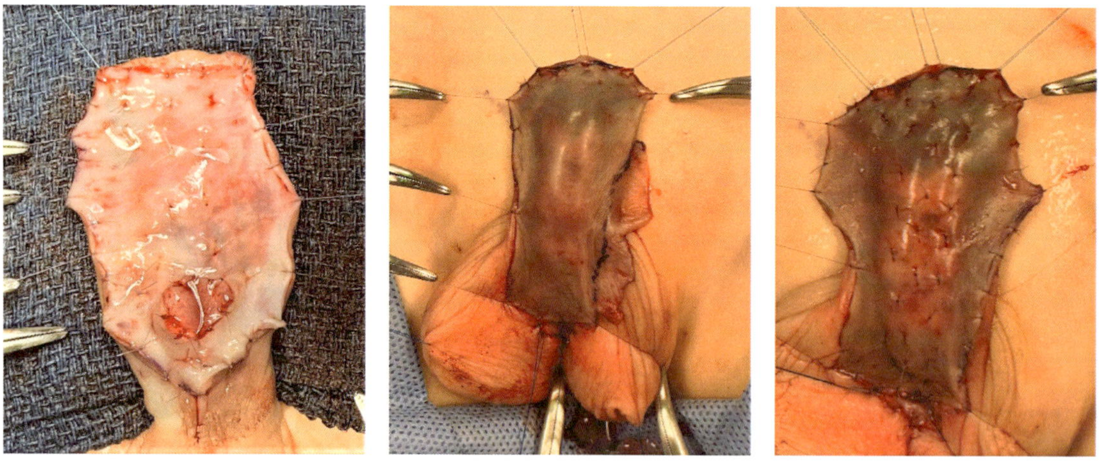

Figure 15. Securing graft to the urethrostomy.
A, the graft was buttonholed to surround the meatus on the proximal shaft. B, Outer prepucial skin graft is advanced within the meatus in a V-shape into the scrotal urethrostomy after spatulating it dorsally. Also note the inner prepuce on the right marked to be trimmed off. C, the same graft trimmed and quilted to the underlying corpora with 7-0 Vicryl sutures.

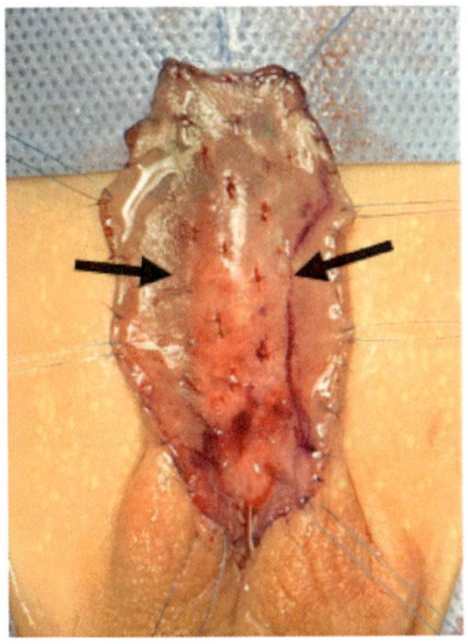

Figure 16. Graft quilting to the corpora.
The shape of the corpora can be seen under the graft (black arrows). The quilting stitches have been placed down the midline of the graft securing it to the midline of the corpora, and then through the graft into the lateral margins of the corpora on either side. Note that this pattern of quilting leaves a margin of graft on both sides free to roll into the neourethra at the next stage. The tie-over bandage will gently compress the lateral graft segments which are not quilted.

Tie-over bandage

The purpose of the bandage is to *gently* compress and immobilize the graft. That adds protection against shearing forces arising from graft movement or fluid collections underneath the graft. We place interrupted simple stitches at intervals across from each other along the graft perimeter approximately 1.5cm apart. These begin with a 6-0 Prolene through the glans wings at the corona and continue proximally using 5-0 Prolene stitches through the shaft skin and graft (Figure 17).

A small weave Vaseline gauze is tightly rolled to place over the graft. We suspect the large square gauzes dry out more rapidly than do the smaller weaves. The rolled gauze should be large enough that the stitches tie over it without coapting the skin edges, since that ensures compression and makes suture removal easier (Figure 18).

The sutures are tied together over the gauze *slightly* snug. It is a technical error to tie them too tight and cause graft ischemia. Remember that the graft and adjacent skin will swell after surgery, which will make

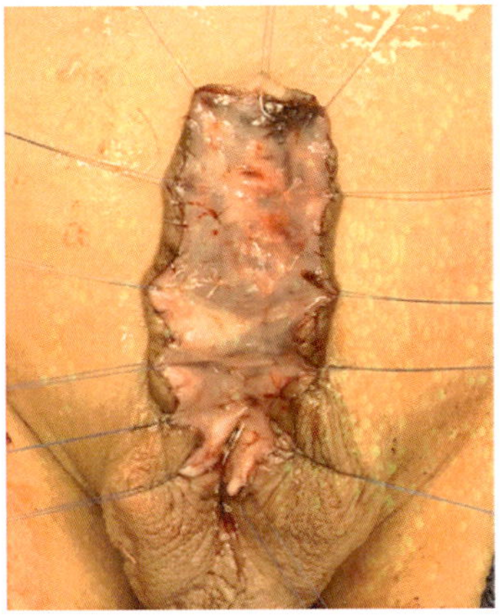

Figure 17. Prolene stays for the tie-over bandage.
The most distal stays are 6-0 Prolene placed though the ends of the corona. Then the remaining 5-0 Prolene stays are placed through graft and penile skin edge at intervals down to the proximal urethrostomy as shown. These are then tied over the rolled Vaseline gauze.

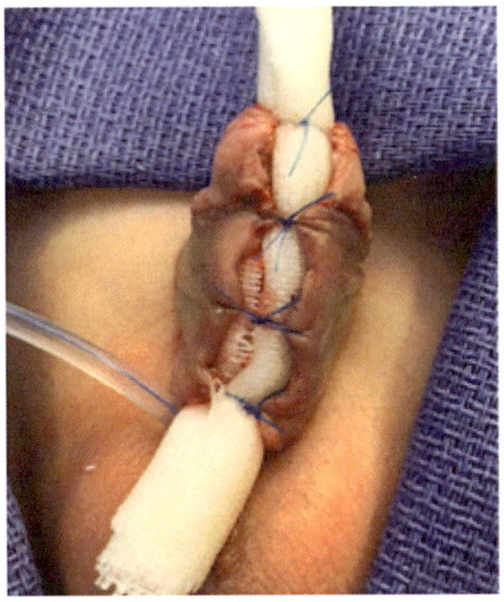

Figure 18. Tie-over Vaseline gauze bandage.
The Prolene stays are tied together snug, but not tight, over the rolled gauze.

the bandage somewhat more tight than when it was secured intraoperatively.

This bandage and the catheter are removed 1 week postoperatively.

Postoperative management

Bedrest

It is *not* necessary to immobilize patients after urethroplasty grafting. Graft quilting and the tie-over bandage provide stabilization during revascularization. In fact, it is not practical to restrict activity in young children, who will kick and scream if that is attempted. We simply discharge them home or to their hotel the day of surgery. Teens and adults are recommended for bedrest for 48 hours after penile surgery, including STAC 2 grafting, in order to avoid scrotal hematomas.

Aquaphor

When the bandage is removed, parents are instructed to apply a generous coating of Aquaphor (petroleum with lanolin) to the graft and skin with each diaper change to keep them moist. This can continue until the next procedure, but probably is most helpful in the initial 12 weeks after grafting.

Topical steroid application

We instruct families to apply betamethasone 0.1% ointment twice daily beginning 1 month postoperatively and continuing for 12 weeks. This should mimic applying sunscreen, and the ointment should coat the entire graft surface and adjacent skin. We use betamethasone cream on prepucial grafts, and betamethasone ointment on oral grafts because the absorbency is slightly different in these tissues.

Wounds have a tendency to contract, and steroid reduces that tendency. It also subjectively helps smooth the junction between skin graft and penile shaft skin.

HBOT

Using paired graft measurements, we have shown hyperbaric oxygen therapy improves graft take in reoperations (Bush and Snodgrass, 2019). It also appears to benefit primary grafts, but with take in those already nearly 95%, it is reserved for those primary patients with known skin risk factors such as penile torsion or single dorsal midline humps of skin.

Details regarding HBOT and graft healing are discussed in Chapter 18.

Initial Graft Appearance

Prepucial grafts can initially appear ischemic when the bandage is taken off (Figure 19), before developing a healthier appearance within a few weeks. It is best to inform parents of this possibility before surgery to decrease their anxiety.

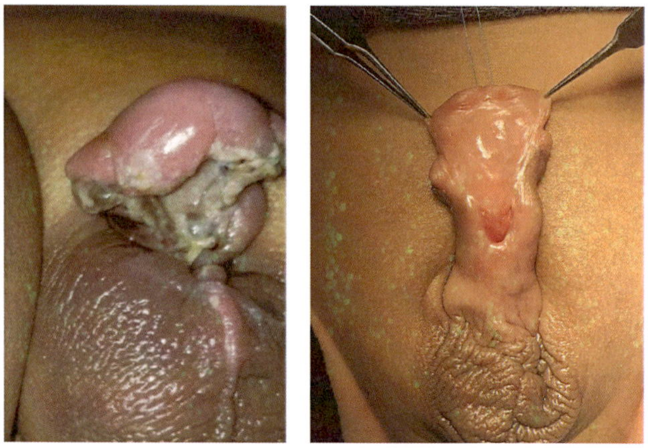

Figure 19. Appearance after prepucial grafting. A, 10 days postoperative appearance following primary prepucial grafting, giving the impression the graft is necrotic. B, same patient 6 months later with no treatment other than Aquaphor and betamethasone ointment.

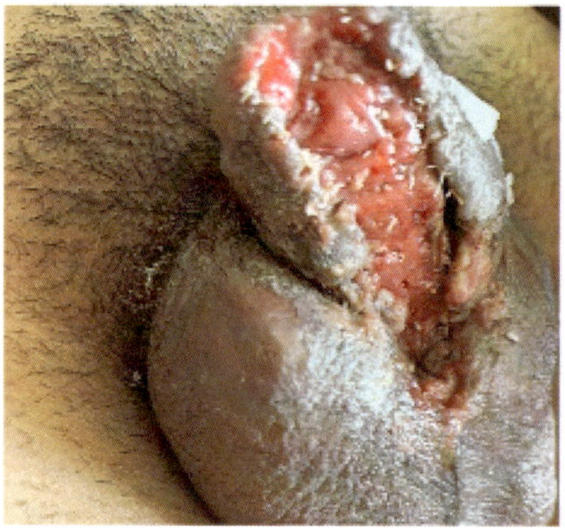

Figure 20. Initial appearance after oral grafting.

Oral grafts typically have a more healthy appearance with the expected red coloration when the bandage is removed (Figure 20).

Factors influencing graft take

Grafts revascularize from the corpora underneath *and* the adjacent shaft skin along their edges. Therefore, the likelihood for successful take is greatest when the graft is placed directly onto intact corpora and sewn laterally to healthy skin. A dartos or tunica vaginalis flap laid onto the tunica albuginea before placing the graft with the thought these would help revascularization will actually hinder that process.

We reviewed STAG repairs and found that graft failure requiring an additional procedure to patch or totally replace it occurred in 9% of those placed onto intact corpora versus a significantly greater 26% to 33% when placed over 1 or more corporotomy incisions covered with dartos.

When we stopped placing grafts onto corporotomy incisions, contractures still developed along the skin margins. We realized that penile skin relocated to cover the ventral shaft needs time to heal before it can reliably support graft take (Chapter 8). Similarly, skin scarred from failed operations may also be unable to support graft healing until it has been repaired and treated with hyperbaric oxygen.

These observations regarding graft healing in both primary and reoperative repairs led to the transition from STAG to STAC, and our systematic incorporation of HBOT in reoperative hypospadias repair.

Graft scars and contractures

Scars generally appear as a line across the graft or as induration in the junction to adjacent skin. Contractures are larger areas of graft loss. Both can be overlooked since scars can be faint and the remaining graft after contracture often appears healthy. One common sign of a graft scar or contraction is a tension band running from proximally into the corona which pulls down the hemiglans (Figure 21). Another is a transverse line across the graft, usually seen at the junction to the urethrostomy (Figure 22), especially when the urethrostomy is at the penoscrotal junction or within the scrotum (Figure 23).

In addition to inspection, stretching the graft at the beginning of the final stage tubularization can detect decreased elasticity from a scar, while contracture is apparent when graft measurements are decreased at the final stage compared to when it was placed.

Because these problems are not always apparent on inspection, we inform parents that the final determination of graft health and its suitability for tubularization is made in the operating room once the procedure is underway.

Adding complexity to this issue is the fact that dartos alongside the graft can be thickened and inelastic, exerting tension along the graft edge and limiting its mobility even though the graft itself is actually healthy. Stretching the cut edge medially reveals that tension, which can then be released by either excising bits of dartos or incising transversely across small

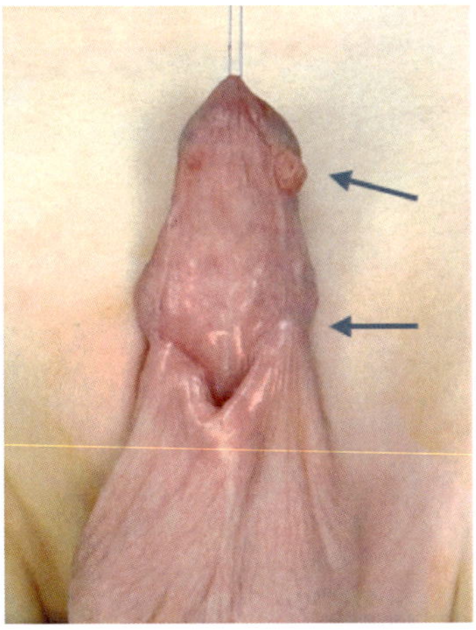

Figure 21. Scar tension band.
There is a visible tension band of scar running along the junction of the prepucial graft to shaft skin which has pulled down the left hemiglans and pulled up the ipsilateral scrotal margin as indicated by the arrows.

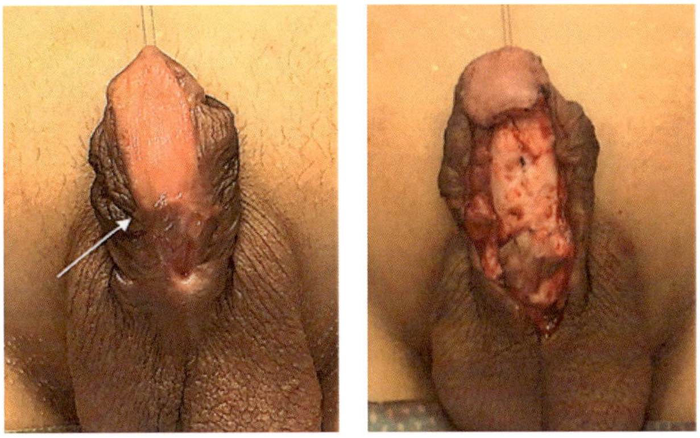

Figure 22. Graft contraction with volume loss.
A, at first glance this graft appears healthy and ready for tubularization. Only a faint line across it at the junction of the graft to the urethrostomy (arrow) indicates there might have been graft contracture. B, incision across the scar reveals the large volume loss from scar contraction. No graft tissue distal to the scar was excised. This case indicates how the appearance of the graft can be deceptive and emphasizes the benefit of measuring grafts when they are placed and before tubularization to help call attention to contractions. This graft had more than 50% shrinkage in area compared to the original graft measurements.

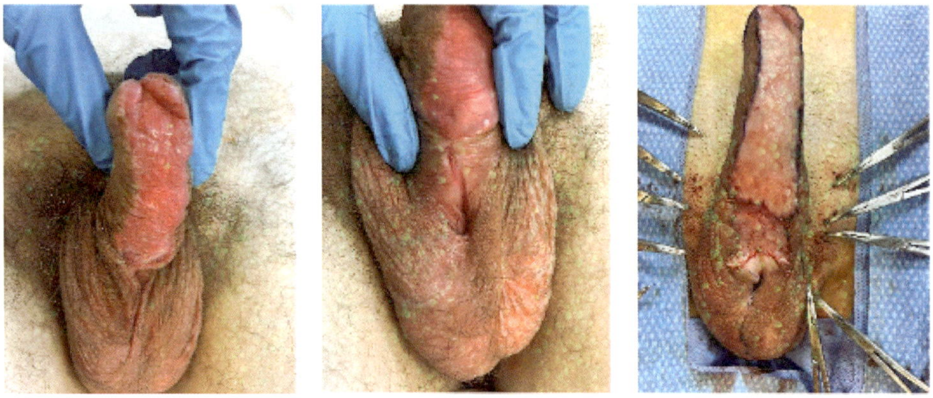

Figure 23. Graft contraction at the penoscrotal junction.
A, at first glance this graft appears healthy and ready for tubularization. B, inspection shows visible scar with graft narrowing at the penoscrotal junction, just above the urethrostomy. C, small patch graft needed in order to avoid incorporating hair-bearing scrotal skin into the neourethra.

tension bands to restore graft elasticity and make tubularization easier. This inspection and release of tension is systematically done along both sides of the graft.

Measuring the Graft

All grafts should be measured when they are placed, and then again at the next operation before tubularization. We measure length from the urethrostomy to the tip of the graft in the glans, and the width at the corona, mid-graft, and at the junction to the urethrostomy (Figure 24), stretching the graft with stays when it is placed and with forceps at the next procedure to capture its full dimensions. These are easy locations to duplicate.

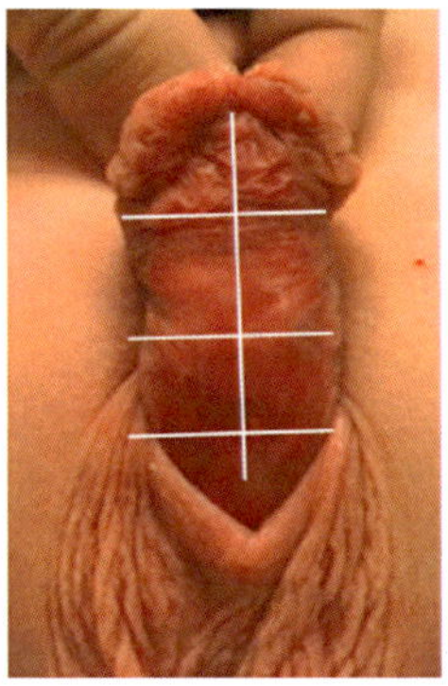

Figure 24. Where graft measurements are taken.
These lines indicate where we measure the graft length and widths (corona, mid-graft, and urethrostomy). The actual measurements are done with the graft stretched to its full extent with forceps.

Managing graft scars and contractures

Often scars can be worked around, for example by moving the skin incision a millimeter or two lateral to a scarred graft edge or notching the edge with a short transverse cut. Decreased graft width from contracture can be restored by inlay grafting, assuming there was little or no loss of length. However, scars in strategic locations such as the corona or within the glans, or those in the scrotum with potential for hair growth if nearby skin is incorporated, may require partial graft excision and patch grafting. Contractions reducing length to the extent that there is longitudinal tension on the remaining graft as shown above in Figure 21, or causing recurrent VC found during artificial erection, similarly require patch or total regrafting.

Graft Margin Scars

The initial skin incision for STAC 3 usually runs within the junction of the graft to skin. When the margin is scarred and there is adequate adjacent penile skin, one option is to make the incision 2mm laterally so that the healthy skin becomes the new graft edge. That usually makes it roll more freely and is easier to suture into a neourethra.

When the graft edge exerts tension pulling down on the ipsilateral hemiglans as shown above in Figure 21, it may be possible to release the tension and lengthen the margin by notching it. The region of greatest

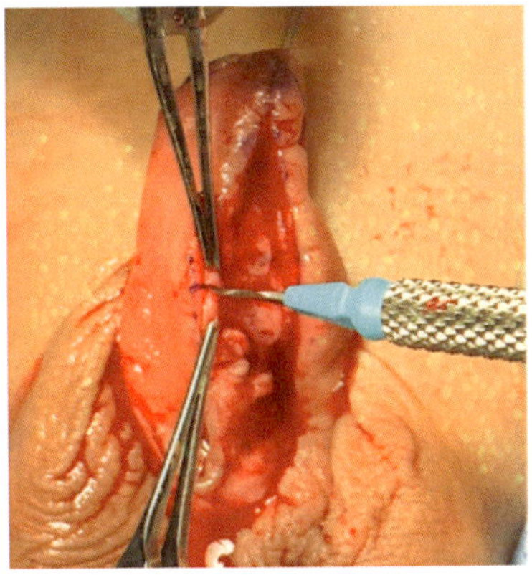

Figure 25. Incising thin scars along the graft margin. Scar seen running along the edge of the graft is cut transversely without incising into the graft epithelium.

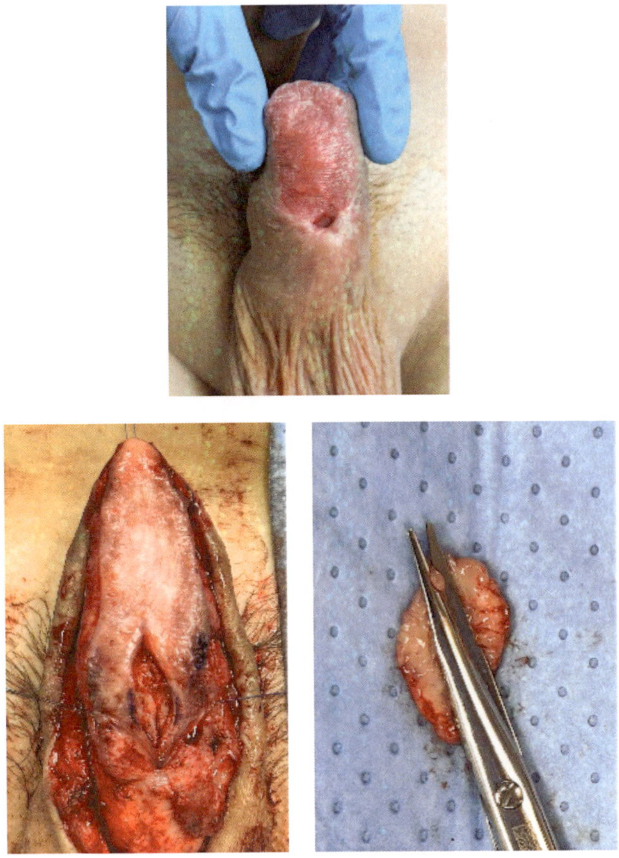

Figure 26. Inlay graft to widen graft narrowing. A, this patient lost some of the graft buttonholed around his proximal urethrostomy, such that it was too narrow to tubularize. B, TIP-like incision is made into the narrowed portion of the oral graft and urethrostomy. C, an inlay graft of an elliptical-shaped portion of lip is harvested, defatted, and sewn into the TIP incision, and the neourethra is tubularized in the same setting.

tension is identified and a small transverse cut is made across the scar (Figure 25). If tension remains it can sometimes be relieved by excising the entire scarred edge with scissors.

These scars occur much less often following STAC than after 2-stage STAG grafts. Nevertheless, checking for them by inspecting and stretching the graft still identifies thickened dartos or small focal scars that can be released to improve the elasticity of the neourethra. This should be a standard procedure during the final stage tubularization.

Graft Contractures

Contractures are scars that shrink the graft. Although it is commonly said that grafts contract 20%, in fact the majority shrink at most a few millimeters, while a few contract 50% or more in length and/or width. We realized reviewing our data that it was the *average* loss which approached 20%, with very few grafts actually having a 20% contraction.

Nevertheless, the belief that grafts shrink 20% is widespread, and has led to recommendations that they be harvested larger to account for this loss. But it is not possible to place a graft that is 20% longer than the distance from the urethrostomy to the tip of the glans, or 20% wider than the distance between the opened glans wings at the corona.

As already mentioned, when graft narrowing occurs and there is excess adjacent shaft skin, the initial incision can incorporate that skin to provide additional width. Alternatively, a TIP incision can be made in the midline of the graft through the epithelium down to near the corpora to widen a narrowed area. When such an incision is < 5mm long it will spontaneously re-epithelialize, but we inlay longer incisions using upper lip oral mucosa, as shown in Figure 26. With all these maneuvers final stage tubularization can proceed.

Otherwise, graft contraction requires a patch or total regrafting, which delays tubularization another 6 months while the new graft revascularizes. Associated VC should straighten when the scarred graft is excised.

Patch and total regrafting

As shown in Figure 22 and 23, graft contractures most often occur near the urethrostomy, leaving the distal graft, especially within the glans, intact. The contracted scar is excised and the resulting space is filled with an oral mucosa patch. These are preferentially harvested from the upper lip or cheek (except when the defect is within the glans), leaving the lower lip intact and available should the patch fail and a longer regrafting become necessary. Figure 27 shows the proximal patch graft for the patient in Figure 22.

Graft contraction within the glans

Much less common is graft contraction within the glans with good healing proximally. These contractions are sometimes recognized because the glans is pulled downwards on one side, but without a tension band running proximally towards the scrotum as

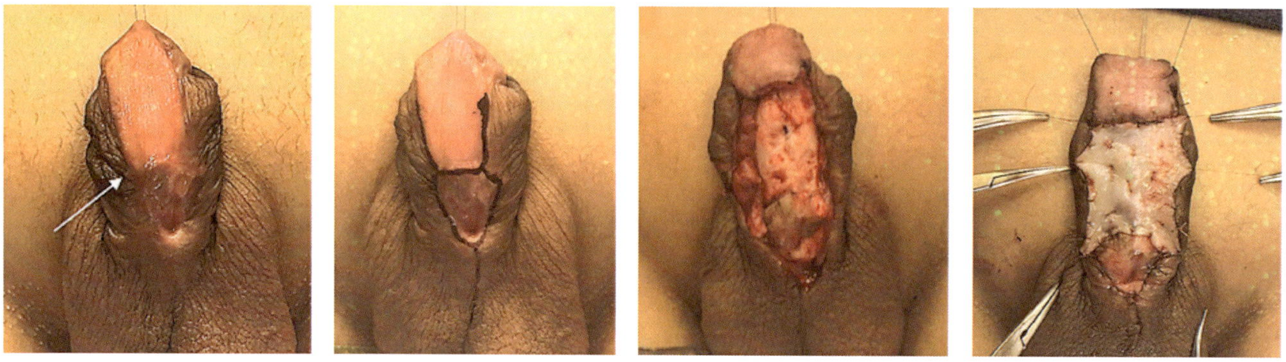

Figure 27. Proximal patch graft using upper lip.
A, an H incision is made along its margin below the corona and across the visible scar. The meatus is released and dissected proximally until healthy tissues are encountered. Similarly, the graft edge is dissected distally until it is freed from the scar reaction. That results in a gap between the urethrostomy and the graft margin which represents the lost graft tissue. Scar on the corporal surface within this gap is meticulously excised. Artificial erection confirms the shaft is straight and then meatus is secured back to the corpora and the defect filled with either upper lip, in this case, or buccal mucosa. Adjuvant HBOT begins postoperatively.

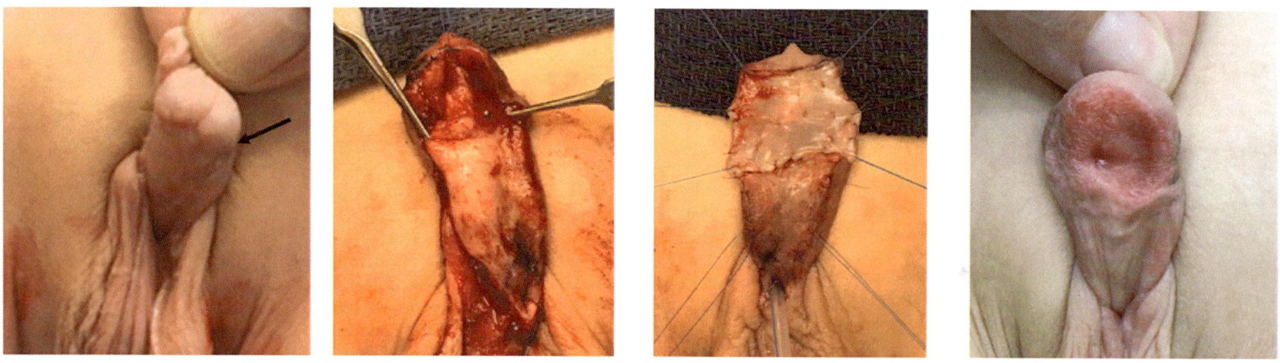

Figure 28. Distal patch re-grafting.
A, the prepucial graft healed with contracture pulling down the left hemiglans (arrow). B, scarred graft within the glans was dissected in continuity with the healthy distal shaft graft. Then artificial erection was done, which showed the penis was straight. Note that the glans wings are now symmetric. The scarred distal portion of the graft was excised, and then the healthy edge was secured to adjacent shaft skin. C, an upper lip graft was placed within the glans and down the distal shaft to meet the remaining graft. D, appearance after healing. The glans is symmetric, and lip graft can be easily distinguished from the lower prepucial skin graft that it is connected to. This neo-plate comprised of oral mucosa and prepuce hybrid grafts can now be tubularized.

shown in Figure 21 above. In other cases there is a visible scar along the graft junction to a glans wings which narrows the graft.

When the remainder of the graft is healthy the distal scarred segment can be excised and patch grafted (Figure 28).

Generalized Contracture

Focal graft contracture is more common than the diffuse contracture shown in Figure 29 with scarring and graft loss within both the glans and the shaft.

Generalized contracture is usually easy to recognize, as the penis is nearly always bent and the graft is visibly and extensively scarred. We first look to see if the glans segment can be salvaged, but when it too is scarred the entire graft is excised. Artificial erection is then done to confirm the penis does not also have recurrent corporal disproportion, which is uncommon but possible. The penis is most often straight and regrafting is done unless the skin is too scarred to support it during revascularization, resulting in a STAC procedure instead. HBOT is always recommended in these cases.

If there is uncertainty regarding the health of adjacent shaft skin it is best to perform a STAC repair with adjuvant HBOT. This reliably lengthens and revitalizes the skin so that subsequent urethroplasty grafting is successful.

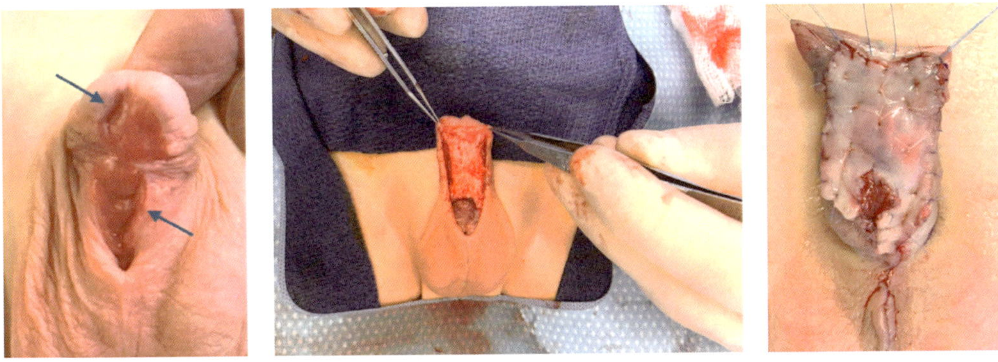

Figure 29. Total regrafting for graft contracture.
A, contracture with loss of graft in both the right glans and left penile shaft shown by the arrows, which also caused recurrent VC. B, after graft excision and dissection of scar from the corporal surface, the penis was straight. C, redo total grafting.

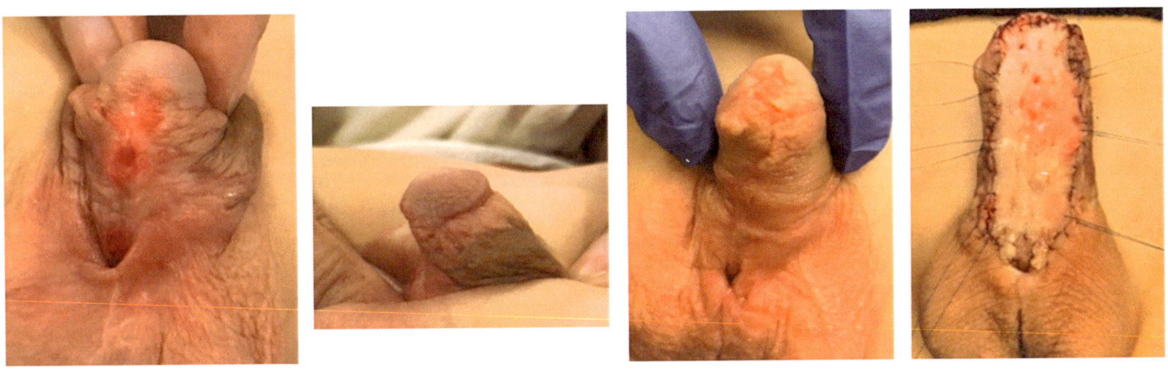

Figure 30. Diffuse graft contracture with recurrent ventral curvature and skin loss.
A, visibly contracted oral graft after a reoperative STAG repair. Note the graft within the glans is also narrowed and deficient, and shaft skin has been drawn up where the graft contracted on the left proximal penile shaft. B, recurrent VC, which is usually due to both ventral skin and graft contracture. C, in this case the penis was still bent more than 30° after removing the graft, and so the prior corporotomies were re-incised and then covered with a dartos flap followed by skin closure in a STAC repair. This is the appearance 6 months later showing the penis is now straight with sufficient supple ventral skin to help support the graft. D, oral mucosa regrafting.

Similarly, in those unusual situations in which curvature ≥ 30° persists after the graft is excised because of recurrent corporal disproportion, repeat corporotomy(ies) are done as needed and covered with a dartos flap in a redo STAC repair (Figure 30).

Oral graft donor site complications

One disadvantage of oral mucosa grafts is the potential for donor site scar contracture, which can prevent full opening of the mouth and/or distort the smile. This can occur after taking grafts from either upper or lower lip or the cheek.

None of these donor sites should be sutured closed. They heal by spontaneous re-epithelialization within a few days and then a scar develops resembling what would be expected had the wound been sutured – a straight line that is indurated (Figure 31).

The scar can then contract and cause tightness and/or lip distortion. Those often resolve before the next operative procedure in 6 or more months. When they persist we release the scar at the next operation (Figure 32). The lip is pulled open to reveal the line of the scar, which is then incised longitudinally in 2 or more locations cutting down to near, but not within, the muscle. Then Kenalog is injected into the wound. A single treatment is most often successful to release tightness or restore a normal smile, although occasionally a repeat release is needed.

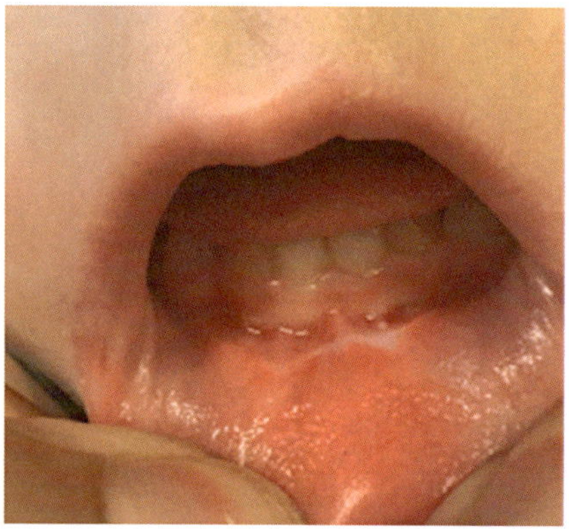

Figure 31. Normal scar after lower lip graft harvest. The arrow points to a fine scar typical of healing 6 months after graft harvest. The lip was not distorted. As with all scars, this will become less apparent with time.

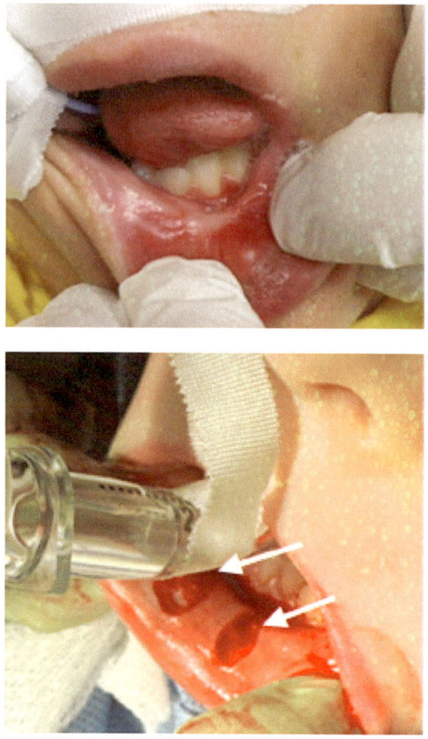

Figure 32. Releasing lip scar contracture.
A, pulling the lip down reveals a tight band of scar.
B, short incisions have been made across the scar to release the tension (arrows).

We are not aware of other specialties harvesting large oral mucosal grafts, which means that few oral surgeons have encountered donor site contractions and consequently may recommend more extensive corrective procedures than necessary. Urologists who harvest oral grafts can easily manage these contractures.

Scabbing over the meatus

Another disadvantage of oral graft urethroplasty is meatal scabbing if the mucosa is exposed to air. Red oral mucosa should not be visible after glansplasty, and problems arise when there is partial dehiscence which then exposes the mucosa (Figure 5). A superficial dry keratin layer can develop, resembling a shedding snakeskin, when oral mucosa is not continuously moist. This then obstructs or deviates the urine stream, especially during the first morning void after the meatus has been dry overnight.

The remedy is to apply Aquaphor directly on the meatus before voiding in the morning or when scab is

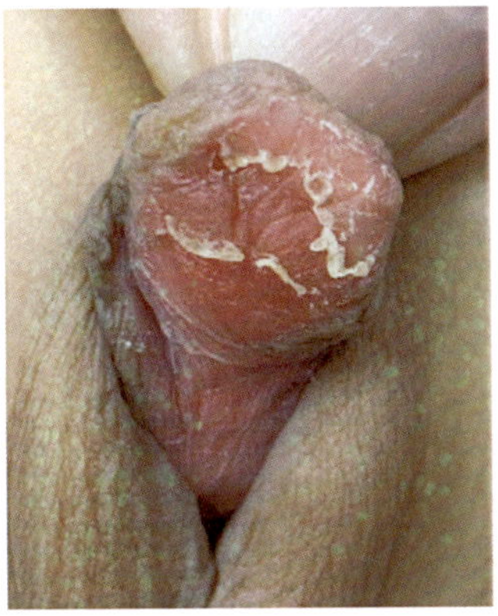

Figure 33. Keratin forms a snakeskin-like film on exposed oral mucosa.
When oral mucosa is exposed to air a film of keratin forms on its surface, resembling a dried snakeskin.

present at other times, which wipes the keratin away. Not all patients with exposed mucosa experience this difficulty, and some who do report that the problem diminishes or resolves over time.

In addition to the unsightly appearance of red mucosa at the meatus when there is partial glans dehiscence, keratin obstructing the meatus is another reason we prefer prepucial graft urethroplasty, and why we save the glanular segment of a prepucial graft when there is contraction proximally that requires patch grafting.

The dried keratin can also usually be seen on grafts before they are tubularized (Figure 33), but is not a problem when the graft is open.

Key Points

Ample data make clear that urethroplasty grafts are superior to skin flaps when the urethral plate must be transected because of VC or scarring from prior surgery. The goal is to make a healthy neo-urethral plate which then can be tubularized into the neourethra.

Prepuce is the best source for urethroplasty grafting, and we have learned that when STAC is done as we describe in Chapter 8, there is nearly always sufficient foreskin to cover the ventral penile shaft and create the neo-urethral plate. No other graft tissue heals as thin and elastic with less induration along its edges as does prepuce.

Lip mucosa is the second choice for urethroplasty grafts, while cheek is rarely needed and should not be placed into the glans because of the increased risk for dehiscence. All oral mucosa grafts share similar disadvantages compared to prepuce, including scar contracture of the donor site, increased reaction at the junction to skin, decreased elasticity after healing, and keratin scabbing when exposed to air. Oral mucosa is best reserved for reoperations when the foreskin has been removed, or when the cultural expectations favor foreskin reconstruction.

Surgeons who repair hypospadias must be able to harvest and manage grafts to provide optimal care, because it is not possible to predict all circumstances when one will be needed. Hypospadias repairs need to be done right the first time regardless of the anatomy found intraoperatively.

Those who are less familiar with grafts can acquire that knowledge. WS did his first graft repair in a reoperation after hearing a lecture by Aivar Bracka, and the lessons he, and we, have learned in subsequent years told in Chapters 8 and 11 should help others significantly shorten the learning curve.

References

Duckett JW: Editorial comment to Hodgson NB: Use of vascularized flaps in hypospadias repair. *Urol Clin North Am* 8: 471, 1981

Rourke K, McKinny S, and St Martin B: The effect of wound closure on buccal mucosa harvest site morbidity: results of a randomized prospective trial. *Urology* 79: 443, 2012

Snodgrass W and Bush N: Staged tubularized autograft repair for primary proximal hypospadias with 30-degree or greater ventral curvature. *J Urol* 198: 680, 2017

Snodgrass WT, Bush N and Cost N: Algorithm for comprehensive approach to hypospadias reoperation using 3 techniques. *J Urol* 182: 2885, 2009

Xu Y, FU Q, SA Y, Zhang J, Jin C, Si J and Song L: Treatment of urethral strictures using lingual mucosa urethroplasty: experience of 92 cases. Chin Med 123: 458, 2010

Chapter 12

Preoperative Testosterone

Proponents of testosterone therapy before hypospadias repair cite 2 advantages: increased vascularity and enlargement of the penis. They consider potential complications such as pubic hair growth to be both rare and transient.

Critics note that there is no high-quality evidence that testosterone either improves outcomes or increases complications.

Adding to the confusion are the lack of objective indications for starting preoperative testosterone, standardized dosing, and defined endpoints for completing treatment. Similarly, there are various androgens available to use orally, topically, or intramuscularly but it is not known if their effects are the same. One related hormone, dihyrotestosterone, is not available in the US or many other countries. Furthermore, the duration of treatment effects is not known, or if it matters when surgery is done afterwards.

Objective Testosterone Therapy

Many urologists use preoperative testosterone for proximal hypospadias when the penis appears small. WS initially did the same, and gave the commonly used 2mg/kg/injection 2 or 3 times before surgery.

Years later, when he realized that boys undergoing proximal TIP had significantly more glans dehiscence than did those who had a distal TIP, we suspected that was explained by the former having a smaller glans. We then began a study measuring glans width and confirmed that the mean width in patients with proximal hypospadias is 12.7mm, versus 14.8mm in similar aged infants with distal hypospadias.

Knowing that testosterone can increase glans width, we next decided to treat those measuring < 14mm with the aim of achieving 15mm. Measurements were repeated 1 month after each injection. We soon observed that the standard 2mg/kg dose stimulated growth to the target size with a single injection in some patients. But the planned regimen of 2 or 3 injections did not achieve the targeted growth in two-thirds of those treated. Therefore, we increased the dose each month when no or inadequate growth was measured, first to 4mg/kg, and then to 8mg/kg, and in one patient to 16mg/kg, to achieve a glans width of 15mm (Snodgrass and Bush et al, 2014).

Once the desired size was reached, patients were scheduled for surgery in approximately 4-6 weeks or after. Those treated had a mean width of 16.6mm, compared to 15.4mm in those who were not treated because they already measured the desired size. We expected surgical outcomes in these 2 groups would be the same since they were operated by the same surgeon using the same technique with the same sutures and had equivalent glans size, but we found that those receiving testosterone had *significantly more* urethroplasty complications than did those not treated, 34% vs 11%. Furthermore, our logistic regression model demonstrated testosterone treatment was an independent risk factor for complications (Snodgrass and Bush, 2016).

Since the goal of therapy was to reduce complications, and not simply to enlarge the penis, we considered testosterone ineffective and stopped using it.

To our knowledge, this remains the only study using objective criteria to select patients for therapy and an objective endpoint to conclude their treatment before surgery.

Not long after we stopped using testosterone, WS traveled to Japan and watched surgeons there operating on proximal hypospadias. He noticed that their dissection of the glans wings was more extensive than his, and learned their rate of glans dehiscence was lower. We made that technical change and our glans dehiscence rate significantly decreased (Snodgrass and Bush, 2016). In fact, the improvement was so great that glans width no longer remained a risk factor for complications.

This experience is another proof that most complications are the result of technical error. The remedy for dehiscence occurring in the smaller glans of boys with proximal hypospadias was *not* to grow it larger with testosterone, but to do a better glansplasty. WS subsequently noticed a photograph of Duckett's glans dissection from one of his papers, and realized it was the same as the Japanese surgeons did. Had WS learned to dissect the glans wings more extensively he would not have encountered so much glans dehiscence and might never have recommended testosterone therapy.

Surveys Regarding Preoperative Testosterone Use

Testosterone use by pediatric urologists before hypospadias repair has not been well-characterized. For example, a survey conducted on the AAP Section of Urology email listserv was answered by only 27 pediatric urologists (Malik and Liu, 2014), which represents less than 10% of certified practitioners. Of those who responded, 78% reported using preoperative testosterone for either all proximal hypospadias or those proximal cases with "a small appearing penis, reduced glans circumference, or reduced urethral plate width." No one answered that they used it for distal hypospadias.

Most ended therapy based on the patient completing the prescribed regimen regardless of the response, while a few considered treatment adequate when the penis appeared sufficiently enlarged. 67% used intramuscular testosterone, and 93% proceeded to hypospadias repair within 1 month or less of ending treatment.

We surveyed members of the hypospadiology.com email group regarding their recommendations for 2

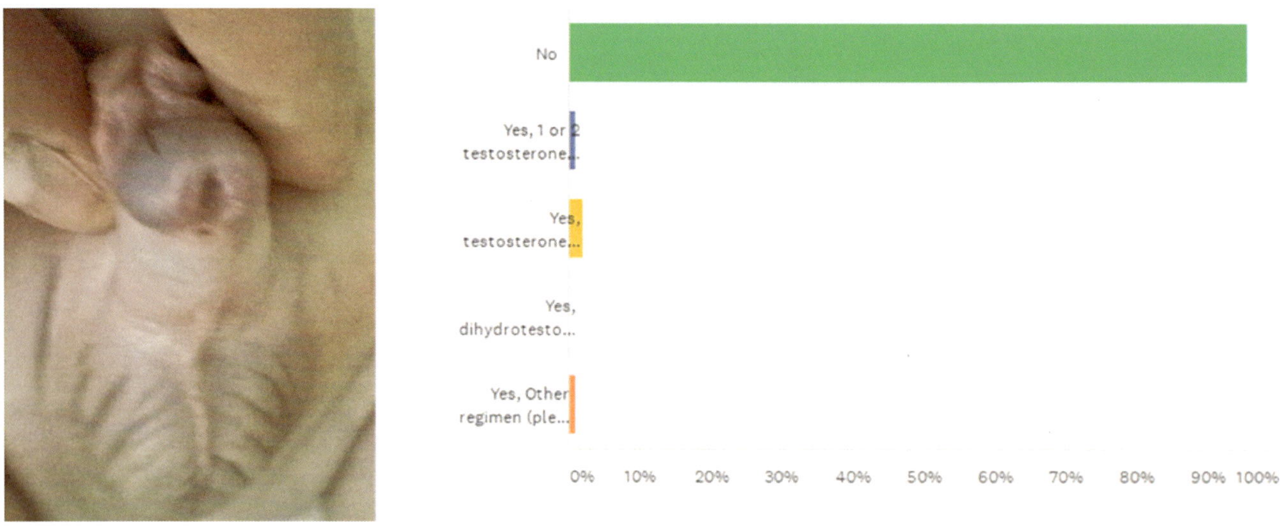

Figure 1. Distal hypospadias survey regarding preoperative hormonal use.
A, picture provided. B, survey options: No (green), Yes 1 or 2 testosterone injections (blue), Yes testosterone cream (yellow), Yes dihydrotestosterone (no respondants), and Yes other regimen (orange).

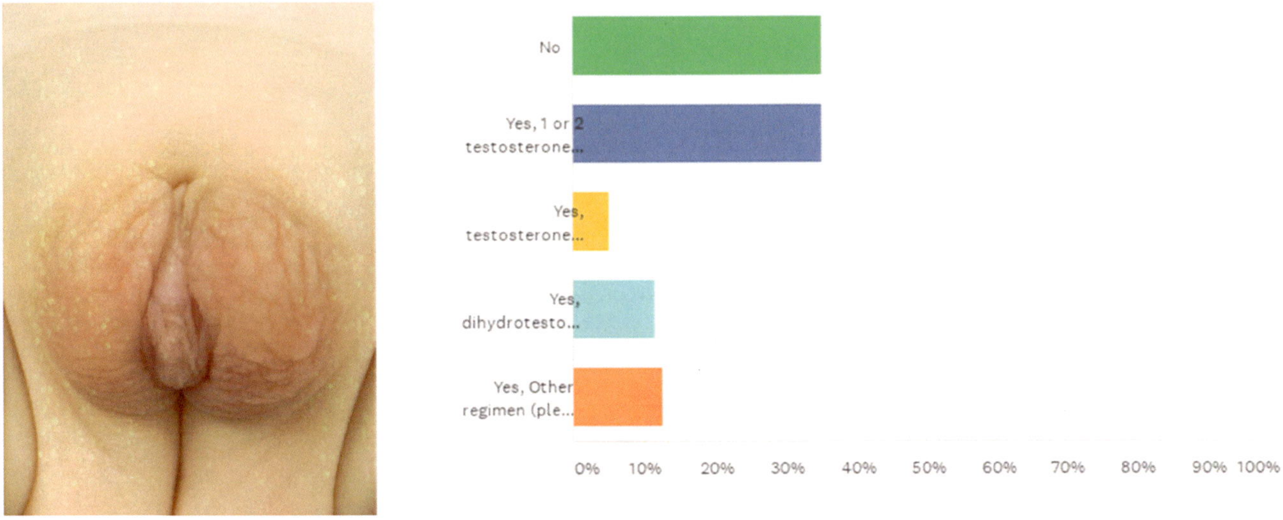

Figure 2. Proximal hypospadias survey regarding preoperative hormonal use.
A, picture provided. B, survey options: No (green), Yes 1 or 2 testosterone injections (blue), Yes testosterone cream (yellow), Yes dihydrotestosterone (turquoise), and Yes other regimen (orange).

sample patients. There were 94 responses from US and international surgeons, comprising 50% of the group at that time (2020).

96% answered they would not recommend testosterone preoperative treatment for this boy with distal hypospadias.

In contrast, 65% responded they would recommend preoperative treatment for his boy. Of those, most would use 1-2 injections of testosterone, while 5% preferred testosterone cream and 12% used dihydrotestosterone, which is not available in the US.

This limited information suggests few surgeons use testosterone before distal hypospadias repair, while a majority do for proximal hypospadias. While some prescribe testosterone for all boys with proximal hypospadias, others use it for a subjectively small appearing penis.

Meta-analysis of Published Results

Several meta-analyses have been published regarding preoperative testosterone therapy before hypospadias repair. These evaluated both retrospective observational studies and RCTs, finding generally low quality with considerable heterogeneity regarding patients and treatment regimens. A standard conclusion is that evidence regarding a potential benefit or harm from treatment requires a well-designed placebo controlled RCT – which has not been reported.

For example, a meta-analysis published in 2017 included 16 trials with 2481 patients, 587 treated with preoperative testosterone versus 1953 not treated. Urethroplasty complications occurred in 34% of those treated and 21% of those not treated, which was not significantly different. However, pooled results from 3 RCTs rated as having moderate quality of evidence showed therapy significantly decreased postoperative complications (Chua et al). Nevertheless, it is noteworthy that most of the patients in 2 of those RCTs had distal hypospadias. The third gave oral testosterone to patients with proximal hypospadias before transverse island repair and stated only 15% of those developed a postoperative complication compared to nearly 40% of those not treated (Chen et al, 2015). Those results, whether with or without testosterone, were considerably better than that more recently reported by the group at CHOP (Long et al, 2017) where the transverse island operation was developed and popularized. But if Chen et al is right that androgens decrease complications by 70%, then every patient with proximal hypospadias undergoing a transverse island repair should receive them.

Four years later, Li et al (2021) evaluated 9 observational studies and 5 RCTs regarding preoperative androgen stimulation. They found that the RCTs demonstrated no effect of androgens on complication rates, whereas the pooled observational studies showed preoperative androgens increased the odds for complications. It is noteworthy that the earlier meta-analysis from the same institution mentioned above (Chua et al) reported analysis of 3 RCTs showed androgen decreased complications, whereas this subsequent review that added 2 more RCTs found it did not impact results.

At the center of this confusion must be the recognition that the widespread use of preoperative androgens must be justified if they cannot be shown to improve the results of hypospadias repair. It is not sufficient to say the treatment causes no harm, especially since there are data that suggest it might.

Side Effects

Proponents of testosterone commonly state that side effects, such as pubic hair growth, are minimal and transient. Although uncommon, we have not found pubic hair growth or other secondary sex characteristics caused by testosterone to disappear after treatment. In addition, the penis enlargement resulting from testosterone stimulation can noticeably exceed normal size for prepubertal boys (Figure 3).

Effect on Wound Healing

Testosterone exerts deleterious effects on wound healing and increases inflammation. In contrast, estrogens promote wound healing, and changes in the balance of sex hormones during aging are thought to partially explain impaired healing in the elderly (Gilliver et al, 2007). The current consensus is that there are no good data showing that increasing testosterone levels improves wound healing (Demling et al, 2020).

Similarly, our database records if a patient was given testosterone and our reviews consistently show those who received therapy have higher urethroplasty complications.

In contrast, there is evidence that anabolic steroids derived from modifying testosterone may directly benefit wound healing (Demling et al, 2020). To date, there are no published studies using anabolic steroids in boys undergoing hypospadias repair.

Effect on Penile Vascularity

To our knowledge, only 1 study reported changes in foreskin vascularization following testosterone stimulation in boys with mostly distal hypospadias. 1% propionate ointment was applied twice daily for 1 month, resulting in an increased number and volume density of blood vessels counted in foreskin specimens (Bastos et al, 2011).

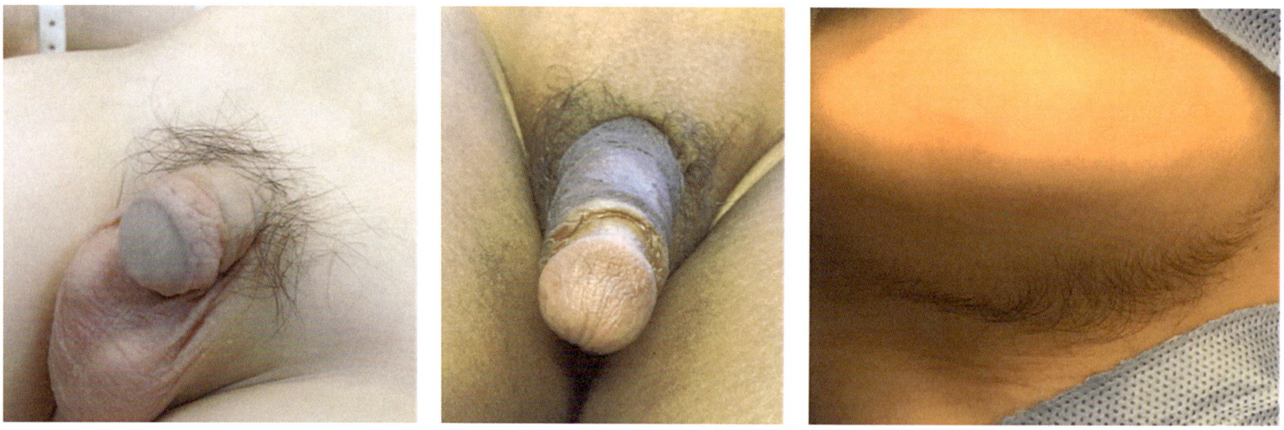

Figure 3. Adverse side effects from preoperative testosterone in boys.
A, coarse pubic hair and penis enlargement inappropriate for age in this 6-year-old after preoperative testosterone. The glans width measured 28mm, the size found in Tanner 4 males. These changes did not regress during 4 years of follow up. B, another boy with coarse pubic hair persisting more than a year after testosterone treatment. C, *4-year old* with a prominent chin and beard after preoperative testosterone.

Should Testosterone Be Used For Microphallic Hypospadias?

Despite casual misuse of the term "micropenis" in boys with severe hypospadias, almost none meet the definition of a stretched penile length < 2SD from the mean, especially after the penis is straightened by 3 corporotomies to lengthen the shorter ventral side to the same length as the longer dorsal side.

The related question is if complications will be decreased by preoperative testosterone for those with the smallest glans width? Those treated in our series described above ranged in size from 9 to 13mm, but testosterone treatment which increased these to 15mm or greater did not diminish complications (Snodgrass and Bush, 2016). Instead, greater glans wings dissection than what we were previously doing has resulted in successful glansplasty in glans as small as 7mm without the use of testosterone.

Should Dihdrotestosterone Be Used For Microphallic Hypospadias?

For the few boys who do meet the definition of a stretched penile length < 2SD from the mean, or those with a glans width significantly smaller than the mean, another option that may have less impact on wound healing than testosterone is dihydrotestosterone (DHT) (Gilliver et al, 2003). This is particularly true for those with known 5 α reductase deficiency and/or alterations/mutations in the androgen receptor gene.

Unfortunately, DHT is not approved for use in the United States and limited data is available. Two studies have shown increased size of the penis after use of DHT transdermal gel (Kaya et al, 2008; Jackson et al, 2024). The study by Kaya et al showed a lower complication rate in the those randomized to receive DHT vs. those who did not, along with penile growth in those treated. Patients had primarily distal hypospadias. In the proximal hypospadias patients treated in the series by Jackson et al, the authors described more glans width growth after DHT (average delta of 9mm) than with testosterone (4mm). This glans width growth was sustained more than 1 year post-treatment in both groups. The study was not designed to compare complication rates between the 2 treatment groups. Additional study using DHT in patients with small glans may be beneficial as a better alternative to testosterone given the known androgen resistance to testosterone in patients with proximal hypospadias, but the impact on wound healing is as yet unknown.

Key Points

The practice of administering testosterone before hypospadias repair lacks a strong evidence-basis and potentially causes harm. The typical regiment of 2mg/kg IM given 2 or 3 times had little effect on glans width in our study, indicating that penis enlargement in boys with proximal hypospadias requires higher doses than usually given. Furthermore, successful treatment that achieves penis enlargement does not necessarily decrease complications. Meanwhile, our finding that testosterone adds another risk factor for complications, plus our successful repair of even the smallest glans sizes convince us to not use it. Those who recommend treatment should prove its value. Until then, informed consent would require parents be informed that it is not known if treatment is of benefit or can possibly cause harm. Additional study using DHT is needed to confirm findings of improved glans width growth compared to testosterone, and to confirm one small study that showed improved results in those who received it.

References

Babu R and Chakravarthi S: The role of preoperative intra muscular testosterone in improving functional and cosmetic outcomes following hypospadias repair: a prospective randomized trial. *J Pediatr Urol* 14: 29e1, 2018

Bastos AN, Oliveira LRS, Ferrarez CEPF, de Figueiredo AA, Favorito LA and Netto JMB: Structural study of prepuce in hypospadias – does topical treatment with testosterone produce alterations in prepuce vascularization? *J Urol* 185: 2474, 2011

Bush NC, Villaneuva C, and Snodgrass W: Glans size is an independent risk factor for complications after hypospadias repair. *J Pediatr Urol* 9:1118, 2013

Chen C, Gong C, Zhang W: Effects of oral testosterone undecanoate treatment for severe hypospadias. *Int Urol Nephrol* 47: 875, 2015

Chua ME, Gnech M, Ming JM, Silangcruz JM, Sanger S, Lopex RI, Lorenzo AJ and Braga LH: Preoperative hormonal stimulation effect on hypospadias repair complications:

meta-analysis of observational versus randomized controlled trials. *J Pediatr Urol* 13: 470, 2017

Demling RH: The role of anabolic hormones for wound healing in catabolic states. *J Burns and Wounds* 4: e2, 2020

Do MT, Kim L, Im YJ, Hahn S, and Park K: Effect of preoperative androgen stimulation on penile size and postoperative complication rate in patients with hypospadias: a systematic review and meta-analysis. *World J Mens Health* 41: 558, 2023

Gilliver SC, Wu F and Ashcroft GS: Regulatory roles of androgens in cutaneous wound healing. *Thromb Haemost* 90: 978, 2003

Gilliver SC, Ashworth JJ and Ashcroft GS: The hormonal regulation of cutaneous wound healing. *Clin Dermatol* 25: 55, 2007

Jackson L, Woodward M, Awad K, Shalaby M: Long-term effects of preoperative testosterone and dihydrotesterone on glans width in boys with hypospadias. J Ped Surg, article in press, 2024

Kaya C, Bektic J, Radmayr C, Schwentner C, Bartsch G, Oswald J: The efficacy of dihydrotestosterone transdermal gel before primary hypospadias surgery: a prospective, controlled, randomized study. J Urol 179(2): 684, 2008

Long CJ, Chu DI, Tenny RW, Morris Ar, Weiss DA,Shukla AR, Srinivasan AK, Zderic SA, Kolon TF, Canning DA: Intermediate-term followup of proximal hypospadias repair reveals high complication rate. *J Urol* 197: 852-858, 2017

Malik RD and Liu DB: Survey of pediatric urologists on the preoperative use of testosterone in the surgical correction of hypospadias. *J Pediatr Urol* 10: 840, 2014

Menon P, Rao KLN, Handu A, Balan L, and Kakkar N: Outcome of urethroplasty after parenteral testosterone in children with distal hypospadias. *J Pediatr Urol* 13: 292e1, 2017

Snodgrass W and Bush N: TIP hypospadias repair: a pediatric urology indicator operation. *J Pediatr Urol* 12:11, 2016

Snodgrass W, Villaneuva C, Granberg C, and Bush NC: Objective use of testosterone reveals androgen insensitivity in patients with proximal hypospadias. *J Pediatr Urol* 10: 118, 2014

Related Conditions

Chapter 13

Preserving the Tunica Vaginalis in Hypospadias Patients With Hernias and Undescended Testes

Both hernias and undescended testes are sometime found in boys with hypospadias, especially those with proximal hypospadias who have an increased likelihood since they are more often born prematurely. The common link between hernias and undescended testes that this chapter explores relates to the availability of tunica vaginalis as a coverage layer over the long neourethra of a proximal repair.

WS published that tunica vaginalis protects better against fistulas than do dartos flaps in proximal TIPs (2011). That likely relates to the relative paucity of dartos in proximal hypospadias plus the need to cover a longer suture line. This is especially true in reoperations in which there may be very little available dartos for a coverage layer.

Hernias

Despite the benefits of tunica vaginalis, we frequently read operative notes by both pediatric surgeons and urologists describing hernia repairs in patients with hypospadias done through an inguinal incision that included bringing the testicle up from the scrotum and stripping off the entire sac to the internal ring. Even when the testicle is not mobilized, traditional dissection of the sac from the spermatic cord in the inguinal canal can result in scarring that leaves the remaining sac too short or insufficiently mobile to make a coverage flap. Furthermore, the tendency for many surgeons to do the procedure bilaterally may ensure that no tunica vaginalis is available for the hypospadias repair. While an external spermatic fascia flap can sometimes be created instead, it is preferable that a different herniorrhaphy technique be used that leaves sac untouched below the internal ring.

Laparoscopic repair of indirect hernias is now well established for young infants. The internal ring can be sutured closed either intra or extra corporeally according to surgeon preference (Figure 1).

When the decision is made to close these hernias in a boy with hypospadias, we recommend the family locate a pediatric surgeon who performs the repair laparoscopically specifically to preserve the tunica vaginalis distal to the internal ring. Occasionally parents have been unable to find a local surgeon to use this method and have instead traveled to our facility to have it done.

Undescended Testes

When necessary, a tunica vaginalis flap can be created from a palpable undescended testis during orchiopexy as part of a final stage proximal hypospadias repair. An example would be a patient with bilateral

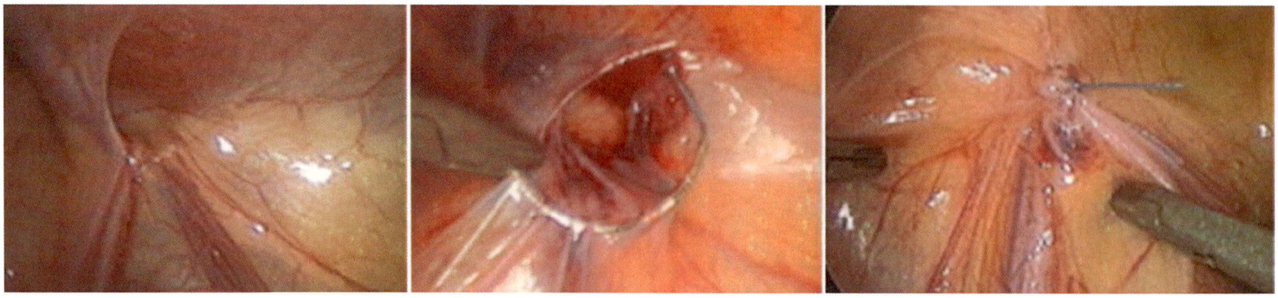

Figure 1: Intracorporeal laparoscopic hernia repair.
A, open right internal ring. B, needle guided around the peritoneum to create a purse-string while avoiding the vas and spermatic cord vessels. C, suture tied intracorporeally to close the internal ring.

undescended testes of which at least one is palpable, or a boy with a unilateral palpable cryptorchid testis who had a contralateral herniorrhaphy that removed the sac.

A tunica vaginalis flap barrier flap cannot be made from an intraabdominal testis. However, we have successfully fashioned a substitute flap by entering a hemiscrotum and dissecting a rectangle of dartos/fatty tissues proximally to near the external ring.

As a general rule we otherwise do not address the undescended testis until a proximal hypospadias repair is completed. In part this is due to the fact that the scrotal transposition often is not fully corrected until the final stage when the meatus is moved from within the scrotum. We have had to relocate testes that were placed by other surgeons into the scrotum before completing scrotoplasty. Furthermore, orchiopexy done during a staged repair before the final operation creates additional reaction around the proximal urethra and urethrostomy, potentially making the hypospadias repair more difficult.

It is not uncommon for a patient with scrotoperineal hypospadias and undescended testes to be recommended for bilateral orchiopexies before the penile reconstruction begins. This removes tunica vaginalis, can create scarring around the proximal urethra and urethral plate, and, as mentioned, sometimes results in a still-malpositioned testes that requires another orchiopexy. At most we perform unilateral orchiopexy during the final stage repair to obtain tunica vaginalis and then plan contralateral orchiopexy 6 months later as an isolated procedure or during repair of a fistula or glans dehiscence. We discourage surgeons from doing orchiopexies in these patients sooner.

References

Snodgrass W and Bush N: Tubularized incised plate proximal hypospadias repair: continued evolution and extended applications. *J Pediatr Urol* 7: 2, 2011

Chapter 14

Hypospadias and Disorders of Sexual Development

Hypospadias and disorders of sexual development (DSD) are separate conditions which sometimes overlap. Few boys with hypospadias also have DSD, while some patients with DSD have hypospadias. Although it is important to identify DSD that occurs in boys with hypospadias, it is also important to realize that boys with hypospadias identify as *boys* (Sandberg et al, 1995).

Traditionally, DSD conditions have been sought primarily in newborns with hypospadias who also have cryptorchidism. In addition, newborns with perineal hypospadias are often labeled as having ambiguous genitalia and evaluated for DSD. Following the 2006 International Consensus Conference on Intersex, these boys are sometimes diagnosed as 46XY "undervirilized males". Finally, males with severe hypospadias are frequently described as having a "micropenis".

Understanding the relationship between hypospadias and DSD requires accurate use of associated terms such as ambiguous genitalia and micropenis, as well as a definition for "undervirilized".

This chapter will review hypospadias and these various additional diagnoses.

Scroto-perineal Hypospadias

Proximal hypospadias ranges from the proximal penile shaft to the perineum, with a penis that most often has VC exceeding 30°. ICD-10 codes list "penile", "penoscrotal" and "perineal" hypospadias, with no separate code for those opening in the scrotum below the penoscrotal junction and above the perineum.

We compared characteristics of 24 consecutive patients with perineal hypospadias to 33 with scrotal hypospadias, finding no differences in the degree of ventral curvature (mean 74.1°, 20-120 vs mean 74.4°, 40-120), mean glans width (12.2mm vs 11.7mm) or mean penile length after ventral straightening (4.5cm vs 4.9cm). Consequently, they can be considered together as having scroto-perineal hypospadias.

Hypospadias and Ambiguous Genitalia

The term "ambiguous genitalia" implies an appearance which is not clearly male or female. However, the subjective nature of this designation leads to such a wide variation in the diagnosis that one study considered genital ambiguity "to be present when a staff pediatric urologist said there was ambiguity" (McAleer and Kaplan, 2001).

"Ambiguous genitalia" should specifically refer to genitalia which could be either male or female.

An example is the masculinized newborn with hypospadias but no palpable testes. That infant can be either a male with hypospadias and undescended testes or a female with CAH; therefore, the genitalia are

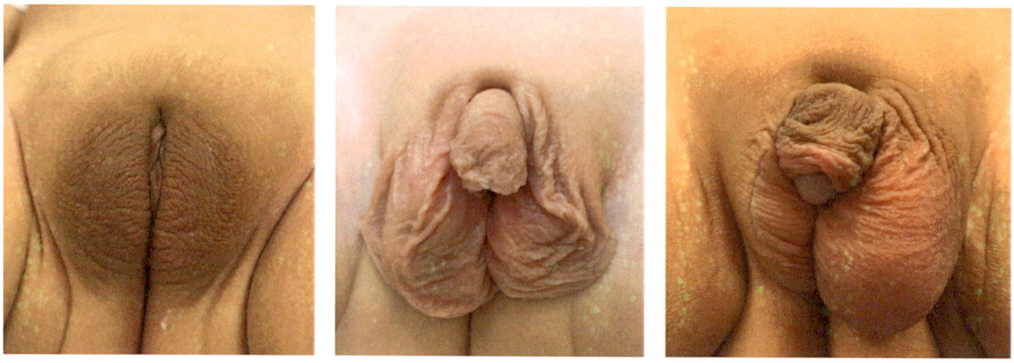

Figure 1. Spectrum of scroto-perineal hypospadias misdiagnosed as ambiguous genitalia.
A, despite the general female appearance, both testes were palpable. Therefore, this child is not female and so does not have ambiguous genitalia. Pictures of his penis are shown in Figure 2 below. B,C, both these newborns were diagnosed as having ambiguous genitalia despite a more masculine appearance than A, with visible and palpable testes. Consequently, neither can be a female and so the genitalia are abnormal, but not ambiguous. That these newborns were all mis-diagnosed with ambiguous genitalia emphasizes that scroto-perineal hypospadias is a rare condition which is not familiar to many providers. The fact that the baby is a boy if there is 1 palpable testicle is a simple and accurate message that pediatric urologists can emphasize.

ambiguous. However, a feminized appearing newborn who has hypospadias and a palpable testis is not female. Consequently, that newborn does not have ambiguous genitalia.

This distinction is very important. When an infant is diagnosed with ambiguous genitalia the parents are informed their child's gender is not certain, causing them significant distress and isolation since they cannot answer the first question of their friends and relatives, "Is it a boy or a girl?" Their concerns regarding gender identity are further increased by the close association between the terms "ambiguous genitalia" and "intersex". Adding to their confusion, endocrinology is frequently consulted and a battery of tests ordered to rule out female CAH, even if both testes are visible.

As mentioned, physical exam that identifies a palpable testicle *excludes* the diagnosis of female gender and, therefore, ambiguous genitalia. *Consequently, the diagnosis of ambiguous genitalia in a newborn with hypospadias should be limited to the very few who also have bilateral nonpalpable testes.* The parents of a newborn with scroto-perineal hypospadias and at least 1 palpable testis can be reassured their baby is a boy with hypospadias, some of whom will undergo additional testing to further evaluate his overall condition in those with a non-palpable testis.

Proximal hypospadias is a rare condition, affecting approximately 1000 newborns per year in the US. Of those, scroto-perineal hypospadias is the least common. Neonatologists and pediatric endocrinologists might not have previously encountered a newborn with the most severe form of hypospadias, and, consequently, are confused by the general appearance of the genitalia. A clear message that a newborn with a palpable testis is male would help reduce this confusion.

Similarly, pediatric urologists also should not label patients with hypospadias and a palpable testis as having ambiguous genitalia. Figure 1 shows examples of patients with varying genital appearance who were incorrectly diagnosed with ambiguous genitalia since each had at least 1 palpable testis.

Hypospadias and Micropenis

Infants with scroto-perineal hypospadias are commonly said to have a "micropenis," or "microphallic hypospadias." Micropenis is defined as stretched penile length (SPL) < 2SD from normal, which is < 2cm in term newborns. However, the VC that averages 70° in boys with proximal hypospadias (Snodgrass and Bush, 2017) complicates determining penile length. An example is shown in Figure 2.

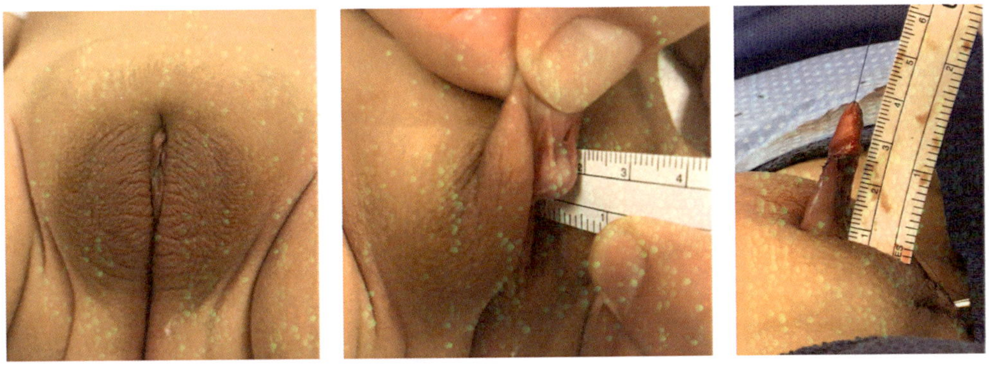

Figure 2. Difficulty measuring stretched penile length before straightening ventral curvature.
A, boy with scroto-perineal hypospadias. B, preoperative stretched penile length from pubis to the tip of the glans is nearly 2cm, but difficult to accurately determine because of ventral curvature which measured 80°. C, repeat measurement in the same patient after 3 corportomies is 38mm, which is within the range of normal for age. This patient should not be diagnosed as having a micropenis despite his initial appearance.

We measured SPL after 3 ventral corporotomies to straighten VC in 57 consecutive boys < 3 years of age with scroto-perineal hypospadias, and found that it averaged 4.7cm. This was greater than the mean of 3.5cm reported in males < 3years (Tomovo et al, 2010). None of these patients in our series met the criteria for micropenis.

We also evaluated 28 adults undergoing reoperation for scroto-perineal hypospadias, using flaccid glans width < 21mm to define a micropenis based on the normal mean of 27mm (SD 0.3) (Chen et al, 2014). Glans width was normal in all patients, averaging 29mm (SD 3.4).

The diagnosis of micropenis is distressing to parents, who worry their son will be inadequate for adult sexual behavior. The diagnosis also may lead to testosterone stimulation to enlarge the penis, which may not be effective in commonly used doses and has uncertain effects on surgical outcomes as reviewed in Chapter 12.

For these reasons, urologists should not refer to boys with hypospadias as having a micropenis unless the SPL is < 2SD *after* ventral lengthening straightens the penis.

46,XY Undervirilized Male

The International Consensus Conference on Intersex added isolated perineal hypospadias to the list of diagnoses included in 46,XY DSD. These patients were recommended to have karyotyping, abdominal-pelvic ultrasound, measurement of 17-hydroxyprogesterone (17-OHP), testosterone (T), gonadotropins (LH and FSH) and anti-mullerian hormone (AMH), with further testing, such as hCG stimulation, as indicated (Hughes et al, 2006).

We reviewed outside medical records in 51 consecutive patients with scroto-perineal hypospadias and found that only 4 (8%) had the complete testing recommended by the Consensus Conference. A karyotype was obtained in 37 patients, and was the only test in 5 of those, while the others had additional evaluations from among those recommended. More than 1 of every 5 had no testing.

Of these, the only conclusively abnormal were 3 karyotypes reporting 45,X/46,XY, 46,XX and 47,XXY. One patient had low T with a subsequently normal stimulation test, while another had an elevated T with low DHT but normal 5 alpha reductase. All other tests performed were normal.

Despite normal evaluations 8 were assigned the diagnosis of "46,XY undervirilized male". Two of those 8 were recommended to be raised female and undergo sex reassignment surgery (despite bilateral palpable testes). The parents of another were told they could choose the gender of rearing. The parents of a fourth were advised to raise their infant as a male, but to defer hypospadias repair until male gender identity could be confirmed. Photographs of a boy initially raised female are shown in Figure 3. All these patients

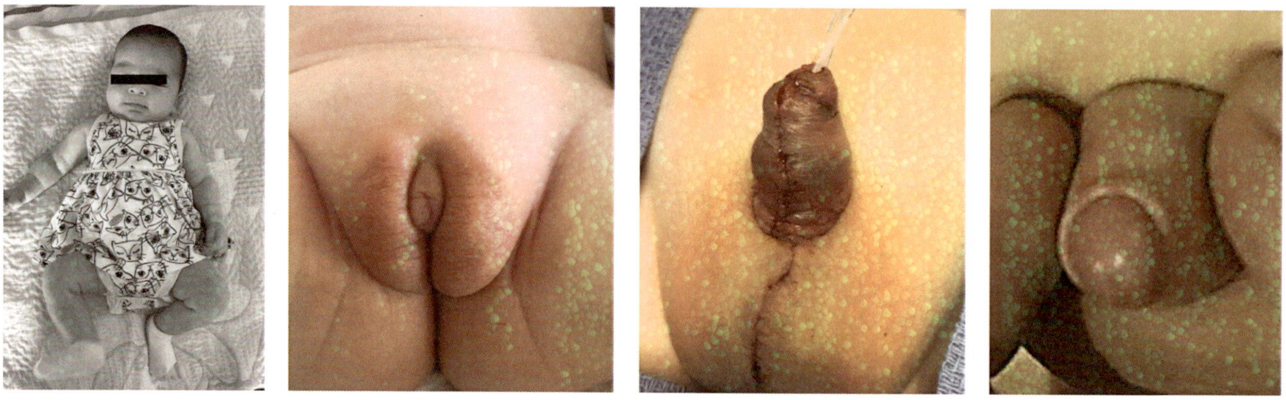

Figure 3. Repair of a boy with scroto-perineal hypospadias initially recommended to be sex-converted to female. A, photo of the patient dressed as a female at age 3 months, as recommended by the DSD team. B, appearance of the genitalia before repair. The glans width measured 10mm. He was not treated with testosterone. C, intraoperative photograph after completing STAC repair. Stretched penile length was a normal 54mm. D, appearance 1 year later.

were evaluated by multidisciplinary DSD teams which included an endocrinologist and a pediatric urologist.

The endocrinologist leading one of these teams that recommended surgical sex reassignment responded that he was not aware of reports that gender dysphoria occurs in males with DSD raised female (Furtado et al, 2012, Reiner, 2005). Meanwhile, we have not found data indicating boys with scroto-perineal hypospadias manifest female gender identity. Rather, a study of boys with hypospadias demonstrated the same masculine behavior as did controls without hypospadias, regardless of the severity of the condition (Sandberg et al, 1995).

Feature	*Score for Yes/No or condition*
EMS	
Scrotal fusion	3/0
Micropenis	0/3
Urethral meatus	
Normal	3
Glandular	2
Penile	1
Perineal	0
Right and left gonad (score for each)	
Scrotal	1.5
Inguinal	1
Abdominal	0.5
Absent	0

Figure 4. External Masculinization Scoring.

An external masculinization score (EMS) shown in Figure 4 has been proposed to standardize physical genital assessment (Ahmed et al, 2000). The authors applied this scale to 423 normal male newborns, reporting 415 scored 12, while the median of those <12 was 11 (9-11.5). Another 202 patients had "ambiguous genitalia" and were assigned male gender. Most of these were diagnosed with partial androgen insensitivity syndrome, dysgenetic testes, and 5 alpha reductase deficiency, and their median EMS score was 3.5 (2-8).

No patient we evaluated with scroto-perineal hypospadias, including the 8 previously diagnosed with undervirilization, had been scored using this scale. Three representative patients who were diagnosed with 46,XY DSD are shown below in Figure 5. Each scores from 5.5 to 6 – meaning they would be considered more virilized than the majority of male patients reported by Ahmed et al to have ambiguous genitalia.

However, these scores of 5.5 to 6 are still less than normal, possibly implying they are "undervirilized" compared to controls. Yet all 8 boys diagnosed with 46,XY undervirilized DSD had normal penile length after straightening their ventral curvature. Each had bilateral palpable testes. All had a normal karyotype, testosterone, LH, FSH and AMH, as well as a normal pelvic ultrasound. HCG stimulation done in 3 was also normal. Records indicated it was the general appearance of the genitalia, and not any specific abnormality, which led to the diagnosis of undervirilization.

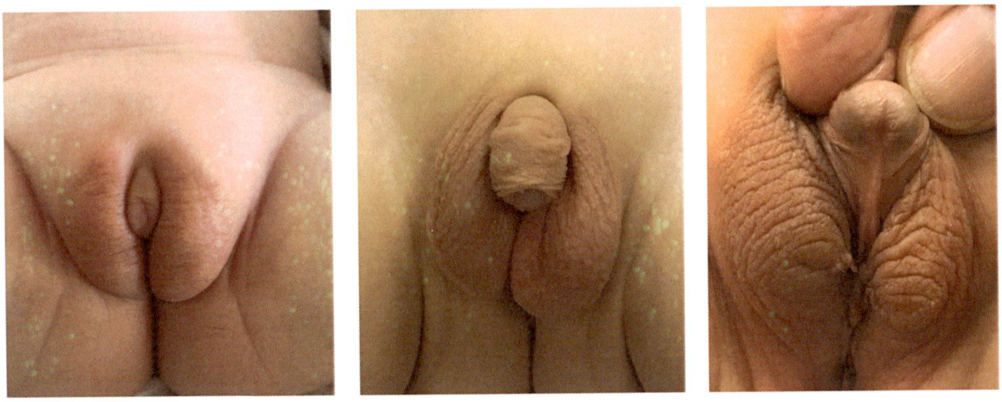

Figure 5. 3 boys diagnosed as having 46,XY undervirilized DSD.
The appearances of these 3 patients are quite different, yet each was diagnosed as undervirilized. Even the first patient with the most feminized general appearance had a normal stretched penis length after 3 corporotomies (shown above in Figure 3) and bilateral palpable testes. These cases demonstrate the subjective nature of this diagnosis as it is currently made.

A diagnosis of undervirilization not only raises questions regarding current management, but also concerns for future genital development including a possible need for testosterone supplementation and risk for inadequate phallic growth at puberty. Yet none of the 28 men we evaluated for scroto-perineal hypospadias required hormonal treatment to initiate or sustain puberty and all had glans width within the normal range.

There are few studies with small numbers of subjects reporting postpubertal penile length in patients with hypospadias. Mean SPL was similar in Tanner 5 males with distal hypospadias and controls (Ryjna et al, 2009; Ortqvist et al, 2015; Moriya et al, 2016). While those with proximal hypospadias measured shorter than controls, all measured normally, meaning none had a length less than 2SD compared to controls (Rynja et al; Ortqvist et al). Therefore, all these men had normal penile length, although the mean of those with proximal hypospadias was on average 2cm shorter.

Moriya et al additionally measured LH and testosterone, finding hypogonadism in 17% of patients, 1/13 (8%) with distal and 4/17 (24%) with proximal hypospadias. All these men were asymptomatic, and none agreed to a trial of testosterone therapy to enlarge their penis.

Together these observations argue against describing boys with scroto-perineal hypospadias as "undervirilized". Not when most have a normal-sized penis, normal hormonal profiles, and enter puberty spontaneously.

Hypospadias Plus DSD

The most common DSD conditions found in association with hypospadias are mixed gonadal dysgenesis (MGD), ovotesticular DSD, and Klinefelter's Syndrome. These are usually diagnosed by karyotyping, often done because the boy has both hypospadias and an undescended testis. The true incidence of these or other DSDs is not well-established because most published reports have not systematically tested patients with hypospadias to determine how many also have one of these conditions.

For example, Kaefer et al (1991) karyotyped only 68% of 79 patients with both hypospadias and undescended testes, finding a DSD in nearly 30%. Those included MGD (14%), ovotesticular DSD (6%), 5-alpha-reducase deficiency (3%), partial androgen deficiency (4%) and Klinefelter's (3%). DSD was more likely in boys with proximal hypospadias and nonpalpable testes.

However, 2 other similar studies obtained karyotypes in 42% and 57% of a total of 157 patients with hypospadias and undescended testes and reported a lower incidence of DSD, comprising MGD in 3% and ovotesticular DSD in 0.06% (McAleer and Kaplan, 2001; Cox et al, 2008).

In the largest of such studies, karyotypes were obtained in a total of 916 patients with undescended testes and/or hypospadias. Only 32 had both conditions, of which 4 (12.5%) had an abnormal karyotype, mostly Klinefelter's (Moreno-Garcia and Miranda, 2002).

More recently, a comparison was made between boys with proximal hypospadias and descended testes (n=91) versus those who also had an undescended testis (n=21). As in these other studies, evaluation was selective, involving only a third of those with descended testes versus all with an undescended testicle. DSD found in 10% with descended testes versus 33% with an undescended testicle (Rowe et al, 2019).

We similarly reviewed karyotypes obtained elsewhere in 37 patients with scroto-perineal hypospadias, of which 3 had bilateral nonpalpable testes and 1 had a palpable undescended testis. An abnormal karyotype (Klinefelter's and MGD) was found in 2/33 (6%) with descended testes versus 1/4 (25%) with an undescended testis who had 46,XX ovotesticular DSD.

Findings by Rowe et al and us that up to 10% of patients with scroto-perineal hypospadias and descended testes have sex chromosome abnormalities supports karyotyping in all newborns with this condition.

Even then, a few boys with a normal karyotype will be discovered during tunica vaginalis harvest to have ovotesticular DSD (Figure 6). When that occurs, the appropriate next step is simply to excise the ovarian tissue and proceed with the hypospadias repair. Since the other gonad can also be abnormal it should either be explored at the conclusion of the operation before the scrotum is closed, or at a subsequent time since retained ovarian tissue can cause gynecomastia during puberty.

Karyotyping, endocrine testing, and surgical examination of the testes do not yield a genetic diagnosis in most patients who might be suspected of having 46,XY DSD. Targeted gene sequencing could potentially establish or exclude a molecular diagnosis in them. However, there are limited data using this technology to evaluate hypospadias. One study of 46 patients with isolated hypospadias considered to have 46,XY DSD found 13% had a variant in an androgen synthesis or action gene and 15% had a variant in a testis development gene (Eggers et al, 2016), but clinical features of these patients were not described.

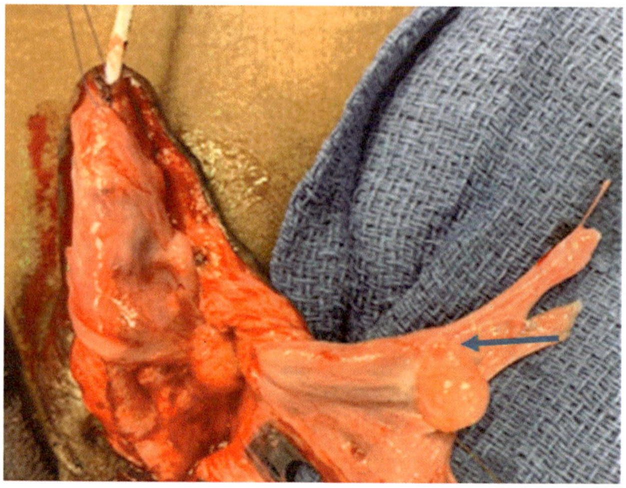

Figure 6. Ovotestis found during hypospadias repair. Arrow points to a cap of ovary affixed to the testicle. This was excised.

In summary, 15 years after the Consensus Conference recommended evaluation of isolated perineal hypospadias, testing remains ill-defined and variable. In the meantime, one unintended consequence of evaluating these boys in DSD clinics has been to unsettle some parents by the implication that their newborn might not be a boy, or could be a boy unable to function as an adult male. Certainly, the advice given to some of these parents that they should consider raising their sons as females, and even to pursue surgical sex reassignment, is also distressing and contrary to the best available evidence regarding gender identity. Given that few boys with scroto-perineal hypospadias are found to have an established DSD using today's technology, their families may feel more comfortable undergoing evaluations in another setting besides a "DSD clinic". Multidisciplinary physicians can reassure parents any additional studies are not to determine gender identity or the sex of rearing in these cases.

Key Points

Few boys with hypospadias have a genetic DSD. The likelihood is greater with proximal hypospadias and an undescended testis, but as many as 1 of every 10 with proximal hypospadias and bilaterally descended testes will have a DSD. Therefore, a karyotype should be done for any hypospadias with an undescended testis, and for all boys with scroto-perineal hypospadias.

Regardless of the genital appearance, a palpable testis excludes the diagnosis of a virilized female and so the patient with a palpable testis does not have ambiguous genitalia and the parents can be reassured despite the genital appearance.

The additional battery of tests recommended by the Consensus Conference appears to adds little information, and, if done, parents should first be reassured the evaluation is not to determine gender or sex of rearing. The same is true regarding gene sequencing, which might provide important and useful information, but does not change the fact that boys with hypospadias are boys. Ideally, DSD teams will collaborate to devise testing protocols for newborns with severe hypospadias to better determine which benefit from what investigations.

Meanwhile, terms such as "undervirilized" and the related diagnosis of "46,XY undervirized male" are best avoided because they are subjective and can create worries about male function which have not been supported by adult follow up.

Similarly, boys with scroto-perineal hypospadias do not have a micropenis, and so this diagnosis should not be made until after penile straightening when an accurate SPL can be measured.

Most parents are confused and upset to learn their newborn has a birth defect of his penis, and that is especially true of for those whose son has scroto-perineal hypospadias. We strongly encourage specialists managing hypospadias to carefully consider the additional distress that terms such as ambiguous genitalia, micropenis, and undervirilization cause them.

Certainly, neither DSD teams nor individual pediatric urologists should recommend sex reassignment to any newborn with testes, even those with the most severe hypospadias.

References

Ahmed SF, Khwaja O, and Hughes IA: The role of a clinical score in the assessment of ambiguous genitalia. *Br J Urol Int*: 85: 120, 2000

Chen XB, Li RX, Yang HN, Dai JC: A comprehensive, prospective study of penile dimensions in Chinese men of multiple ethnicities. *Int J Impot Res:* 26: 172, 2014

Cox MJ, Coplen DE and Austin PF: The incidence of disorders of sexual differentiation and chromosomal abnormalities of cryptorchidism and hypospadias stratified by meatal location. *J Urol* 180: 2649, 2008

Eggers S, Sadelin S, van den Bergen JA, et al: Disorders of sex development: insights from targeted gene sequencing of a large international patient cohort. *Genome Biology* 17: 243, 2016

Furtado PS, Moraes F, Lago R, Barros LO, Toralles MB, and Barroso U, Jr: Gender dysphoria associated with disorders of sex development. *Nat Rev Urol* 9: 620, 2012

Hughes IA, Houk C, Ahmed SF, and Lee PA: Consensus statement on management of intersex disorders. *Arch Dis Child* 91: 554, 2006

Kaefer M, Diamond D, Hendren WH, Vemulapalli S, Bauer SB, Peters CA, Atala A, and Retik AB: The incidence of intersexuality in children with cryptorchidism and hypospadias: Stratification based on gonadal palpability and meatal location. *J Urol* 162: 1003, 1999

McAleer IM and Kaplan GW: Is routine karyotyping necessary in the evaluation of hypospadias and cryptorchisim? *J Urol* 165: 2029, 2001

Moreno-Garcia M and Miranda EB: Chromosomal anomalies in cryptorchidism and hypospadias. *J Urol* 168: 2170, 2002

Moriya K, Nakamura M, Nishimura Y, Kitta T, Kanno Y, Chiba H, Kon M and Shinohara N: Factors affecting post-pubertal penile size in patients with hypospadias. *World J Urol* 34: 1317, 2016

Ortqvist L, Fossum M, Andersson M, Nordenstrom A, Frisen L, Holmdahl G and Nordenskjold A: Long-term followup of men born with hypospadias: urological and cosmetic results. *J Urol* 193: 975, 2015

Reiner WG: Gender identity and sex-of-rearing in children with disorders of sexual differentiation. *J Pediatr Endocrinol Metab* 18: 549, 2005

Rowe CK, Adam MP, Ahn JJ and Merguerian PA: Yield of modern genetic evaluation for patients with proximal hypospadias and descended gonads. *J Pediatr Urol* 15: 527, 2019

Rynja SP, Wouters GA, can Schaijk M, Kok ET, de Jong TP and de Kort LM: Long-term followup of hypospadias: functional and cosmetic results. *J Urol* 182: 1736, 2009

Sandberg DE, Meyer-Bahlburg HFL, Yager TJ, Hensle TW, Levitt SB, Kogan SJ and Reda EF: Gender development in boys born with hypospadias. *Psychoneuroendocrinology* 20: 693, 1995

Snodgrass W and Bush NC: Staged tubularized autograft for primary proximal hypospadias repair with 30-degree or more curvature. *J Urol* 198: 680, 2017

Snodgrass W and Bush NC: unpublished data, 2020

Tomova A, Deepinder F, Robeva R, Lalabonova H, Kumanov P and Agrawal A: Growth and development of male external genitalia: a cross-sectional study of 6200 males aged 0 to 19 years. *Arch Pediatr Adolesc Med* 164:1152, 2010

Chapter 15

Hypospadias and BXO

Balanitis xerotica obliterans (BXO), also known as lichen sclerosis, can affect both uncorrected and previously operated hypospadias. We calculated that it occurred in 0.8% of our hypospadias patients in 2 age groups: boys at a mean age of 6 years and men at a mean age of 36 years (Snodgrass and Bush et al, 2016). BXO is thought by some to be a chronic auto-immune skin condition, but the etiology is still unknown.

Presentation and Diagnosis

BXO presents as white scarring involving the foreskin, penile shaft skin, scrotum, urethral meatus, and /or the urethral plate (Figure 1). Following hypospadias repair, it can develop at the tip of the reconstructed prepuce causing secondary phimosis, or around the meatus after circumcision creating meatal stenosis. Inadequately treated, the disease can progress along the urethra and produce obliterative strictures.

Patients we evaluated with the condition in non-operated hypospadias were asymptomatic. Those who developed BXO following hypospadias repair presented with dysuria, stranguria, and/or a deflected stream after an asymptomatic interval. All tissues regularly used in hypospadias urethroplasty were affected, including the urethral plate, prepucial flaps and grafts, and oral mucosa.

It is important to emphasize that patients who present with the new onset of dysuria, stranguria, and/or a deflected stream after initially successful hypospadias repair have potentially acquired BXO. Usually the diagnosis is obvious during physical examination,

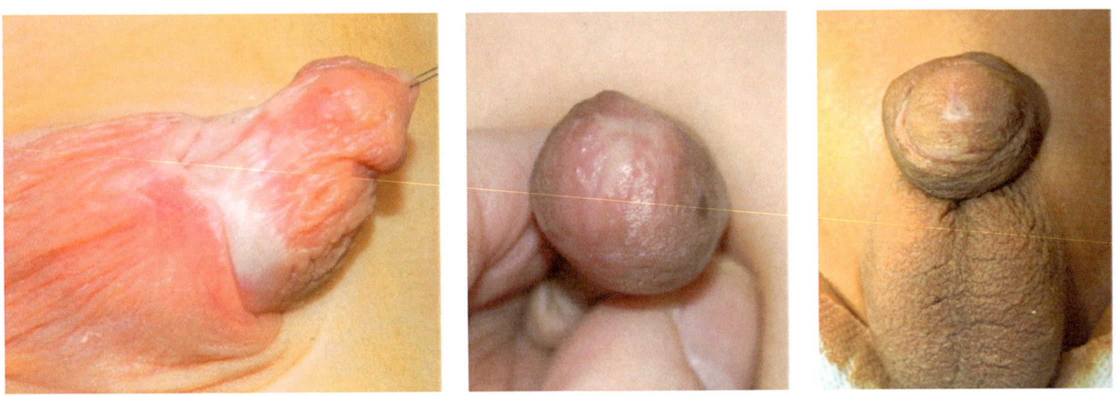

Figure 1. BXO in hypospadias patients.
A, uncorrected hypospadias with BXO involving the penile shaft skin, scrotal skin, and the urethral plate. B, BXO creating secondary phimosis after prepucioplasty. C, BXO causing new meatal stenosis several years after distal hypospadias repair.

when the white cicatrix and skin discoloration, or less commonly peri-meatal ulceration, is present. But some have these symptoms without the characteristic white appearance shown above yet respond to clobetasol with resolution of their complaints.

Ideally, biopsy is done to confirm the diagnosis. However, it can be difficult in some cases to obtain a sliver of representative tissue, while in others with typical symptoms and clinical appearance of BXO, histology is inconclusive. We nevertheless manage these patients under the presumption that they have the condition.

Management

WS was taught that BXO is primarily a surgical condition, requiring affected urethral tissues be removed and replaced with oral graft, which was said to be resistant to the disease. Recurrences around the meatus, where there inevitably is a junction between genital skin and oral mucosa, could be managed with betamethasone. However, nearly half of his patients had recurrences after 2-stage oral grafts that did not respond to betamethasone and were thought to require another 2-stage oral graft repair. When 1 of those patients balked at that recommendation and continued using betamethasone and then tacrolimus to control symptoms for another year before agreeing to surgery, WS encountered BXO invading down the distal urethra, with biopsy proving BXO involvement within the oral mucosa (Figure 2).

He spoke with Paul Anderson, an adult reconstructive urologist in the UK, over dinner during an AUA meeting who told him that betamethasone is ineffective, while ultrapotent steroids such as clobetasol are potentially curative.

Clobetasol

Class I ultrapotent topical steroids such as clobetasol are the first line treatment against both primary and recurrent BXO. Clobetasol 0.05% is applied once daily for 6-12 weeks. When the meatus is involved, a metal dilator or feeding tube is used to push the steroid into the distal urethra. Complete disease regression occurs in approximately half of patients, with improvement in symptoms for others (Lewis et al, 2018). Maintenance therapy may be necessary in some patients.

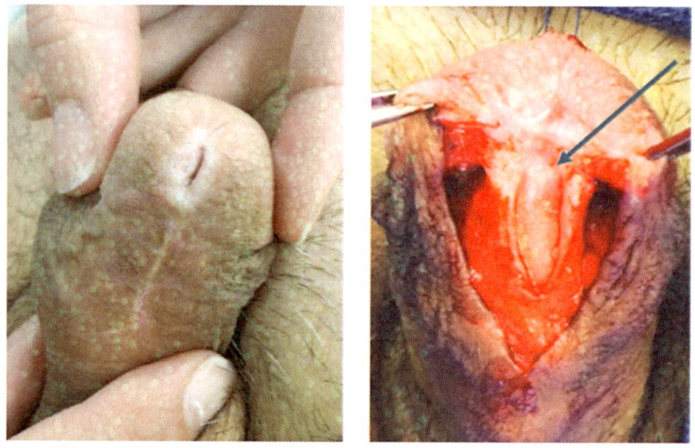

Figure 2. Recurrent meatal BXO invading oral mucosa inside the neourethra.
A, typical white discoloration where skin of the glans meets oral mucosa at the meatus. B, BXO invading down the neourethra below the corona within oral mucosa (arrow).

Betamethasone is a Class III steroid which does not have sufficient potency to effectively treat BXO and should not be used.

Clobetasol has also been found to be more effective than tacrolimus, which is no longer recommended. Topical androgens are no longer recommended, either.

aWhen topical ultrapotent steroids are not effective surgery is required. For example, a trial of clobetasol for disease involving the reconstructed prepuce can be given, but persistent or frequently recurrent BXO should be removed by circumcision. The glans underneath is then often found to be involved, in which case adjuvant treatment with clobetasol is necessary.

Disease at the meatus causing stenosis which persists despite clobetasol can next be managed by a dorsal meatotomy (to avoid re-creating hypospadias by a ventral incision) plus triamcinolone injection, a Class II highly potent steroid. If that fails, then excision of all visible BXO with lip graft STAG urethroplasty is done.

Similarly, BXO extending down the neourethra can first be treated with clobetasol insertion. The traditional option when surgery is needed for stricturing is complete excision of the BXO-involved tissues with replacement using lip mucosa in a STAG repair. However, because of the risk for recurrence, and to avoid a 2-stage repair, single stage oral mucosa inlay grafting

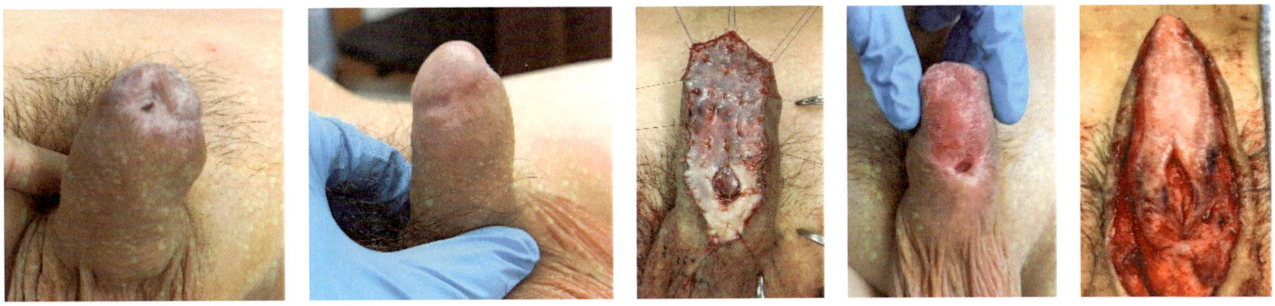

Figure 3. Patient with BXO showing glans obliteration at initial surgery, and graft contracture at follow up requiring inlay grafting.
A,B this teen had BXO that developed 10 years after his original distal hypospadias repair, unrecognized by his original surgeon, who performed 2 cut-backs for urinary retention but did not treat with any steroids, despite the characteristic white discoloration. C, STAG oral graft at the time of his BXO excision since the penis was straight. D, loss of the buttonholed portion of his graft, such that it was too narrow to tubularize. E, TIP-like incision is made into the narrowed portion of the oral graft and urethrostomy and an inlay graft was placed. White skin near urethrostomy was excised and he will be monitored lifelong for additional BXO skin changes and/or neourethral stricture.

has been reported to have similar results (Dubey et al, 2005; Levine et al, 2007; Kulkarni et al, 2009). In either 1-stage or 2-stage procedures, there are significantly fewer recurrences in oral mucosa than in genital skin grafts, which should not be used (Trivedi et al, 2008).

Results

We reported treatment in 12 patients with meatal BXO. Initially, betamethasone and tacrolimus were used with minimal response. Later, when we changed to clobetasol, 2 of 3 treated patients had complete resolution of symptoms and disappearance of the white lesions.

10 patients next had excision of BXO with a 2-stage oral graft replacement urethroplasty. 40% recurred at a median of 26 months (22-105), while the others remained disease-free with similar follow up. Of the 4 with recurrences, 3 underwent another 2-stage oral graft repair and 1 of those had recurrent disease within 6 months which responded to clobetasol.

These outcomes support guidelines emphasizing first line treatment with clobetasol, which is the only medical therapy potentially achieving complete remission. Clobetasol can also be used for recurrences after 1 and 2-stage urethroplasties to avoid additional surgery.

We have no experience with dorsal meatotomy plus triamcinolone injection as yet, but would use that as the second treatment if clobetasol alone was not effective for meatal BXO with stenosis.

If these measures fail, 2-stage oral graft repair with complete excision of BXO is done when the disease has obliterated the meatus and /or urethra leaving little or no normal tissue to augment with an inlay graft. The option of a 1-stage inlay oral graft remains for patient with less severe disease.

We have seen glans obliteration and even significant graft contracture in patients with BXO (Figure 3), and recommend perioperative HBOT for those undergoing penile reoperation to decrease risk for graft contracture. Studies are ongoing to evaluate other treatment modalities such as platelet-rich plasma therapy and/or various laser/light therapies which are currently being utilized in women with vulvar disease.

Key Points

The late onset of dysuria, stranguria and/or defection of the urinary stream after previously successful hypospadias repair potentially indicates BXO, even when the characteristic white appearance is not seen. Typical findings include new phimosis of previously retractable reconstructed foreskin, or new meatal stenosis.

Medical therapy, specifically with clobetasol and *not* betamethasone, is the first treatment and can achieve complete remission in up to half of patients.

Surgery is needed for persistent disease despite clobetasol. A key lesson we have learned is that BXO is not cured by simply excising the lesion and replacing it with oral mucosa. Therefore, meatotomy with steroid injection, and inlay grafting using oral mucosa, are potential options before complete excision and staged oral mucosa graft repair.

References

Dubey D, Sehgal A, Srivastava A, Mandhani A, Kapoor R, Kumar A. Buccal mucosal urethroplasty for balanitis xerotica obliterans related urethral strictures: the outcome of 1 and 2- stage techniques. *J Urol* 173:463, 2005

Kulkarni S, Barbagli G, Kirpekar D, Mirri F, Lazzeri M. Lichen sclerosis of the male genitalia and urethra: surgical options and results in a multicenter international experience with 215 patients. *Eur Urol* 55:945, 2009

Levine LA, Strom KH, Lux MM. Buccal mucosa graft urethroplasty for anterior urethral stricture repair: evaluation of the impact of stricture location and lichen sclerosis on surgical outcome. *J Urol* 178:2011, 2007

Lewis FM, Tatnall FM, Velangi SS, Bunker CB, Kumar A, Brackenbury F, Mustapa MFM and Exton LS: British Association of Dermatologists guidelines for the management of lichen sclerosis 2018. *Br J Dermatol* 178: 839, 2018

Snodgrass W, Blanquel JS, and Bush NC: Recurrence after management of meatal balanitis xerotica obliterans. *J Pediatr Urol* 13: 204, 2017

Trivedi S, Kumar A, Goyal NK, Dwivedi US and Singh PB: Urethral reconstruction in balanitis xerotica obliterans. *Urol Int* 81: 284, 2008

Complications and Reoperations

Chapter 16

Urethroplasty Complications and Recurrent Ventral Curvature

Every surgeon who repairs hypospadias encounters complications after some of those operations. The question is why?

In an earlier era, after the MAGPI was described followed by a host of other methods to repair distal hypospadias, Duckett taught that most complications occurred because the surgeon chose the wrong operation for the anatomy of the patient (Keating and Duckett, 1995).

Today there are fewer repairs in common use, yet complications continue. Rather than choosing the wrong operation for the anatomy, **the most common reason for complications is that the surgeon made a mistake while performing the repair.** We know this because half of our practice is reoperations after unsuccessful surgery done by pediatric urologists, and their records describe technical errors which directly relate to the complication(s) the patient developed. Nevertheless, the patient, or his mother, are often blamed; for example, the boy's constipation caused a fistula (yes, we have read this explanation in clinic notes!), or he was too active and dehisced his wound because his mother was inattentive.

A related reason is that the penis is bent. Most of the patients we reoperate for routine complications, including fistulas, glans and wound dehiscence, meatal stenosis, urethral strictures and diverticula, also have persistent or recurrent VC exerting tension in the region where the complication occurred.

These are sobering observations, as is the fact that no other surgery done by pediatric urologists harms more children than does hypospadias repair. But these observations are also *encouraging*, because surgeons can significantly decrease their complications by improving how they do the key steps in TIP and STAC repairs.

This chapter focuses on mistakes made during urethroplasty and glansplasty, emphasizing how to avoid them. Preventing complications is another way of saying surgeons need to do it right the first time. That cannot be over-emphasized, since the risk for additional complications *doubles* when the first operation is not successful (Snodgrass and Bush, 2017).

Persistent or Recurrent Ventral Curvature

The most common cause of urethroplasty complications after proximal, and many distal, repairs is persistent or recurrent VC ≥ 30°. In fact, we reported this was found in an astonishing 85% of patients who presented to us with otherwise typical complications including fistulas, glans dehiscence, meatal stenosis and urethral strictures after proximal repairs done elsewhere. Furthermore, 100% of patients with persistent or recurrent VC also had urethroplasty complications (Snodgrass and Bush, 2019).

This curvature averaged 50°, and was diagnosed at a mean of 22 months postoperatively in 83% of patients

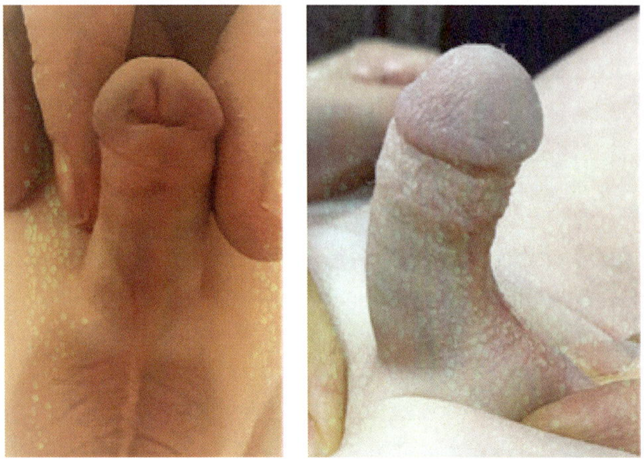

Figure 1. Glans dehiscence with recurrent ventral curvature.
This boy was originally diagnosed as having "distal hypospadias with mild chordee" and was managed by dorsal plication and TIP repair. Tension from recurrent VC that measured 35° after the skin was released contributed to or caused glans dehiscence.

whose initial straightening was done by chordee excision, 70% after dorsal plications, and 33% following single ventral corporotomy with corporal grafting.

Although persistent or recurrent VC is more common in boys born with proximal hypospadias, we also encounter it in patients with unsuccessful distal repairs, as shown in Figure 1.

This curvature exerts tension on the ventral aspect of the penis which pulls on the repair with each spontaneous erection postoperatively, leading to complications and resisting attempts to correct them until the penis is straightened. In fact, recurrent complications nearly always indicate underlying VC.

Therefore, it is important for surgeons to recognize signs of persistent or recurrent VC. The typical appearance is shown in Figure 2. In addition to the hunched-over shape, VC resists lifting the glans cephalad such that the scrotum pulls with it and then the penis snaps back down as soon as it is released.

Regardless of the preoperative examination, *every* patient undergoing reoperation for a hypospadias complication must also have an artificial erection to verify that the penis is straight. This is true even when the penis was originally reported straight, or natural erection in the clinic appears to show it straight. For example, WS observed a straight erection in a school-age boy with a recurrent penoscrotal fistula after 2 prior attempts to close it by another, very experienced, senior surgeon. Intraoperatively we found him to have VC at the penoscrotal junction just below the fistula (Figure 3). He was successfully repaired with 3 ventral corporotomies in a reoperative STAG procedure. Most likely, the first surgeon wrapped a tourniquet around the junction before doing artificial erection, which obscured the bend. The first artificial erection should be done *without* a tourniquet to avoid this mistake. He healed fistula-free after successful correction of this curvature.

Management completely changes when curvature is found. Rather than a simple fistula closure or a reoperative TIP for glans dehiscence, the finding of ventral curvature ≥ 30° converts the repair to a reoperative STAC.

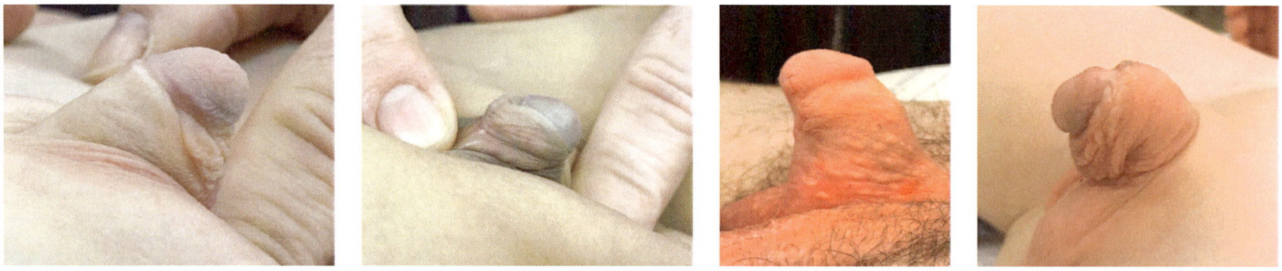

Figure 2. Examples of postoperative ventral curvature.
Each of these patients has postoperative VC, giving the penis a "hunched-over" appearance. In addition, there is resistance to lifting the glans cephalad, and the penis snaps back to this position when it is released.

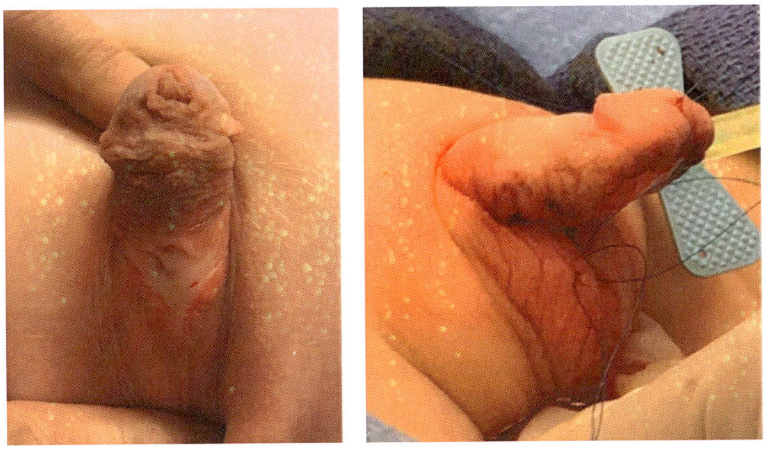

Figure 3. Recurrent fistula with penoscrotal ventral curvature.
A, recurrent penoscrotal fistula in a penis observed preoperatively to have a straight spontaneous erection. B, VC was found at the penoscrotal junction below the fistula, where a tourniquet was likely placed by the first surgeon performing artificial erection.

Common Technical Errors During Urethroplasty

Technical errors made in the key steps of hypospadias repairs can cause urethroplasty complications even when the penis is straight, or add to the likelihood for a complication when there is also tension from a bent penis during erections.

In this section we define urethroplasty complications and review those errors which cause them. Reoperations to correct complications are described in the next chapter.

> *Fistula: a leak of urine from the neourethra anywhere below the meatus.*

It is a technical error increasing the risk for fistulas to:

1. tubularize the urethral plate or graft neo-plate in a single layer.
2. not cover the neourethra with a barrier flap.

In addition, we published that the first layer of the neourethra in a proximal repair, either TIP or STAC, should be sewn using *interrupted* subepithelial stitches to best align the edges and maintain even tension on the long suture line. We also found that tunica vaginalis provides greater protection against fistulas in proximal repairs than does a dartos flap (Snodgrass and Bush, 2011).

While it is commonly believed that fistulas result from distal obstruction, in fact, we rarely encounter that even though we always calibrate the neourethra with an 8Fr sound to check for it (Snodgrass and Bush et al, 2015).

Some fistulas are noticed almost immediately after the catheter is removed. Although it is tempting to replace the catheter hoping the fistula will close, we are not aware of published data indicating that happens. Similarly, parents are sometimes advised to dilate the meatus to encourage a fistula to close, but we believe dilations should never be recommended in boys.

Occasionally a fistula will close spontaneously, presumably when edema within the neourethra adequately subsides. There are also published experiences applying cyanoacrylate to close the leak. One reported successful closure in 4 of 6 fistulas diagnosed and treated in the outpatient clinic within 3 days of catheter removal, using from 1 to as many as 5 applications (Prestipino et al, 2011). Topical cyanoacrylate has also been reported effective in closing long-standing fistulas, as discussed in Chapter 17.

Fistulas can occur even years after hypospadias repair, but, like most complications, are usually found within the first 6-12 months (Snodgrass and Bush et al, 2014; Castagnetti et al, 2013).

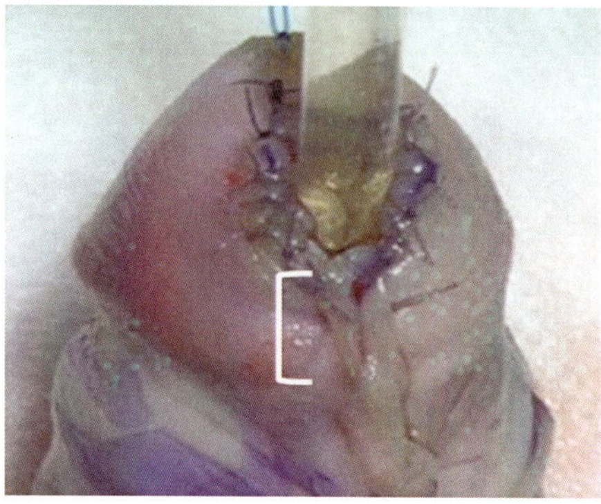

Figure 4. Inadequate glans fusion caused by suturing the glans wings to the urethral opening.

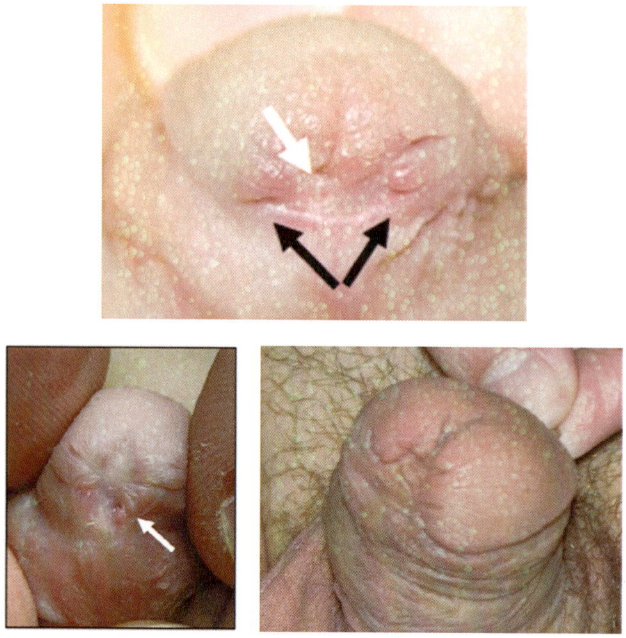

Figure 5. Examples of glans dehiscence.
A, white arrow points to the meatus at the corona, while the black arrows show the completely separated glans wings. Note also the transverse scar in both glans wings where sutures cut through the epithelium as they pulled apart. B, the white arrow shows a subcoronal meatus with the glans wings totally separated. C, the glans wings separated completely, but with a thin band of skin between them giving the illusion of a normal meatus. This adult complained of urine spraying which resolved with reoperative glansplasty providing normal glans fusion. He also has transverse scars in the glans wings resulting from mattress sutures cutting through them as they dehisced. Because of this risk, glansplasty sutures should *never* be placed through the surface epithelium.

Most fistula closures are successful. A recurrent fistula is a warning to the surgeon that there likely are additional contributing factors, usually persistent or recurrent VC and/or poor vascularity needing HBOT. In fact, the first patient we treated with HBOT had a recurrent fistula with visibly ischemic tissues whose closure was finally successful with this adjuvant therapy.

> *Glans Dehiscence: separation of the glans wings leaving fusion < 2.5mm*

It is a technical error increasing the risk for glans dehiscence to:

1. not dissect the glans wings sufficiently to ensure tension-free approximation over the neourethra.
2. sew the glans wings to the opening in the neourethra when that results in short glans fusion, as seen in Figure 4.
3. not preserve inner prepuce to create a ventral mucosal collar.
4. close the mucosal collar and/or ventral shaft skin with tension on the glansplasty.
5. leave a large catheter which can create tension on the glans wings.

Two complications can result from suturing the glans wings to the neourethra opening. The surgeon may not achieve normal glans fusion together below the neomeatus, as shown here with less than 2mm approximation. Or, to close the glans with normal fusion the surgeon will tubularize the neourethra farther distally and risk creating meatal stenosis. We *never* suture the end of the tubularized urethral plate or graft neo-plate directly to the glans wings for these reasons.

Glans dehiscence is one of the most common complications after hypospadias repair, and the one least commonly recognized and reported (Figure 5). Many patients we evaluate with failed distal repairs, and the majority with proximal hypospadias complications, have glans dehiscence. Their records almost never mention it, or instead describe dehiscence as a "large" or "retracted" meatus.

Glans dehiscence is an important complication for 2 reasons. First, the abnormal anatomy increases the risk for abnormal function, specifically urine spraying since the glans does not properly enclose the meatus and focus the stream like a nozzle on a hose. We reported that over 90% of men with glans dehiscence reported spraying. In fact, this is such a reliable association that we know there is glans dehiscence before we perform an examination when a patient mentions spraying.

Second, the penis does not look normal when the meatus is not encircled by glans. Differences in appearance concern teens and young adults, creating body image worries that can discourage them from developing sexual relationships.

All this is true when the glans wings separate completely, or nearly so leaving fusion < 2.5mm. Lesser separation with fusion > 2.5mm, which usually means the most distal of the 3 glans approximation stitches came apart, still leaves normal anatomy.

Glans dehiscence almost always occurs between 10 and 14 days postoperatively (Figure 6). There are usually no signs of inflammation or infection accounting for it. Rather, the glans which appeared normal one day is dehisced the next. Occasionally parents report the boy suddenly had unexplained pain and the glans was found open and revealing more of the catheter than at the last diaper change.

We first noticed that proximal TIP had more glans dehiscence than distal TIP, despite the same surgeon doing the same surgery with the same glansplasty

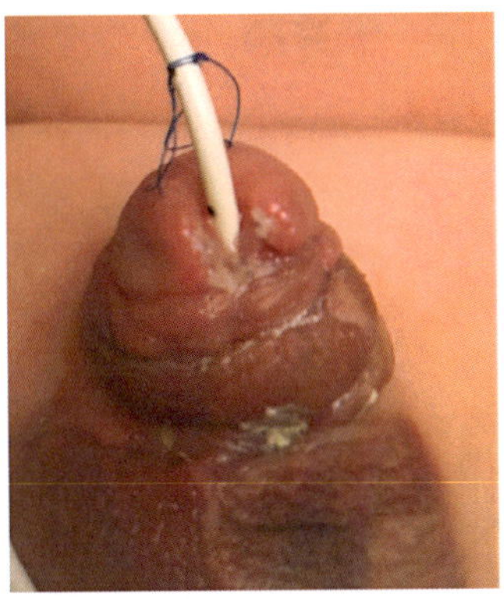

Figure 6. Typical glans dehiscence 10 days postoperatively.
The glans wings have separated completely to the corona after hypospadias repair, exposing the portion of the stent that was previously inside the distal neourethra. There are no signs of infection or trauma.

(Snodgrass and Bush et al, 2011). This led us to measure glans width to confirm that the diameter is significantly smaller in proximal hypospadias than normal boys or those with distal hypospadias, finding it averaged 12.9mm versus 14.8mm, respectively (Bush and Snodgrass et al, 2013). In addition, we found the width did not significantly change from age 3 months, when mini-puberty subsides, to 10 years, before adolescent puberty begins, meaning there is little somatic growth and no benefit to delaying surgery hoping the glans will enlarge (Bush and Snodgrass et al, 2017).

Knowing that testosterone increases glans size, we embarked on a study treating boys with glans width less than 14mm using preoperative injections as discussed in Chapter 12. However, despite successfully increasing the glans width to at least 15mm, the average size in distal hypospadias where dehiscence is less frequent, testosterone therapy did not decrease the risk of glans dehiscence.

Rather, we learned that more extensive dissection of the glans wings than what WS was taught (Figure 7) reduced glans dehiscence to the extent that small glans diameter was no longer a risk factor for complications (Snodgrass and Bush, 2016).

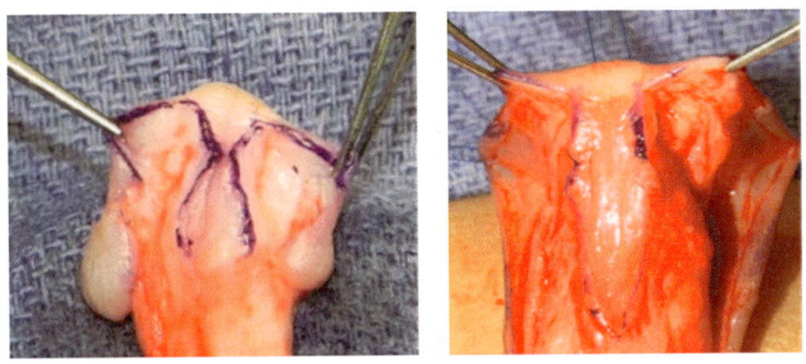

Figure 7. Extensive glans wings mobilization to reduce glans dehiscence.
A, "standard" dissection of the wings laterally to 3 and 9 o'clock. This may be adequate, especially for distal hypospadias, as long as there is no tension on the subsequent closure. B, more extensive dissection superiorly at 3 and 9 o'clock frees the wings a few more millimeters off the corpora, reducing tension when they are approximated medially. Once we realized that greater dissection of the glans wings reduced complications, our "standard" dissection became more extensive than it was previously, even when the glans is 14mm or greater in diameter.

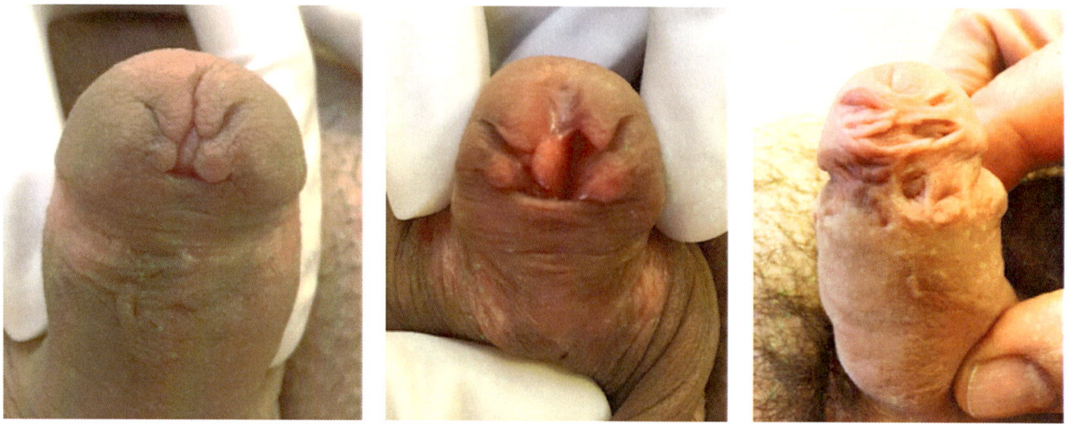

Figure 8. Glans scars from mattress stitches.
A,B, deep cuts to the glans wings made by mattress sutures as they dehisced. C, disfiguring wounds from mattress sutures even though the glans did not dehisce. Mattress stitches can create large scars which do not occur when subepithelial sutures are used to approximate the glans wings. These scars are sometimes impossible to revise. There is *no reason* to use mattress stitches for glansplasty, or to place any stitches through the glans epithelium.

Subsequently we observed that tension exerted on the glansplasty from short ventral shaft skin and an absent mucosal collar also causes glans dehiscence. This taught us that the mucosal collar is important not only for aesthetics, but also to provide a buffer between the glansplasty and shaft skin closure. This observation also emphasized the role that tension, whether from VC or short penile skin, plays in urethroplasty complications.

WS was taught to close glans wings with interrupted mattress stitches, which some surgeons still do, thinking it will prevent dehiscence. However, when proper dissection is done there should not be tension on the wound necessitating mattress sutures, and those sutures will likely not prevent dehiscence when there is tension.

A major problem with mattress stitches is that they can cut through the glans wings to make disfiguring scars, whether or not the glans dehisces (Figure 8). Therefore, these should *never* be done. As described in the chapters on TIP and STAC repairs, we successfully approximate the glans wings with a single subepithelial layer.

Finally, use of a large catheter such as 10-12Fr is associated with a higher rate of urethroplasty complications such as glans dehiscence than use of a smaller catheter (6-8Fr) (personal communication, 2024, van Der Toorn). This may be from increased tension on the glansplasty repair by the larger catheter. Since the main job of the catheter is simply to divert the urine, and not to "form" the neourethra, we have always used a smaller catheter – 6Fr in those with glans 14mm and larger, 5Fr feeding tubes in those with glans ≤ 13mm, and 12Fr catheters in Tanner V patients.

When dehiscence occurs despite a straight penis with healthy shaft skin, reoperative glansplasty is done, supplemented with HBOT. That is successful in 80%, but if the glans dehisces a second time we do not offer third glansplasty since our success in those patients was less than 50%.

Meatal Stenosis: Meatus < 8Fr with obstructive urinary symptoms (stranguria, retention) and/or UTI

It is a technical error that can lead to meatal stenosis to:

1. not incise the urethral plate deeply to the underlying corpora in TIP repair.
2. tubularize the urethral plate or graft neourethra too far distally.

Meatal stenosis is *not* a small-appearing meatus with a fine stream, especially during the first months postoperatively when edema at the neomeatus and within the neourethra can create these impressions. Rather, the diagnosis is made in a boy who is straining to void and usually not emptying his bladder. These patients

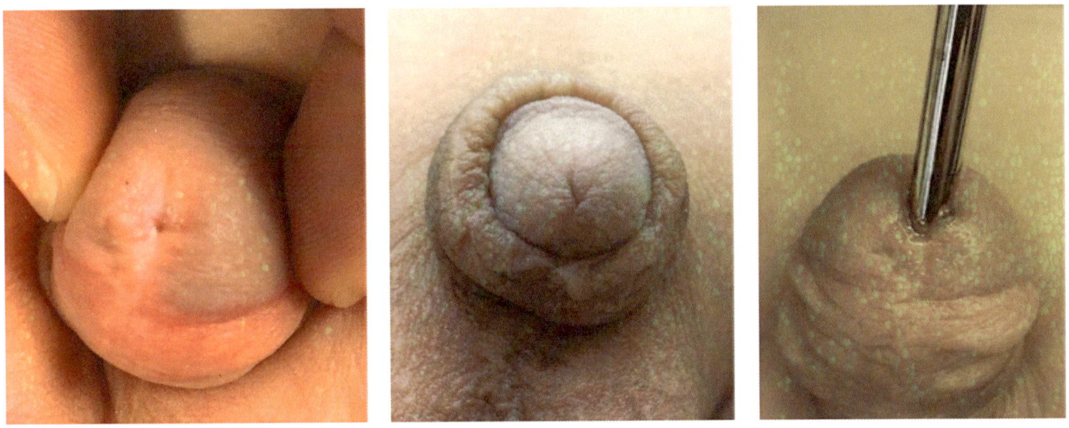

Figure 9. True meatal stenosis versus a small-appearing meatus.
A, this neomeatus is visibly scarred and only accepted a lacrimal duct probe, indicating true meatal stenosis. B,C, a small-appearing meatus without anatomic constriction or obstructive voiding symptoms does not define meatal stenosis, as seen in this case in which an 8Fr sound passed easily.

may strain so hard that they stool. They often present urinating in droplets and may have urinary infection. Elevated post-void residual is common. An unsuccessful attempt to pass an 8Fr sound confirms the diagnosis (Figure 9).

Hesitance to incise the urethral plate down to the tunica albuginea of the underlying corpora can create a neomeatus that is too small. Ironically, surgeons who worry that the TIP incision will scar and cause obstruction actually increase the likelihood for stenosis by not incising deeply enough!

Surgeons who want to mature the urethral opening to the glans wings as they learned to do with flaps may continue rolling the urethral plate or graft neo-plate too far distally to make it easier to sew to the glans. To avoid this, we recommend beginning urethral tubularization distally and placing the first stitch at the level of the midglans, no closer than 3mm to the end of the plate (Figure 10). We then perform glansplasty over the neourethra *without* sewing glans wings to the neourethra opening.

Meatal stenosis is an anecdotal diagnosis in our practice, which means that it is not the inevitable result of scarring from TIP incision. A surgeon who encounters meatal stenosis as defined above more commonly is making a technical error which can be corrected.

This is fortunate, since a meatotomy done ventrally can re-recreate the hypospadias defect, and a failed

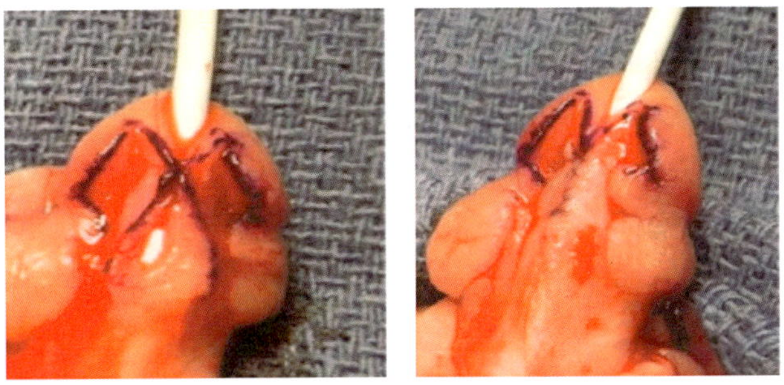

Figure 10. Correct location of the most distal tubularizing stitch.
A, the first and most distal stitch should be located at about the midglans, halfway between the distal end of the urethral plate or neoplate and the corona, as indicated by the arrow. B, angled view after tubularization is complete showing how wide open the end of the plate is. This protects against meatal stenosis, which should be a rare complication. Subsequent closure of the glans wings also begins at the midglans, and is done *over*, and not to, the neourethra as described for both TIP and STAC glansplasties.

meatotomy leads to a reoperative STAG repair to remove the scarred tissues and replace them with a healthy graft. There are no reports describing the operative procedure and results of meatotomy or "meatoplasty" for true meatal scarring after hypospadias repair, and it is likely that "success" in many cases comes from incising a meatus that already has a normal caliber and/or was still resolving postoperative edema. The operative reports we have reviewed after hypospadias meatotomy rarely mention first calibrating the meatus to confirm the anatomic diagnosis.

We perform meatotomy *dorsally*, and specifically search for a transverse scar at the meatus that can be incised to give a Heinike-Mikulicz enlargement. Then we inject the meatus with Kenalog to inhibit additional scarring.

We *never* use postoperative dilations to prevent or to manage meatal stenosis.

If meatal stenosis recurs after meatotomy, healthy tissue has to be imported to the meatus. Dorsal incision through the stenosis and into normal glans distally would be needed for a single stage inlay graft repair to place the wide center of the graft across the stenotic region. For that reason we have not used inlay grafts, but instead rely on STAG repair to excise the distal scar and replace it with lip mucosa. This is discussed in the next chapter.

> *Neourethra Stricture: Narrowing of the neourethra to < 8Fr proximal to the meatus*

It is a technical error that can result in neourethra stricture to:

1. not incise the entire urethral plate deeply in TIP repair.
2. tubularize a neo-urethral plate narrowed by graft contraction.
3. fail to correct VC.

A stricture of the neourethra is a rare complication after either TIP or STAC repairs. As with meatal stenosis, failure by a surgeon to deeply incise the entire urethral plate before tubularizing it can make a small-caliber neourethra. Similarly, if a graft contracts in width and the surgeon does not either TIP or inlay graft the constricted area, or incorporate adjacent penile skin with the graft to make the neourethra wider, the caliber might not be adequate.

Otherwise, strictures usually indicate an area with decreased vascularity. WS encountered that when he mobilized the urethral plate from the corpora as a straightening maneuver combined with proximal TIP. Nearly 1 of every 5 of those patients developed a focal stricture early postoperatively (Snodgrass and Bush et al, 2013).

Similarly, flap repairs have a higher risk for strictures and meatal stenosis because the ends of the flaps have less reliable blood supply (Duckett, 1981). These strictures sometimes are not recognized for many years until the lumen narrows sufficiently that the patient develops stranguria and/or urinary infections.

Some surgeons continue to use flap repairs, believing their blood supply must be more reliable than revascularization of a graft. While that makes sense intuitively, the fact is that published complication rates after graft repairs are consistently less than after flap repairs in similar patients (Snodgrass and Bush, 2017). We have used SPY technology to examine the blood supply after graft healing, and found that it typically has increased vascularity compared to the penile skin from which flaps are derived (Figure 11).

We have also seen strictures at the site of persistent/recurrent VC, presumably from tension on the neourethra at this site. Repair in this circumstance involves reoperative STAC repair to straighten the penis, and then later grafting the resulting defect.

Imaging and Cystoscopy

We never obtain urethrography or VCUG in boys suspected to have a stricture after hypospadias repair. These are difficult to perform when there is a stricture, and the information gained is not worth the discomfort to the boy.

Similarly, there is little reason to perform a separate cystoscopy when a stricture is suspected. We know

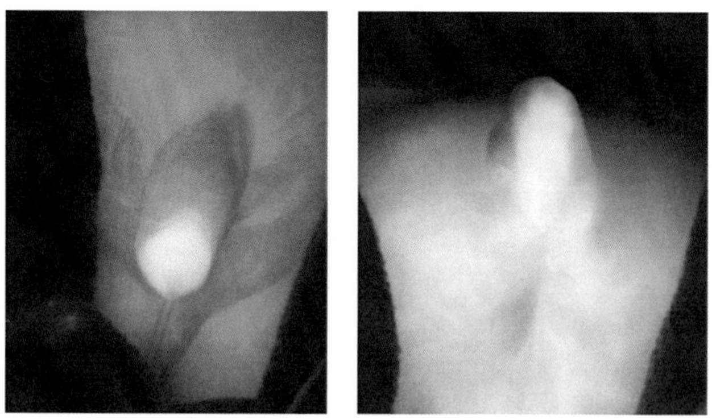

Figure 11. Oral graft neovascularity.
A, dorsal shaft skin perfusion as seen using SPY. B, ventral view in the same patient showing increased vascularity of the lip graft compared to surrounding penile skin.

the operation when a stricture is encountered will be an inlay graft versus a STAG repair (assuming the penis is straight), and also that the stricture will most often occur at or distal to the original meatus. No other information is needed preoperatively to justify another anesthetic for cystoscopy.

Management

Once a stricture has developed dilations will not keep the neourethra open. Furthermore, dilations are painful for the patient and distressing for his parents to perform. Therefore, we *never* manage a stricture, even temporarily, with dilations.

We also do not perform direct vision internal urethrotomy, because its 2-year success rate is low and the procedure can extend the stricture and cause additional scarring in the tissues around the incised region. Some of the most intense scars we have encountered within and around the neourethra developed after DVIU.

Husmann and Rathburn studied strictures after hypospadias repair, limiting their investigation to those measuring 1cm or less, which all underwent DVIU. Overall success was 24% at 2 years. Those that occurred after TIP or onlay flaps fared best, with success in 66%. Repeat DVIU in those that failed initially was never successful, meaning this procedure should not be done twice. Hypospadias patients who underwent DVIU, especially repeated DVIU, were at increased risk of erectile dysfunction (Husmann 2021).

Open surgical management depends on the extent the neourethra is obliterated. If sufficient lumen remains so that a TIP incision leaves enough urethra on either side to stitch, inlay grafting can be used for a single stage repair. Recurrent strictures develop in <10% (Ye et al, 2008; Snodgrass and Bush et al, 2009).

Otherwise after verifying the penis is straight, STAG is done, excising the scarred neourethra and replacing it with an oral mucosa graft, subsequently tubularized at a second stage. Focal obliterative strictures with a healthy distal neourethra and normal neomeatus can be repaired by removing the obstruction and then grafting between a proximal and distal urethrostomy.

As with all urethroplasty complications, an artificial erection should always be done when a stricture is encountered. We have observed that tension generated during natural erections apparently impacts perfusion to the neourethra and can create a stricture. When that curvature is 30° or more, then 3 corporotomies for straightening with a STAC repair should be done.

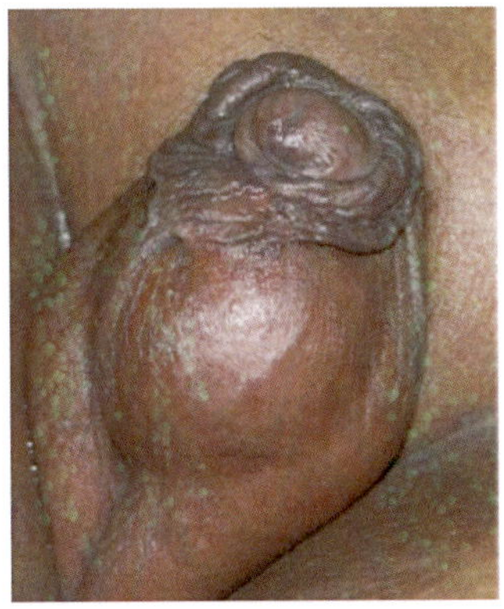

Figure 12. Diverticulum of the neourethra following a Byars flap repair.
Diverticula are more common when a flap urethroplasty is combined with a glansplasty that creates normal glans fusion, as seen in this case. Because the foreskin adheres better to the corpora in graft repairs. diverticulum are much less common despite a glansplasty providing normal glans fusion.

Diverticulum: Visible ballooning of the neourethra during voiding

It is a technical error that can cause a diverticulum to:

1. create the neourethra in proximal hypospadias using a flap, especially when a terminal meatus is created.
2. make the neourethra on the penile shaft significantly wider than it is at the corona.

This complication almost never occurs after TIP or STAC repairs. For example, the meta-analysis of TIP repair for distal and proximal hypospadias by Pfistermuller et al did not report diverticula. We encountered 1 (2%) after STAG repair (Snodgrass and Bush, 2017), as did Pippi-Salle et al and Ferro et al. An example of a diverticulum in a patient who had undergone flap repair is shown in Figure 12.

Diverticula are more common after proximal flap repairs, despite using the same foreskin as for grafts. Those occurred in from 6% to 14% in 3 recent reports of Byars flaps (Stanasel et al, 2015; McNamara et al,

2015, Long et al, 2017), and in 9% to 12% of transverse island prepucial flaps (Weiner et al, 1997; Long et al, 2017).

In contrast, 55% of the patients that WS repaired using a combination of Byars flaps with distal TIP developed large diverticula. These patients had TIP glansplasty, meaning they had normal glans fusion. We suspect that normal glans enclosure increases resistance to urine flow since the glans is less distensible than the urethra. This relative resistance combined with turbulent flow through an irregular flap neourethra causes the foreskin to dilate. Grafts, which have better fixation to the corpora and make a straight neourethra, are much less susceptible to this complication.

The difference in the increased incidence of diverticula WS found compared to other Byars flaps and transverse island series likely relates to the difference in glansplasties – as routine flap repairs may have less, often subnormal, glans fusion. Some surgeons in the series cited above deliberately left the meatus at the corona, which would decrease the impetus for ballooning, although at a likely cost of future urine spraying.

It is unusual for a diverticulum to recur after excision (Vallasciani et al, 2013).

Hair in the Neourethra

It is a technical error that can result in hair in the neourethra to:

1. tubularize *any* scrotal skin into the neourethra.
2. incorporate hair follicles around the proximal meatus or urethrostomy into the neourethra.

Hair in the urethra results when skin with follicles is incorporated into the urethroplasty. It can occur in proximal TIP if the surgeon does not specifically exclude skin at the penoscrotal junction from the urethral plate tubularization. Similarly, proximal shaft skin or scrotum sewn to a urethrostomy can bring hair follicles into the neourethra if the incision at the final stage does not intentionally exclude that skin.

Though less common today, this complication also develops from tubularizing a midline scrotal cleft in proximal hypospadias repairs, which has sometimes been done from a deep scrotal or perineal meatus to the penoscrotal junction to join a tubularized prepucial flap. Some surgeons still advocate using "shiny" midline scrotal skin in the urethroplasty, assuming it will not grow hair at puberty. However, the consequences if hair does grow can be severe, usually requiring excision of the involved neourethra and replacement with an oral mucosa graft, and so this should not be done. It is never *necessary* to incorporate scrotal skin into a neourethra.

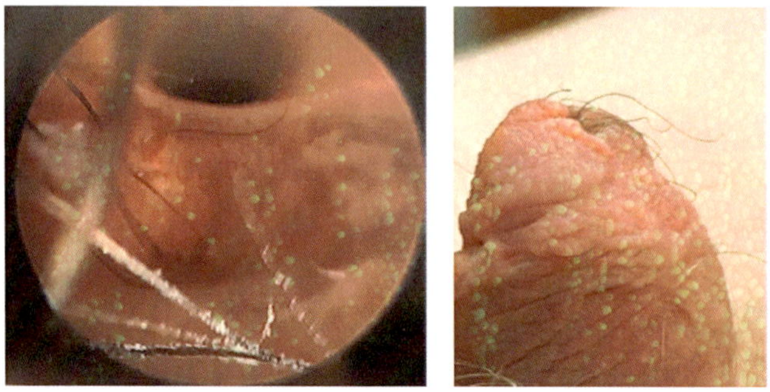

Figure 13. Hair in the neourethra.
If skin follicles were incorporated into the neourethra during repair hair will grow at puberty. A, in this case a proximal TIP included penile shaft or scrotal skin at the penoscrotal junction. B, hair growing out the meatus after prepubertal skin flap urethroplasty.

During puberty hair begins to grow and acts as a foreign material within the urethra (Figure 13), inciting urinary infection and/or dysuria. Stones can also form on the hair. This hair can also protrude from the meatus, which is particularly distressing to the patient.

While urethroscopic laser depilation can be attempted when there are few hairs, aiming the laser directly at the base of the follicle and destroying it can be difficult. As with other depilations, several sessions may be needed directed at the anagen (growth) phase in order to eradicate the follicle.

Definitive therapy when endoscopic treatment fails, or encounters too many hair follicles to manage, requires the hair-bearing segment to be excised and replaced with oral mucosa in a reoperative STAG repair.

Penile Torsion: Twisting of the penis outside the normal range from 5:30 to 6:30 o'clock

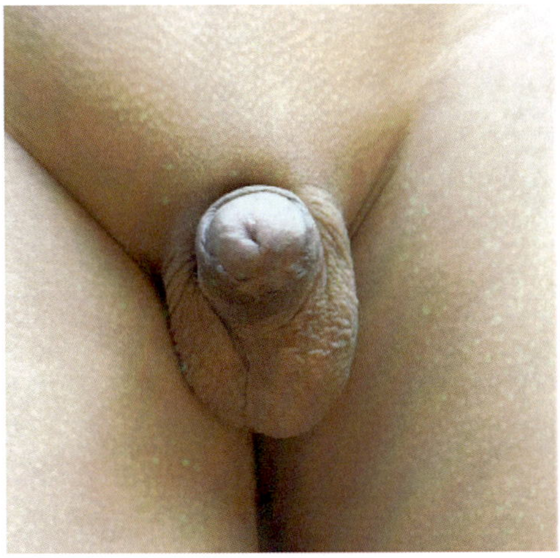

Figure 14. Acquired penile torsion.
The penis is twisted to the left at approximately 4:30 o'clock, resulting from partial contraction of a left tunica vaginalis flap.

It is a technical error which can cause penile torsion to:

1. shorten the ventral penile skin on one side during skin closure.
2. inadequately mobilize the base of a dorsal dartos flap.
3. insufficiently mobilize a tunica vaginalis flap up to the external ring.

A twisted penis looks abnormal, and, if torsed outside the narrow range of normal orientation from 5:30 to 6:30 o'clock, can cause the urine stream to miss the toilet.

Some patients with distal hypospadias also have congenital penile torsion, which should be corrected during repair by releasing dartos attachments around the base of the penis. In this section we refer to acquired penile torsion, either from an error in sizing the penile shaft skin symmetrically during closure, or from not mobilizing neourethra coverage flaps sufficiently (Figure 14).

A trial of Betamethasone 0.1% cream application to the ventral/lateral shaft skin twice daily for 12 weeks combined with massage and stretching the penis (physiotherapy) may decrease skin asymmetry. If the twist persists, surgical skin revision is required - sometimes with penile skin grafting - to correct the ventral shaft shortage.

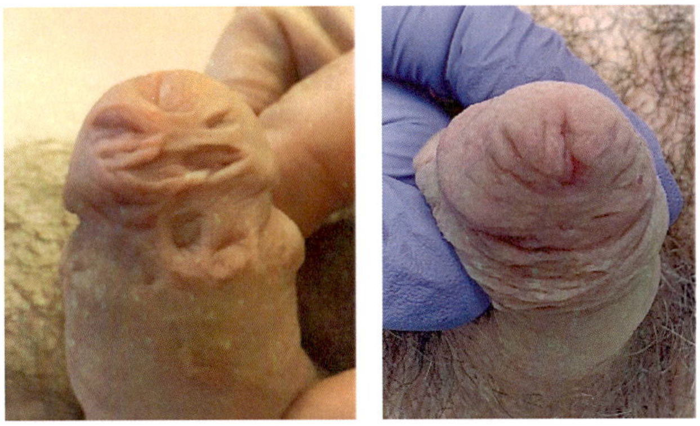

Figure 15. Glans scars from sutures.
These unsightly deformities of the glans are the result of technical error, sewing through the glans epithelium with simple or mattress sutures. There is no need for epithelial stitches, and so this complication is completely preventable.

Similarly, stretching and massaging the penis might reduce torsion from a short barrier flap. Otherwise, if torsion persists after 12 months, an incision made at the base of the penis over the flap gives access to simply transect it, since the flap will have performed its function to reduce fistulas and the distal end will have been vascularized by local tissues.

Glans Scars: Transverse scars in the glans

It is a technical error that can cause glans scarring for the surgeon to:

1. approximate the glans wings with mattress sutures through the epithelium.
2. sew the glans surface with stitches through the epithelium.

This complication results from surgeons performing glansplasty with either mattress or simple sutures through the surface epithelium. There should be no tension on the glans wings when they are approximated; therefore, mattress sutures are not needed to hold them together. If mattress sutures are used anyway, the suture can cut though the epithelium as illustrated above in Figure 8.

Similarly, simple stitches through the glans epithelium can create visible scars (Figure 15). We have not closed the epithelium of the glans as a separate layer in more than 15 years.

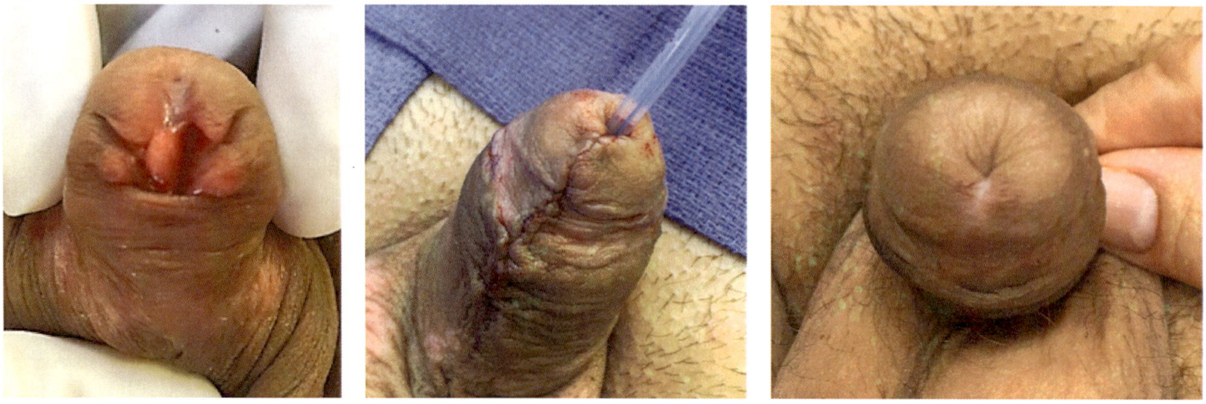

Figure 16. Repairing glans scars.
A, deep, disfiguring glans scars from mattress sutures through the epithelium. B, in this case, most of these deep cuts could be excised, with the remaining portions de-epithelialized and sutured during this single stage reoperative TIP repair. C, appearance 3 months postoperatively. However, not all glans scars can be repaired, emphasizing that surgeons must avoid making them in the first place.

Some glans scars can be excised during reoperations (Figure 16). Or the cut can be de-epithelialized and the edges sutured back together. This should be done at the first operation when multistaged procedures are done so that the wounds can heal before glansplasty.

However, not all these epithelial scars can be repaired to restore the normal, smooth appearance to the glans. These defects then last a lifetime, reminding the man every day that he was born with a birth defect of his penis - even if hypospadias repair was otherwise successful.

Skin Incision Scars and Suture Tracts: Irregular scars in the circumcision line, and epithelialized tunnels filled with keratin

It is a technical error that can cause irregular scars and suture tracts in the circumcision line and median raphe to close wounds with epithelial stitches (Figures 17,18).

It is not necessary to suture the circumcision line or median raphe through the epithelium. The skin edges are smoother and less apparent when they are closed with subepithelial stitches. Although some surgeons claim that PDS sutured through the epithelium does not produce irregular "baseball" stitch scars, any suture through the skin carries that risk. The main reason surgeons stitch through the epithelium is to save a few minutes of time, but when scars develop the patient must live with them for his lifetime - unless

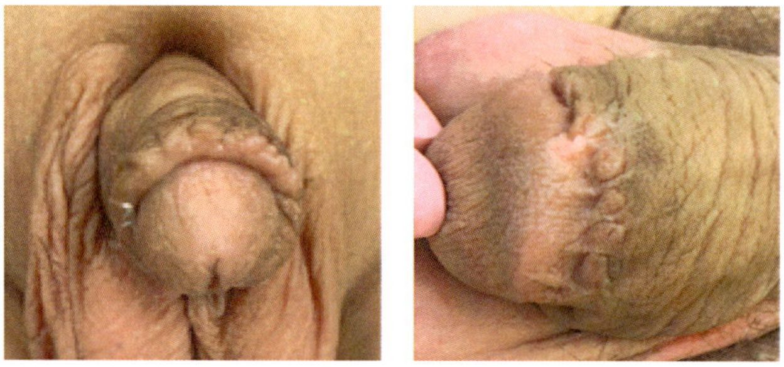

Figure 17. Baseball stitch scars from epithelial skin closure.
A, irregular scars from epithelial suturing, in this case using PDS. B, adult with scars and insufficient remaining skin to allow them to be excised.

there is sufficient remaining shaft skin to allow the scars to be excised and the edges reapproximated using subepithelial stitches.

Suture tracts are more likely to occur when stitches are placed through the epithelium, although they can also develop with subepithelial stitches when the needle passes through a skin appendage such as a gland or a hair follicle.

These tracts never resolve and will always produce keratin that can have a foul odor when it is expressed. We begin all reoperations looking for these tracts and unroofing them with a fine, sharp tipped iris scissor (Figure 18). No additional treatment is needed and these do not recur.

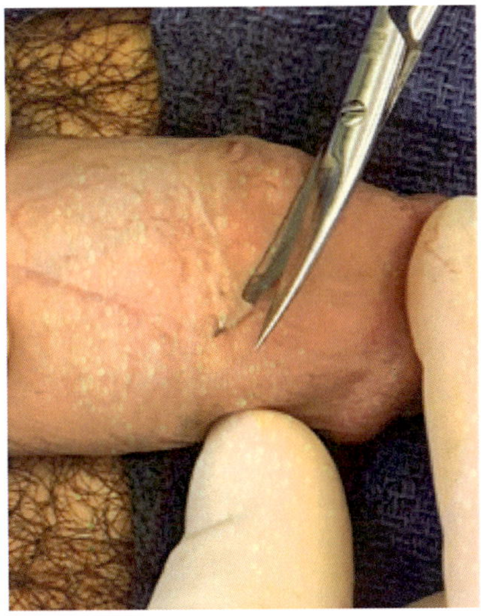

Figure 18. Suture tract.
Unroofing a suture tract using sharp-pointed iris scissors.

Suture tracts can also be unroofed in the outpatient clinic after first applying topical EMLA for local anesthesia.

Key Points

We have emphasized throughout this chapter that most urethroplasty complications result from technical errors made by the surgeon. Not every boy whose neourethra is closed in a single layer or is not covered with a barrier flap will develop a fistula. But the risk is increased, and some will suffer a complication and need another operation to fix it which could have been avoided by using better surgical technique the first time.

WS originally tubularized proximal TIPs with a single running epithelial stitch, mimicking the method he learned to make tubularized prepucial flaps. Mike Mitchell happened to watch that step and commented there would be fewer fistulas if he closed in 2 layers using subepithelial stitches. But WS was not convinced and continued this technical error for a several more years, until he reviewed his data and found 33% fistulas despite covering every neourethra with dartos. Then he started closing as Mitchell, and other reports on urethroplasty, recommended and the rate of fistulas decreased by two-thirds. Many boys would have been spared this complication and its repair had he improved his surgical technique sooner.

Similarly, nearly all the operative reports we review in patients with complications after repairs done by pediatric urologists describe technical errors relating to those complications. We encourage all surgeons to review their own outcomes, and those who find complications occurring more often than what the best series publish should compare how they do key steps to how those with better results do them.

We also emphasize that many urethroplasty complications are themselves signs of other underlying problems, usually VC. Accordingly, artificial erection should be done during every hypospadias reoperation to make certain the penis is straight.

Finally, this chapter reminds us all again that it is important that each step of a hypospadias repair be done right the first time.

References

Bush N, DaJusta D, and Snodgrass W: Glans penis width in patients with hypospadias compared to normal controls. *J Pediatr Urol* 9:1188, 2013

Bush NC and Snodgrass W: Pre-incision urethral plate width does not impact short-term tubularized incised plate urethroplasty outcomes. *J Pediatr Urol* 13: 625, 2017

Bush NC and Snodgrass W: Hyperbaric oxygen therapy improves oral graft take in hypospadias staged tubularized autograft reoperations. *J Urol* 202: 1, 2019

Castagnetti M, Zhapa E and Rigamonti W: Primary severe hypospadias: comparison of reoperation rates and parental perception of urinary symptoms and cosmetic outcomes among 4 repairs. *J Urol* 189: 1508, 2013

Duckett JW: Editorial comment to Hodgson NB: Use of vascularized flaps in hypospadias repair. *Urol Clin North Am* 8: 471, 1981

Ferro F, Zaccara A, Spagnoli A, Lucchetti MC, Capitanucci L, Villa M: Skin graft for 2-stage treatment of severe hypospadias: back to the future? *J Urol* 168: 1730, 2002

Husmann DA: Erectile dysfunction in patients undergoing multiple attempts at hypospadias repair: Etiologies and concerns. J Pediatr Urol 17(2): 166, 2021.

Husmann DA and Rathbun SR: Long-term followup of visual internal urethrotomy for management of short (less than 1cm) penile urethral strictures following hypospadias repair. *J Urol* 176: 1738, 2006

Keating MA and Duckett JW: Failed hypospadias repair. In Cohen MS and Resnick M (Eds): **Reoperative Urology.** Boston, Little Brown and Co, 1995, p. 188

Long CJ, Chu DI, Tenny RW, Morris Ar, Weiss DA,Shukla AR, Srinivasan AK, Zderic SA, Kolon TF, Canning DA: Intermediate-term followup of proximal hypospadias repair reveals high complication rate. *J Urol* 197: 852, 2017

McNamara ER, Schaeffer AJ, Logvinenko T, Seager C, Rosokliga I, Nelson CP, Retik AB, Diamond DA, and Cendron M: Management of proximal hypospadias with 2-stage repair: 20-year experience. *J Urol* 194: 1080, 2015

Pfistermuller KL, McArdle J and Cuckow PM: Meta-analysis of complication rates of the tubularized incised plate (TIP) repair. *J Pediatr Urol* 11: 54, 2015

Pippi Salle JL, Sayed S, Salle A, Bagli D, Farhat W, Koyle M, Lorenzo AJ: Proximal hypospadias: a persistent challenge. Single institution outcome analysis of three surgical techniques over a 10-year period. *J Pediatr Urol* 12: 28e, 2016

Prestipino M, Bertozzi M, Nardi N, Appignani A: Outpatient department repair of urethrocutaneous fistulae using n-butyl-cyanoacrylate (NBCA): a single-centre experience. *BJUI* 108: 1514, 2011

Snodgrass W and Bush N: Extensive glans wings mobilization reduces hypospadias repair complications. Abstract presented to SPU, 2016b

Snodgrass W and Bush N: TIP hypospadias repair: a pediatric urology indicator operation. *J Pediatr Urol* 12:11, 2016

Snodgrass W and Bush NC: Staged tubularized autograft repair for primary proximal hypospadias with 30-degree or greater ventral curvature. *J Urol* 198: 680, 2017b

Snodgrass W and Bush NC: Persistent or recurrent ventral curvature after failed proximal hypospadias repair. *J Pediatr Urol* 15: 344e1, 2019

Snodgrass WT, Bush N and Cost N: Algorithm for comprehensive approach to hypospadias reoperation using 3 techniques. *J Urol* 182: 2885, 2009

Snodgrass W, Cost N, Nakonezny PA and Bush N: Analysis of risk factors for glans dehiscence after tubularized incised plate hypospadias repair. *J Urol* 185: 1845, 2011

Snodgrass WT, Granberg C and Bush NC: Urethral strictures following urethral plate and proximal urethral elevation during proximal TIP hypospadias repair. *J Pediatr Urol* 9: 990, 2013

Snodgrass W, Grimsby G and Bush NC: Coronal fistula repair under the glans without reoperative glansplasty or urinary diversion. *J Pediatr Urol* 11: 39, 2015

Snodgrass W, Villanueva C and Bush NC: Duration of follow-up to diagnose hypospadias urethroplasty complications. *J Pediatr Urol* 10: 208, 2014

Stanasel I, Le HK, Bilgutay A, Roth DA, Gonzales ET, JR, Janzen N, Koh CJ, Gargollo P and Seth A: Complications following staged hypospadias repair using transposed preputial skin flaps. *J Urol* 194: 512, 2015

Vallasciani S, Berrettini A, Nanni L, Manzoni G and Marrocco G: Observational retrospective study on acquired megalourethra after primary proximal hypospadias repair and its recurrence after tapering. *J Pediatr Urol* 9: 364, 2013

Wiener JS, Sutherland RW, Roth DR and Gonzales ET, Jr: Comparison of onlay and tubularized island flaps of inner prepucial skin for the repair of proximal hypospadias. *J Urol* 158: 1172, 1997

Ye WJ, Ping P, Liu YD, Li Z and Huang YR: Single stage dorsal inlay buccal mucosal graft with tubularized incised urethral plate technique for hypospadias reoperations. *Asian J Androl* 10: 682, 2008

Chapter 17

Hypospadias Reoperations

Decision-making for hypospadias reoperations follows the same principles as for primary repairs. The choices are largely determined by penile curvature and available shaft skin, more so than by the location of the meatus.

Regardless of the presenting urethroplasty complication, by far the most common underlying finding in hypospadias reoperations, especially those for proximal hypospadias, is persistent or recurrent VC (Snodgrass and Bush, 2019). This fact derives from a general lack of understanding of why the penis is bent and how it should be straightened, as discussed in Chapter 2. It also emphasizes the need to perform an artificial erection in all patients undergoing reoperation.

This bending creates increased tension along the ventral penis during natural erections, which then pulls at repairs to open fistulas or dehisce the glans and wound, or decreases perfusion and contributes to meatal stenosis and strictures. Records we review indicate that many surgeons focus on the failed urethroplasty, often proceeding to an oral graft reoperation without considering these underlying reasons the earlier repair failed. Consequently, fistulas and dehiscence or partial obstructions recur despite what otherwise might have been technically correct operations.

Deficient and scarred penile skin is another near universal finding after unsuccessful surgery. With the exception of MIP, all hypospadias presents with ventral skin deficiency which persists in many patients needing a reoperation. Furthermore, in reoperations the skin deficiency can also involve the dorsal skin because of prior Byars flaps. This is one reason that reoperations should begin *without* completely degloving the penis – because detaching the dorsal skin can make closure even more difficult, and exposure is sufficient through a ventral incision.

Like VC, deficient skin exerts tension on repairs which contributes to urethroplasty complications. Scarred skin also may not be able to provide neovascularity along the edges of urethroplasty grafts. As in primary repairs, deficient and unhealthy skin benefits from STAC lengthening and rehabilitating it before urethroplasty to avoid tension on the neourethra and glans and the need for a Cecil maneuver, scrotal flap or skin graft to close the penile shaft. This skin rejuvenation is aided by perioperative HBOT. Nevertheless, in a few patients the skin is so deficient and/or damaged that it must be replaced with an external penile skin graft before the urethroplasty.

Accordingly, decision-making for reoperative urethroplasty is similar to primary repairs. A straight penis with satisfactory skin can undergo TIP unless these is gross scarring of the urethral plate from prior surgery. In that situation, either an inlay graft repair or excision of the scarred tissues with staged oral grafting can be done. Patients with VC ≥ 30° should have STAC repair.

There is the additional consideration of wound healing after prior unsuccessful surgeries. It has been consistently reported that reoperations have more complications than primary repairs using the same surgical technique. In fact, we previously published that the first reoperation has *double* the risk for complications as did the primary repair, and that risk increases to 40% with 3 or more reoperations (Snodgrass and Bush, 2017). This emphasizes again the importance of getting the first operation right.

But it also says that surgeons need to think beyond the technical details of their reoperations for strategies to improve tissue health. Given the penis is an end-organ deriving its blood supply from vessels entering at the base whereas most the critical surgical intervention is done at the most distal end, improving vascularity damaged by prior surgery should be an integral part of these repairs. The best therapy currently available to improve vascularity and wound healing is HBOT, which we incorporate into our management of nearly all failed hypospadias repairs.

Finally, surgeons must consider the emotional and psychological impact of failed surgery on patients and families, especially when they are told several more operations must be done. We find it helpful to focus caregivers on the final result rather than the number of procedures needed to achieve it. Specifically, boys with hypospadias want to grow into men with a normal penis and so their parents should keep that goal at the forefront. We also highly recommend older children, teen and adult patients seek care with a licensed therapist, as well as family members of younger patients who are having anxiety and/or stress regarding additional surgery.

Furthermore, surgeons must keep in mind that it is the patient and his family who are suffering when complications occur. We learned from them that their worries are magnified when surgeons tell them that "this almost never happens in my patients," which concerns them that something rare has happened that might not be able to be fixed. Surgeon guilt after complications is an issue that should be addressed with a variety of coping mechanisms beyond the scope of this chapter.

Magnitude of the Problem

Approximately 1 of every 10 primary distal repairs develops a complication, and the Dutch Hypospadias Study showed the rate is most likely higher, averaging nearly 1 out of every 5 repairs and ranging to nearly 1 of every 2 (van der Toorn et al, 2015). In the US, there are approximately 9000 primary distal hypospadias repairs done each year, meaning at least 1800 boys are likely to have complications afterwards. Another 1000 primary proximal hypospadias repairs are done annually, and reports from Texas Children's, Boston Children's, and CHOP indicate that from 50% to 70% of these will have complications. Together these add to at least 2300 reoperations a year, not counting the additional surgeries generated when some of those reoperations fail.

If these reoperations are evenly shared by the more than 1000 certified pediatric urologists in the US, each will do approximately 2 a year. Some of these will be relatively less complex fistula closures, but the remainder involve complex urethroplasties where the stakes are much higher. We have already explained that most these complications result from mistakes the surgeon made—and is likely to repeat in the next operation. For that reason, we strongly recommend that centers designate a surgical team to care for these patients, and then review the team's outcomes on a regular basis.

Impaired Wound Healing

Surgeons in all specialties typically focus more on the technical performance of an operation than on the subsequent healing of the tissues, even though both are important for a successful outcome. Because of that, there is relatively little information regarding non-technical factors that influence healing such as genetics, nutrition, and vascularity.

We suspect that some families are predisposed to greater scarring, which could predict an increased likelihood for skin or graft contractures. Today we systematically inquire about unusual wound healing in both patients and families hoping for greater insight into these complications. Similarly, we document whether a patient has eczema to determine if that inflammatory skin disease is a risk factor for abnormal healing. We also document the presence of intra-uterine growth restriction, preoperative testosterone use and intrauterine exposure to progesterone so that future studies can help evaluate whether or not any of these factors influence wound healing.

Abnormal nutrition is known to impair wound healing but seems less a factor in otherwise healthy patients in the US. We do, however, verify positive weight gain in infants born with IUGR and other medical conditions which might impact their nutrition before scheduling hypospadias repair.

There are no readily available clinical tests of tissue vascularity, but it is reasonable to assume it is decreased after prior surgery. To our knowledge, the only therapy currently available to increase vascularity is HBOT. After initial anecdotal success we wanted to objectively document its benefit, and decided oral graft outcomes determined by paired length and width measurements could be a surrogate for local vascularity and general wound healing. We added HBOT in those undergoing oral mucosa grafting who already had 3 or more prior repairs and used as controls similar patients with less than 3 repairs. There was significantly less graft contraction in those receiving HBOT, even though they were at greater risk because of more failed surgery (Bush and Snodgrass, 2019). Realizing that, we changed our protocol and now recommend perioperative HBOT for nearly all reoperations, especially those involving grafts.

While we objectively showed HBOT improves graft take, it is more difficult to demonstrate its other wound healing benefits. Nevertheless, we have observed there is usually less subcutaneous scarring after its use, and some patients with terrible scar contracture have it significantly reduced by treatment. HBOT is used as a known adjuvant therapy in patients with keloiding and/or hypercontractile wound healing. This includes improved penile skin health, and so skin deficiency and scarring after prior repair is another indication for HBOT.

The postoperative skin and graft care we recommend using Aquaphor and betamethasone are another example of nonsurgical wound management, directed at keeping healing skin moist and counteracting the natural tendency for wounds to contract. It is also beneficial to stretch and massage healing tissues in the penis, and inside the mouth when oral grafts are harvested, often referred to as physiotherapy.

Timing of Reoperations

Reports describing the earliest hypospadias surgeries indicate that both planned stages and reoperations were scheduled after only brief intervals for healing. Today it is widely accepted that at least 6 months should elapse between operations to give tissues adequate time for recovery. Some advocate longer waiting periods, although we are not aware of data suggesting delays of a year or more improve results over reoperations done at 6 months.

Reoperations when VC is ≤ 30°

The following sections discuss repairs of complications when the penis is straight or has VC measuring less than 30°. It is impossible to overemphasize that artificial erection should be done at every reoperation. That is especially true when complications are recurrent. For example, fistula closure is so reliable that a recurrent fistula should immediately raise concerns that there is underlying VC which has been overlooked. Failure to check an artificial erection is a technical error even if no VC was detected at the prior operation and a reoperation is otherwise done optimally.

When artificial erection finds VC of 30° or more, reoperative STAC should be done as described below.

Fistula Closure

The neourethra distal to the fistula is calibrated with an 8Fr sound to confirm there is no distal anatomic obstruction, and fluid is injected into the meatus to verify the location of the fistula(s). Artificial erection is also done to determine if the penis is straight.

The general principles of fistula closure when the penis is straight include excision of the tract, suture closure of the opening in the urethra, and flap coverage over the repair to avoid overlapping suture lines between the urethral and skin closures.

Coronal Fistulas

Many surgeons are taught that a fistula at the corona requires a reoperative glansplasty. However, the most common complication of opening a well-healed glans and redoing the urethroplasty and glansplasty is another fistula. So WS decided to try closing coronal fistulas without opening the glans when it had fusion of 3mm or more, and found that approach was successful in 95% of a series of patients who had fistulas 2mm or smaller (Snodgrass and Bush et al, 2015).

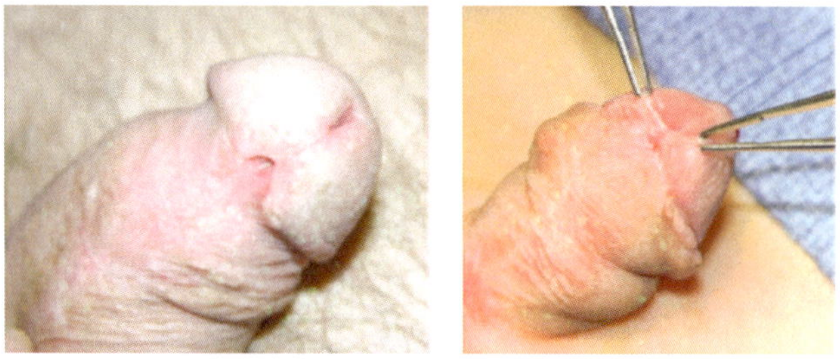

Figure 1. Coronal fistula vs glans dehiscence.
A, fistula below a well-healed glans with normal fusion of the wings. The fistula should be closed without reopening the glans wings. B, fistula below a narrow web of skin between separated glans wings held by the forceps. This patient has glans dehiscence and needs a reoperative urethroplasty and glansplasty.

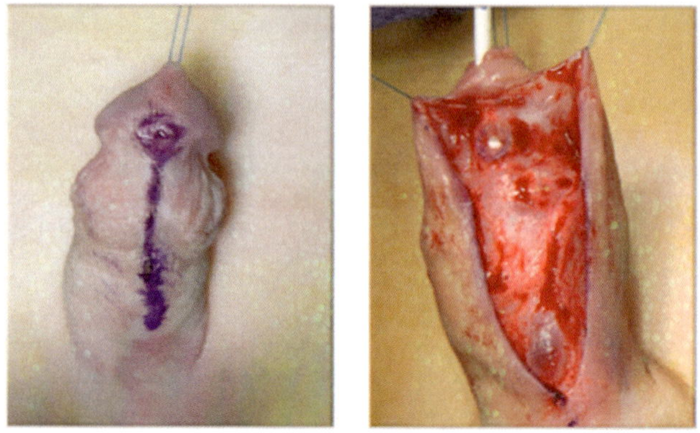

Figure 2. Coronal fistula closure.
A, an incision is made around the fistula and down the median raphe, giving excellent exposure to close the leak, cover the repair with a dartos barrier flap, and revise any redundant ventral shaft skin. A shorter incision is satisfactory when skin revision is not needed. B, cephalad retraction of the skin and glans improves exposure to dissect the fistula tract off the glans, close the urethral defect, and then advance a dartos coverage flap over and past the repair.

Surgical Technique

When the 8Fr sound is passed at the beginning of the operation, glans fusion is also evaluated. Fistula closure is done when there is normal glans fusion of 3mm or more, while reoperative TIP is required when there is dehiscence leaving less than 3mm glans fusion or a thin web of skin bridging between totally separated glans wings (Figure 1).

Visualization is critical and so we first inject 1:100,000 epinephrine around the fistula. The incision circumscribes the skin close to the fistula, and then continues down the median raphe to give better exposure and facilitate making a dartos coverage flap. The skin is dissected laterally, preserving dartos on the ventral penile shaft. Distally, dissection releases the tract from the glans, taking care not to enter the urethra. Stays on the corners of the skin lift the glans edge and expose the fistula (Figure 2).

During this process, bands of scar tissue, dartos, or skin exerting tension on the region of the fistula are sought and released. WS was taught to repair fistulas through the smallest possible circumferential incision, but a tiny incision which just exposes the tract does not give adequate visualization to detect and release bands of tension which might have pulled open the leak in the first place.

Next, the tract is excised just above the wall of the urethra, which is sutured closed using interrupted subepithelial 7-0 or 9-0 Vicryl. The fistula is preferably closed in 2-layers, although sometimes only a single layer can be placed without adding tension or narrowing the urethral lumen. The urethra is again distended with fluid to be certain there are no leaks.

Then a flap is created from the dartos proximal to the fistula and moved to cover the entire repair. This flap extends past the closure onto the underside of the glans and is sutured there with 9-0 Vicryl.

The stays are released to allow the glans to return to its normal position. When the fistula was at the corona, the exposed glans margin is reapproximated with interrupted subepithelial 6-0 Vicryl. The shaft skin immediately over the closed fistula is approximated with epithelial 9-0 Vicryl to minimize suture reaction around the repair.

Next, any excess ventral shaft skin is excised and the edges closed using interrupted subepithelial 7-0 Vicryl stiches. Throughout this process, the skin is checked to be certain it is not being closed under tension. Because there is an underlying dartos flap, shaft skin is closed down the median raphe without creating an eccentric skin flap to place over the fistula.

We do not use urinary diversion after fistula closure.

Results

We reported this repair was successful without post-operative urinary diversion in 95% of patients at a mean of 18 months follow up (Snodgrass and Bush et al, 2015).

As mentioned, fistula closure is so reliable that a recurrent fistula most often means there are additional underlying problems. While distal obstruction is occasionally found associated with fistulas, tension from missed VC, deficient skin, or subepithelial scar is the most common explanation for failed fistula repair.

Coronal Fistula with Glans Dehiscence

A coronal fistula can occur just below a thin band of skin extending between separated glans wings, as shown above in Figure 1B. These patients actually have glans dehiscence and should be managed by reoperative TIP repair as discussed in the next section.

Other Fistulas

In our reported series cited above nearly two-thirds of the fistulas were coronal. The remainder occurred at various locations on the penile shaft or in the scrotum. The same principles apply to them, and, generally, these are less technically demanding to close. The most important considerations are to be *certain* the penis is straight and that the repair is not under tension. As with coronal fistulas, a midline incision that includes the leak should be made large enough for good exposure and to cover the repair with a barrier flap. We have not found it necessary to cover a fistula with a tunica vaginalis flap. We have seen fistulas recur despite coverage with a tunica vaginalis barrier layer when persistent VC was missed by the operating surgeon. This makes subsequent repair of the long urethroplasty after STAC repair more difficult and thus, we recommend avoiding this when penile or scrotal dartos is an option for barrier layer coverage.

Repairing Glans Dehiscence

Glans dehiscence is corrected by reoperative TIP or inlay graft (G-TIP) when the penis is straight or has less than 30° VC, or by STAC when there is VC measuring 30° or more. Most patients presenting with glans dehiscence had it occur after their primary repair. Recurrent glans dehiscence is a warning sign that there is VC ≥ 30°, and/or tension from short ventral skin.

TIP vs G-TIP

When the penis is straight the main decision is whether to do reoperative TIP or G-TIP. Glans dehiscence after the primary repair accounts for nearly 90% of our patients undergoing reoperative TIP. Many of these initially had a distal TIP, but others had Mathieu or onlay prepucial flaps done elsewhere. In all these situations the urethral plate most often is still supple and without gross scarring. We always begin the procedure intending to do a reoperative TIP, but in the occasional patient whose incised plate is not normally elastic we do a G-TIP.

The other reason to G-TIP glans dehiscence is when the urethral plate was removed at an earlier repair and a graft neo-plate or a prepucial flap was tubularized. Although a TIP incision into a previous graft or prepucial flap might heal similarly to an incised urethral plate, we inlay graft when the incision into a neo-plate is 5mm or longer.

Surgical Technique: Reoperative TIP

After the skin incision, all the key steps for reoperative TIP are done in the same way as they are for primary TIP repairs.

Initial skin incision

A Y-shaped incision is marked running along the junction of the glans wings to the urethral plate, below the meatus, and down the median raphe (Figure 3). 1:100,000 epinephrine is injected into the glans wings before incision. There is usually no reason to deglove the entire penis since sufficient exposure is gained working ventrally, and skin irregularities can usually be revised through this ventral incision. Complete degloving can even make the situation worse, especially when the dorsal skin is deficient and is not easily stretched back into place.

Skin dissection

The skin is dissected laterally preserving dartos on the penile shaft, and subcutaneous scar tissue is released.

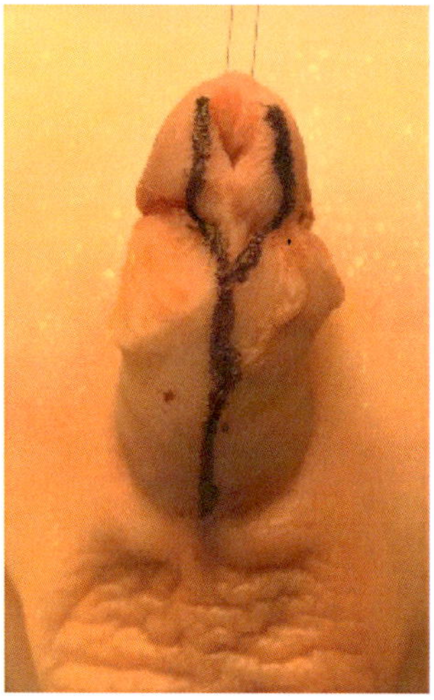

Figure 3. Incision lines to repair glans dehiscence. The glans wings are marked along their visible junction to the urethral plate, and then the incision continues down the median raphe. It is rarely necessary to deglove the penis entirely.

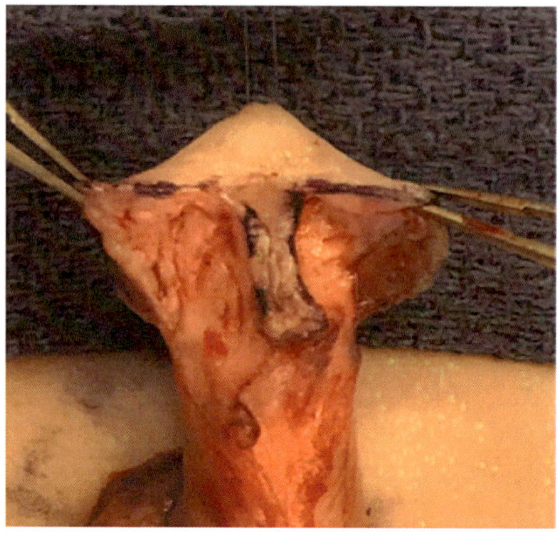

Figure 4. Glans wings dissection for glans dehiscence. It is especially important to completely release tension from the glans wings during reoperative TIP repair for glans dehiscence. Here the glans wings have been dissected first to 3 and 9 o'clock, and then superiorly until they opened horizontally and no further tension was felt.

Artificial erection

Then artificial erection is done to confirm the penis is straight.

Dissecting the glans wings

Next, the glans wings are dissected along the surface of the corpora to 3 and 9 o'clock and superiorly on each side as needed to release tension resulting from scars after prior repair (Figure 4). This extended dissection is especially important in a reoperation for glans dehiscence to achieve a tension-free closure.

In addition, scar found on the undersurface of the opened glans wings is incised or excised, which also lengthens them and relieves tension that might otherwise pull the repair back open.

If a Mathieu or onlay flap procedure was done previously we remove the flap, because the incised urethral plate will make a normal neourethra and the superior glans fusion from TIP potentially increases the risk for a flap diverticulum (Figure 5).

TIP Incision

Counter-traction is held along the sides of the urethral plate while it is incised deeply to near the underlying tunica albuginea of the corpora. As in primary TIP repairs, this incision extends into the meatus proximally and stops distally at the junction between the plate and the glans.

Urethral Plate Tubularization

A 5 or 6Fr stent is passed into the bladder and tied to the glans traction suture. The smaller stent is used when the glans measures 13mm or less to avoid adding tension to the glans wings approximation.

Tubularization of the urethral plate begins distally at approximately the midglans, at least 3mm from the end of the plate. The first stitch is placed epithelially, using 7-0 Vicryl. While we sometimes close the urethral plate with continuous sutures, more often interrupted subepithelial stitching is done in reoperations.

Dartos Flap

Next, a ventral dartos flap is created and advanced distally to cover the entire neourethra (Figure 6), suturing it to either side of the opening with 9-0 Vicryl.

Glansplasty

The glans wings are first aligned at their midpoint using an epithelial 9-0 Vicryl stitch. Then 3 interrupted subepithelial 6-0 Vicryl stitches are placed, the first under the 9-0 stitch, the 3rd at the corona

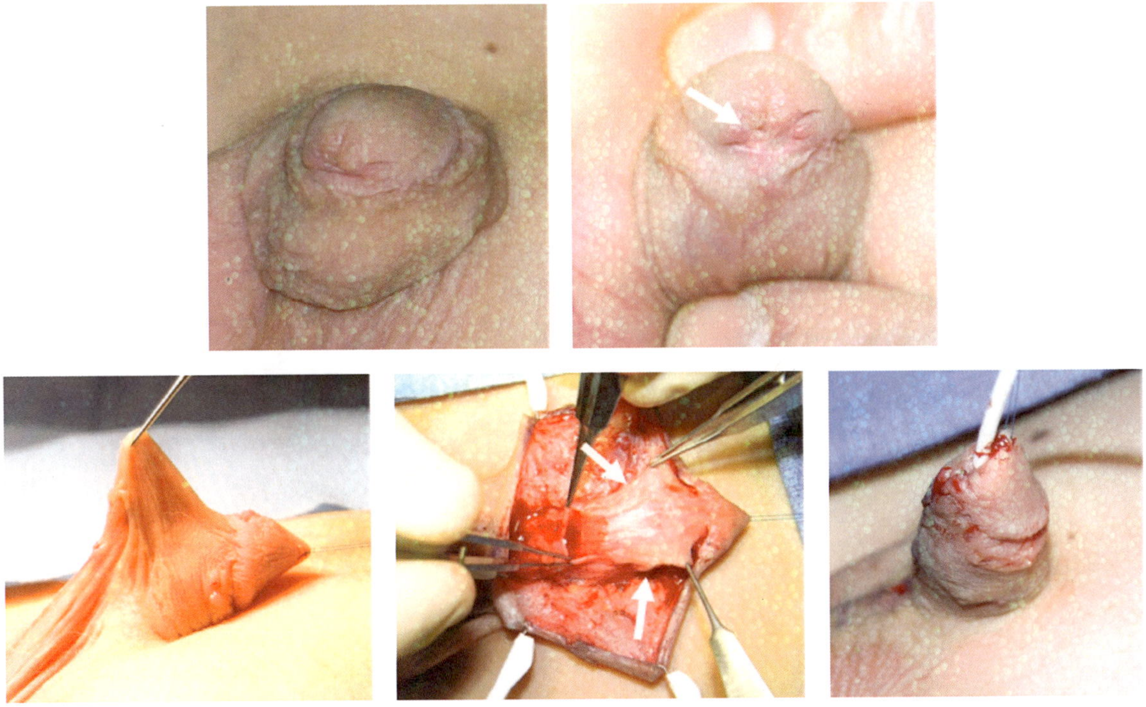

Figure 5. Reoperative TIP for glans dehiscence with removal of onlay flap.
A, pyramidal appearance after distal shaft onlay prepucial flap repair. B, complete glans dehiscence with a coronal meatus (arrow). Note also the transverse cuts in the left glans wings from epithelial suturing. C, excess ventral skin contributing to the abnormal appearance. D, exposure achieved by ventral midline incision without total degloving. Incision down the neourethra split the onlay flap into halves. The arrows indicate these flaps which will be excised from along each side of the urethral plate. There is no visible scar in the urethral plate. E, normal glans fusion and cylindrical appearance of the penis after TIP reoperation.

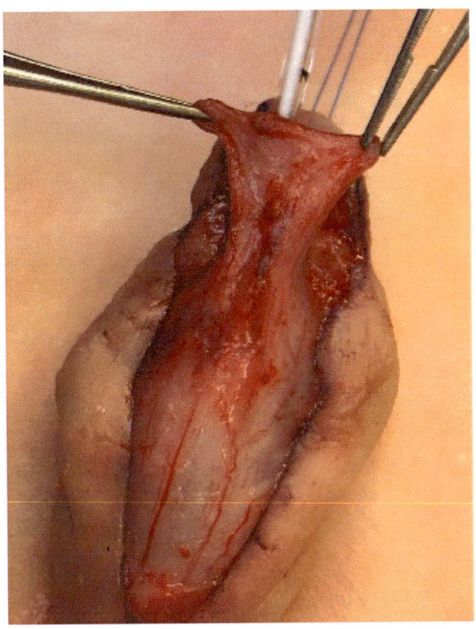

Figure 6. Ventral dartos flap.
Ventral dartos preserved on the corpora during degloving is fashioned into a flap used to cover the neourethra.

and the 2nd midway between the first stitch and the 3rd. The second stitch also catches a bite of the dartos flap to hold it in place. As with primary TIP, the glans is closed over, but not sutured to, the neourethra. There should be no tension on the approximated glans wings.

Mucosal Collar and Skin Closure

The mucosal collar is first checked for scar tissue to excise. It is important that the collar not exert tension on the glansplasty. It is approximated using 9-0 epithelial stitches just below the corona, and then completed using interrupted subepithelial 7-0 Vicryl stitches.

The shaft skin is also carefully inspected and stretched looking and feeling for tension bands. Scar along the incision edge can be excised, which will lengthen the skin (figure 7). Smaller bands can be released by superficial transverse incisions under the epithelium.

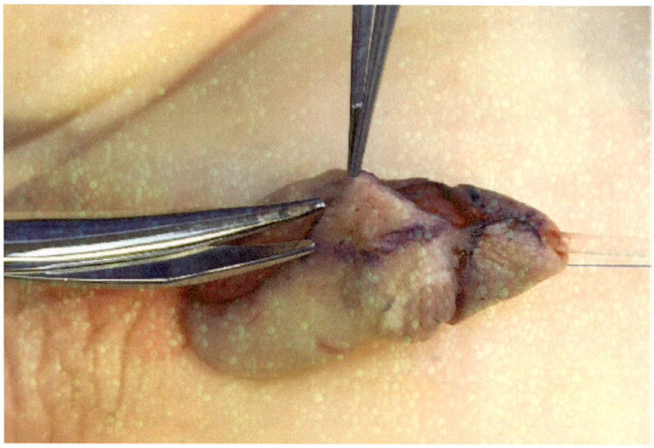

Figure 7. Excising scarred skin.
Excess skin is excised. When the skin edge is scarred, this excision also lengthens the shaft skin and reduces associated tension.

When scar and bands of tension have been released, the skin is sewn with interrupted subepithelial 7-0 Vicryl.

Postoperative Management

Postoperative care is the same as described in Chapter 6 for primary TIP repair. TIP reoperations are all done as ambulatory surgery without hospitalization. Urinary diversion is used for 1 week. The same bandage used in primary TIP is placed and falls off spontaneously. Routine medications include hydrocodone with acetaminophen, ibuprofen, oxybutynin, and sulfamethoxazole/trimethoprim.

Perioperative HBOT helps with healing of both the urethroplasty and shaft skin and is an integral part of management described in detail in Chapter 18.

Results

We reported that glans dehiscence recurred in 10% after reoperative TIP in patients with mostly distal hypospadias (Snodgrass and Bush et al, 2009). In the past, we offered a 3rd glans closure, but found that over half of those dehisced again. Thinking these prepubertal boys might have a successful outcome if glansplasty was delayed until puberty when the glans is at least twice larger, we followed a small number of patients and then did a final repair at that time. However, none of these teens had a successful glansplasty and 1 sustained loss of glans volume.

Today we do a single reoperative TIP for glans dehiscence, but no more if this repair also dehisces. We emphasize again that a recurrent complication often indicates there is also VC or tension from short ventral skin. When dehiscence recurs in the absence of these factors, repeated glansplasties are not likely to be successful and can damage the glans.

While observing these patients, we found that boys and teens with repeat glans dehiscence after repairs that placed the meatus in the correct location at the tip of the glans usually have a compact stream and void standing. This is in contrast to other patients in whom the surgeon intentionally made a coronal or subcoronal meatus, who are much more likely to spray and may have to sit to void.

Most importantly, we have significantly decreased both primary and reoperative glans dehiscence by greater dissection of the glans wings and greater diligence to identify and release bands of skin tension.

Surgical Technique: Reoperative G-Tip

Key steps in this procedure are identical to those described above for TIP, except that the TIP incision is grafted before tubularizing the urethral plate. It is important to extend the incision proximally into healthy urethra. After incising the plate, 7-0 PDS stays are placed in the outer edges at its midportion on both sides to hold it open.

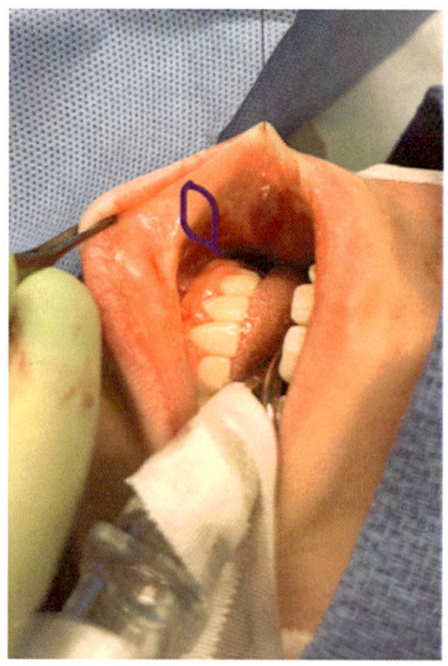

Figure 8. Left upper lip elliptical graft for G-TIP.
Small grafts should be taken from the upper lip, not lower.

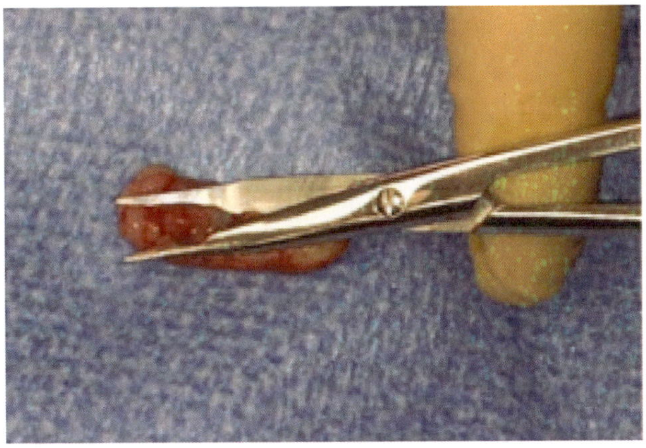

Figure 9. Defatting a small upper lip graft for G-TIP reoperation.
Small grafts are not easy to defat balanced on a fingertip or pinned to a board. It is easiest to dampen a spot on a towel or the surgical drape to hold the graft and then defat using scissors as shown here.

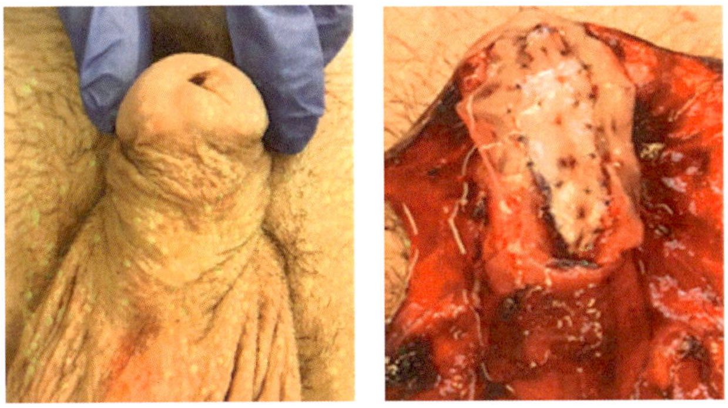

Figure 10. G-TIP (inlay graft) reoperation.
A, eccentric meatus from a tunneled prepucial tube repair. B, TIP incision was made through the narrowed neourethra with upper lip inlay grafting as shown.

Graft Harvest

A first-generation cephalosporin is given intravenously, then the visible margin of the *upper* lip is marked. 5-0 Prolene stays hold the lip upwards. A damp gauze is packed in the throat next to the endotracheal tube. The elliptical-shaped graft is outlined with a marking pen, taking care to make it sufficiently wide to account for the dip from the epithelial surface down to the corporal made by the TIP incision (Figure 8).

1:200,000 bupivacaine with epinephrine is injected. Then the graft is removed, dissecting in a plane superficial to the underlying fat and muscle. The donor site is *not* sutured or otherwise treated.

These small grafts are most easily further defatted by placing them onto a damp spot on the drapes, which will hold the graft without needing a pin board (Figure 9).

Surgeons should *never* take these smaller grafts from the lower lip. That region should always be reserved in the event that a longer graft is needed at a future date.

Inlay Grafting

The graft is then sewn into the defect, beginning proximally using 7-0 Vicryl (Figure 10). We continue sewing around the perimeter with epithelial interrupted stitches, taking care not to pull the edges too taut. At least 1 quilting stitch is placed in the middle of the graft, but if the graft is long enough, additional quilting stitches anchor it to the corpora proximally and distally to the middle stitch. The graft is trimmed as needed as sewing proceeds distally.

Plate Tubularization

Following graft placement, urethral plate tubularization is done in 2-layers with subepithelial stitches; the first using interrupted 6-0 Vicryl and the second a continuous 6-0 PDS.

Postoperative Management

Care after G-TIP is the same as described above following reoperative TIP repair. No special care is needed for the lip donor site, and these patients do not need hospitalization or bed rest. The catheter provides urinary diversion for 10 days.

Results

We reported 7% recurrent glans dehiscence in a series of 15 boys after reoperative G-TIP done for glans dehiscence before we learned to dissect glans wings not only laterally but also superiorly off the corpora (Snodgrass and Bush et al, 2009). Another series included 16 patients with wound dehiscence, and G-TIP was successful in each (Ye et al, 2008).

Surgeons should have a low threshold to graft the TIP incision in reoperations, especially when there has been more than 1 failed operation. If there is any question that the urethral plate is sufficiently elastic or supple to expect good wound healing, it is better to graft the TIP incision.

On the other hand, if the incised urethral plate or neoplate remains stiff or has downward tension that is not released by TIP incision, the plate should be excised and a staged graft repair done.

Correcting Meatal Stenosis

As discussed in the preceding chapter, meatal stenosis is over-diagnosed after hypospadias repair when the surgeon concludes that a small-appearing meatus and a fine stream indicate a need for intervention without calibrating to prove it is less than 8Fr. In addition, we are not aware of a report on outcomes from meatotomy in a series of patients after hypospadias surgery.

Meatotomy

The records from other pediatric urologists that we review show that most cut the meatus open down its ventral side when they believe there is stenosis. Knowing that incision must continue through all scarring and into normal urethra, this incision often leaves insufficient glans fusion - meaning the hypospadias is re-created with an increased risk for urine spraying.

We have limited data on meatotomy since meatal stenosis occurs in <1% of our own primary patients, and most of those coming to us with true stenosis also have other complications that are best managed by STAC. When we do an isolated meatotomy we first look to release bands of scar just within the meatus using small transverse cuts with a knife. Then we incise the meatus *dorsally* as in TIP repair. Most often there is sufficient adjacent mucosa to suture back to the meatus and cover the defect without creating tension.

G-TIP

We have no experience inlay grafting for meatal stenosis. When there is scarring at the end of the neourethra, an inlay graft of oral mucosa would have to extend well beyond that point and into normal glans to add sufficient width to the meatus, leaving an unsightly red mark on the glans. Therefore, if a meatotomy does not succeed we perform reoperative staged graft repair.

STAG

Excising the scarred tissue and replacing it with healthy oral mucosa is the most reliable way to correct true meatal stenosis, i.e. a scarred neomeatus <8Fr, when a meatotomy is not effective. A 2-stage STAG repair is done when the penis is straight.

Surgical Technique: Reoperative STAG

Skin Incision and Artificial Erection

The diagnosis of meatal stenosis is confirmed by the inability to pass an 8Fr sound, which normally should traverse the neomeatus easily. Then a midline incision is made from the corona down the penile shaft and the skin is dissected laterally. Next, artificial erection is done.

Glans Wings Dissection

After verifying that the penis is straight, the midline of the glans is injected with 1:100,000 epinephrine. Then it is incised and glans wings are created bilaterally while simultaneously excising the scarred meatus and glanular urethra. The wings are dissected from the corpora to 3 and 9 o'clock and superiorly as needed so that the glans is open like the middle of a book without tension. 6-0 Prolene stays are placed at the corona on each side to hold the wings apart.

Moving the Urethral Meatus Proximally

The urethra now must be cut back onto the distal shaft, so that the meatus is approximately 1cm below the corona to make room for an adequate graft. It is a technical error to leave the meatus closer to or at the corona (Figure 11). Remaining distal urethra or neourethra is excised.

The urethra is spatulated, and then its floor is sewn to the corpora at 11, 12 and 1 o'clock using 7-0 Vicryl. Next, adjacent shaft skin is sutured to the ventral aspect of the urethra to complete the urethrostomy as shown in Figure 10. More recently, our preference is to button-hole the graft to surround the meatus or the urethrostomy. Sometimes the penile skin will contract some around the urethrostomy site, and the subcoronal to midshaft region is a difficult place to have skin deficiency. Button-holing the graft around the urethrostomy leaves the skin intact, and the

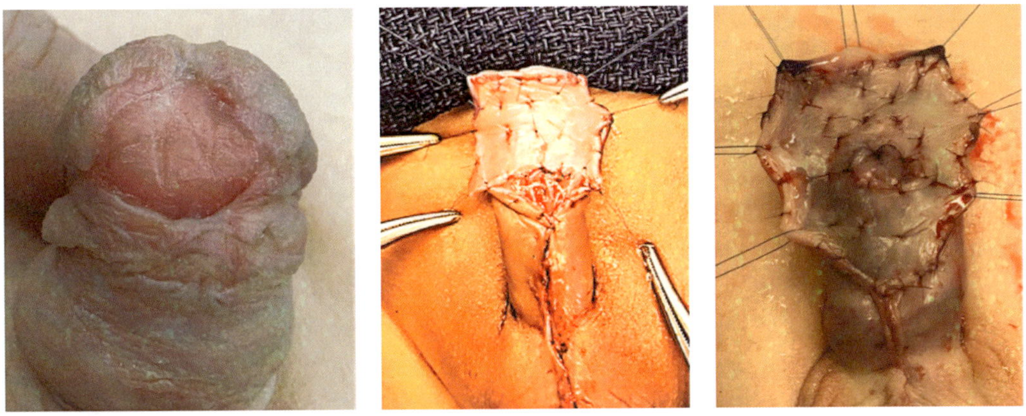

Figure 11. Graft done without moving the urethral meatus proximally.
A, this oral mucosa graft done elsewhere is too short and thick (it was performed with cheek mucosa) to successfully roll into the neourethra and close the glans wings. B, re-grafting was done after moving the meatus further proximally onto the distal shaft. C, we now buttonhole a graft around the subcoronal urethrostomy instead of sewing it adjacent to the urethrostomy as in B

excess oral graft around the ostomy can be excised at the time of tubularization.

Upper Lip Grafting

Upper lip graft is harvested as described in the preceding section and shown in Figure 11. For meatal stenosis, a rectangular-shaped graft is harvested, taking care to avoid injury to Stenson's duct. Upper lift graft is able to extend up to approximately 3.5cm in length when some of the cheek is also utilized. The upper lip is incised just lateral to the frenulum, and this upper lip portion is placed in the glans, with some of the thicker cheek part of the graft utilized along the shaft and for the buttonhole. Once the graft is fit into the defect, from the urethrostomy to the tip of the glans, it is first secured with 7-0 Vicryl to the corona next to the Prolene stays. Additional interrupted 7-0 Vicryl stitches are placed through the skin and graft around the perimeter. Distally, the graft is secured to the end of the glans with subepithelial stitches to avoid visible suture marks at the future neomeatus.

During this process it helps to hemostat every other perimeter stitch to maintain the graft's width, as otherwise there is a tendency to narrow it by stretching it lengthwise.

It is easiest to quilt thicker oral grafts to the corpora using a 6-0 Vicryl on an RB1 needle. We begin distally in the midline and sew the graft to the corpora

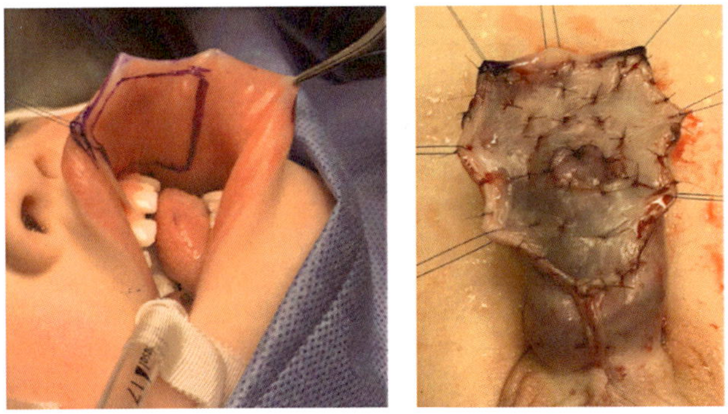

Figure 12. Upper lip graft.
A, graft outlined on the inner upper lip. B, graft sewn around the perimeter and quilted into place. Note it was buttonholed to surround the proximal urethrostomy.

at 5mm intervals down to the urethrostomy. An additional row of stitches is placed to either side of this first one. We keep the graft moist with saline throughout this process.

We now prefer to buttonhole grafts so that they surround the proximal urethrostomy, as shown in Figure 12.

After the graft is sutured, 5-0 Prolene stays are placed at approximately 1.5cm intervals from the corona to the urethrostomy on each side. Graft length and its width at the corona, midsection, and junction to the urethrostomy are measured and recorded.

An 8Fr foley catheter is passed into the bladder and the balloon inflated. A tightly rolled Vaseline gauze is laid on top of the graft, and then the stays are tied together over it to hold the roll in place and provide gentle, not tight, compression. Additional gauzes are laid over the penis and held with large Tegaderm™ bandages.

Postoperative Management

There is no special wound care for the lip donor site. Older boys can use compounded Magic Mouth Wash containing lidocaine, Benadryl and Maalox as needed for discomfort. The outer gauzes fall off spontaneously and are not replaced. The catheter and tie-over bandage are removed at 1 week.

HBOT

Because HBOT improves oral graft take (Bush and Snodgrass, 2019), it is always used for reoperations. Our current protocol with grafting calls for 20 dives perioperatively, with 1-5 done immediately before surgery and the remainder after surgery.

Results

STAG is the most reliable means to resolve meatal stenosis since it excises all scarred tissues and replaces them with well-vascularized labial mucosa. Our labial graft take using HBOT is the same as prepucial graft take in primary repairs (Ahmed et al, 2024). This is better than the less reliable vascularity of random skin flaps, such as Mathieu or onlay repairs done using previously operated skin (Jayanthi et al, 1994).

Repairing Neourethral Strictures

Urethral strictures usually indicate tissue ischemia resulting in scarring. As with other complications it is important to first determine that the penis is straight, since ventral curvature ≥ 30° can induce strictures in the region where maximum tension develops during spontaneous erections. Patients found to have this extent of curvature should be managed by 3 corporotomies and STAC. When the penis is straight, strictures are repaired in a single stage with an inlay graft or in 2-stages by STAG.

The choice between inlay and STAG is determined by the extent the neourethra is narrowed. Lesser degrees are managed with an inlay, but strictures that nearly obliterate the lumen require excision of the affected segment with replacement 2-stage grafting. In addition, a stricture in a neourethra that ends on the penile shaft is managed by STAG to relieve the stricture and extend the meatus to the tip of the glans.

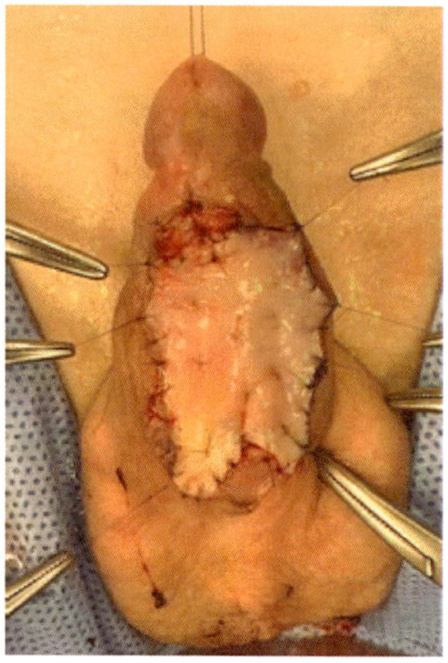

Figure 13. Focal stricture excision with Johansen-type STAG repair.
In the unusual situation that a focal obliterative stricture develops in the midportion of an otherwise healthy neourethra with a normal terminal meatus, the scarred region can be excised preserving the healthy distal meatus and a labial graft placed between a proximal and distal urethrostomy, indicated by the arrows.

A focal stricture between a healthy distal and proximal neourethra is manage by either inlay grafting or a STAG with a Johansen modification (Figure 13). When a staged repair is deemed best the affected area is excised, leaving the healthy distal neourethra and creating 2 stomas. Assuming the adjacent shaft skin is healthy, an oral graft taken from the upper or lower lip, depending on the length needed, is placed between the stomas and subsequently tubularized in 6 or more months after it revascularizes. Despite theoretical concerns for a stricture forming at either stoma or a diverticulum between them, we have encountered neither of these complications to date.

Dilations

As stated in the preceding chapter, dilations do not cure strictures and are painful. We *never* recommend them, even as a temporizing measure.

Direct Vision Internal Urethrotomy

We also do not use DVIU to manage hypospadias strictures. If a surgeon chooses to try DVIU, he or she should first do an artificial erection to determine that the penis is straight, as incising the stricture will not be effective when it is bent. Furthermore, DVIU for hypospadias strictures should be limited to a single treatment of those developing after TIP or onlay procedures (Husmann and Rathbun, 2006). As mentioned in Chapter 16, some of the worse periurethral scarring we have encountered followed unsuccessful DVIU. If a stricture recurs after DVIU, another DVIU should *not* be done. DVIUs in hypospadias patients are also associated with erectile dysfunction (Husmann, 2021).

Dorsal Inlay Graft vs STAG

The decision whether to inlay graft or do STAG is made intraoperatively after opening the urethra. We have not found urethroscopy to help make this decision when done either as a separate procedure or at the beginning of the repair.

Surgical Technique

Localizing the stricture

A stent is placed down the urethra until it reaches the stricture. The skin incision is made in the median raphe over this region, extending both above and below the constriction to provide good exposure. Surrounding tissues are released to expose the surface of the urethra.

Artificial erection

Artificial erection is always done next, regardless of the results of prior erections and irrespective of whatever means was used to previously straighten the penis. Even if a prior operative note states the penis was straight with artificial erection, in the event of a stricture it still needs to be checked as we have found such reports either unreliable, or that some patients contract.

Opening the Stricture

Once the penis is confirmed to be straight, the urethra is entered on its ventral side distal to the stricture, and this incision is continued proximally through and beyond it so that there is healthy urethra exposed above and below the lesion.

Inlay Graft vs STAG

If the urethra is nearly obliterated as shown in Figure 14, or there is obvious longitudinal tension on the region of the stricture, then excision of the scarred area with a Johansen-modified STAG repair is done. If the neourethra does not end with a terminal meatus, the scarred abnormal urethra is completely excised and replaced with an oral graft reaching to the tip of the glans.

On the other hand, if it appears there is sufficient width of the neourethra to supplement with an inlay graft, TIP incision is made dorsally through the stricture down to the tunica albuginea of the corpora. This incision also continues 2-3mm into normal urethra distally and proximally.

Inlay Grafting

As discussed above, the sides of the urethra are held open with 7-0 PDS stays, and the needed length and width of graft to fill the defect is harvested from the upper lip. The donor site is *not* sutured closed.

The graft is defatted and then sewn around the perimeter and quilted down the midline of the defect using 7-0 Vicryl interrupted stitches. Then the urethra is closed over a 6Fr stent passed into the bladder using interrupted subepithelial 7-0 Vicryl, and a second layer of continuous 6-0 or 7-0 PDS.

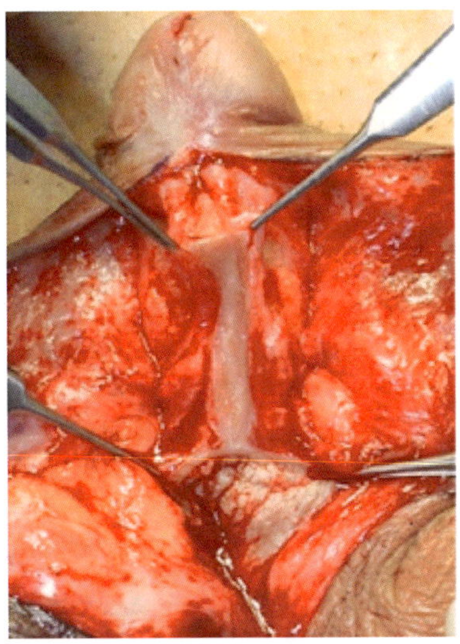

Figure 14. Obliterative neourethral stricture. The entire neourethra made from a foreskin flap is reduced to a strip no more than 3mm wide. Excision with STAG repair using lip graft is the best treatment.

Next, a dartos flap is created to cover the entire repair. If suitable dartos is not available, a tunica vaginalis flap is used instead, as described for proximal TIP and STAC repairs.

Postoperative Management

The catheter is removed 10 days after repair. No special care is given to the lip donor site other than Magic Mouthwash for older boys and adults.

Results

In a series of 37 patients with strictures after hypospadias repair, recurrent strictures after inlay graft repair occurred in 3 (8%). These recurrences were at the junction of neourethra to native urethra (Ye et al, 2008), and may have developed because of a technical error of not sufficiently incising proximally into normal urethra.

STAG Repair

The focal obliterative stricture is excised. The proximal and distal ends of the healthy urethra are made into urethrostomies and labial graft is placed between them, buttonholed around both urethrostomies whenever possible. 6 months later the graft is tubularized to restore urethral continuity.

If the distal urethra ends below the normal meatal location on the glans and/or with abnormal glans fusion, then the entire distal urethra is excised and replaced with graft so that the final operation will create a normal meatus.

A catheter is passed down the proximal urethrostomy into the bladder, and a rolled Vaseline gauze used for a tie-over bandage onto the graft.

Results

Despite the theoretic risk for stricture at the graft-to-urethrostomy junctions, or development of a diverticulum in the interposed segment, we have not observed either of these complications in our series of these repairs.

Total graft replacement of the neourethra avoids that potential risk for recurrent stricture but is not necessary when the distal segment ends in a normal meatus, and risks glans dehiscence if a previously healed glansplasty is reopened.

Repairing Diverticulum

Most boys with diverticula do *not* have distal obstruction from meatal stenosis or a stricture, but the surgeon still must verify that by passing an 8Fr sound. More often, a diverticulum results from dilation of a more elastic native urethra or segment of neourethra proximal to a less distensible segment of neourethra – a situation analogous to a megaureter developing above a normal-sized and patent but inelastic ureterovesical junction.

Either a stricture or a relatively rigid segment of neourethra can result from the tension exerted by VC, and so artificial erection must also be done to determine if the penis is bent.

Assuming no VC, diverticulum repair involves either imbrication, or excisional tapering of the enlarged neourethra plus inlay grafting of the distal, non-dilated neourethra when there is a stricture or that segment is relatively inelastic.

Surgical Technique

Skin Incision and Artificial Erection

Incision is made in the ventral median raphe from the corona down into the scrotum past the end of the diverticulum. The shaft skin is dissected laterally from the redundant neourethra, preserving dartos to make a barrier flap later.

Artificial erection is done to confirm the penis is straight.

Imbricating the diverticulum

Fusiform dilation of the neourethra can be reduced by imbrication. We perform this in 2-layers using interrupted subepithelial 6-0 PDS sutures to taper it to a similar size as the non-dilated urethra. After imbrication, the neourethra is pressurized with saline to ensure a smooth appearance.

Excisional tapering

Large diverticula are best managed by excising the excess tissue. The diverticulum is opened throughout its length, usually along one side off the midline to avoid overlapping suture lines with the penile skin during closure. The urethra distal to the diverticulum

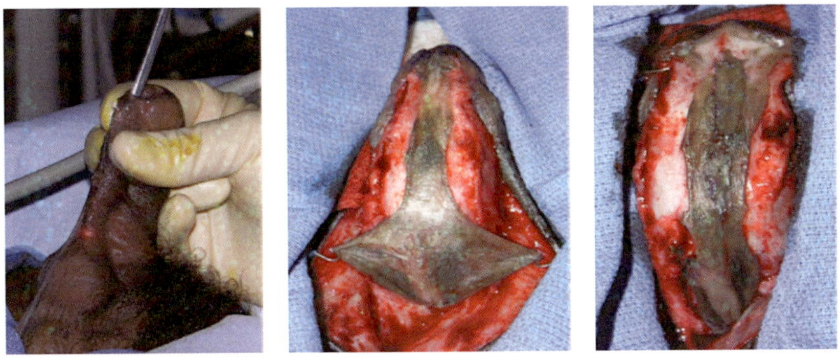

Figure 15. Diverticulum repair with inlay grafting.
A, a sound is passed in a patient with a proximal diverticulum, demonstrating there is no meatal stenosis or stricture. B, the neourethra is opened, showing the discrepancy in size of the distal segment and suggesting that it is less distensible. C, tissue excised from the diverticulum is used to inlay graft the distal segment so that the entire neourethra has a uniform caliber.

is also exposed and opened for a short distance so that the repair will result in a smooth and uniform neourethra. The excess tissue is excised, taking care not to remove so much that the remaining urethra ends up with too small a caliber. The repaired urethra rarely expands again and so the diverticulum should not be overly narrowed thinking that it might recur otherwise.

A 6Fr stent is passed into the bladder, and then the edges of the urethra are closed in 2 layers using subepithelial stitches, the first with interrupted 7-0 Vicryl and the second with 6-0 or 7-0 PDS. A dartos flap is made to cover the repair, and if that is not possible a tunica vaginalis flap is used. A catheter provides urinary diversion for 10-14 days.

With distal inlay grafting

Even though calibration shows there is no stricture, a "normal" sized distal urethra is presumed to be stiff and contributing to the diverticulum. TIP incision is made in the distal urethra, and the excised diverticulum tissue is inlay grafted into it to make the neourethra uniform (Figure 15).

Results

Diverticula occurred in 27% of proximal repairs in one series, mostly after onlay and tubularized preputial flaps. Only 1 of the 13 was found to have a distal stricture. A recurrent diverticulum occurred in 1 (8%) after excision and closure (Snyder et al, 2005). Another report of 5 diverticula also found that recurrence is uncommon after excision (Vallasciani et al, 2013).

Reoperations for VC ≥ 30° and/or Multiple Complications

Many patients presenting with complications after hypospadias repair have more than one of the problems described above. Most of those also have underlying VC ≥ 30° and are best managed by reoperative STAC repair. They present with deficient, scarred shaft skin in combination with multiple or large fistulas, wound dehiscences, meatal stenoses, obliterative strictures, or symptomatic hair in the neourethra (Figure 16).

Those with multiple complications whose penis is straight often still need STAC reoperations because the shaft skin is scarred and needs time to rejuvenate before the urethroplasty is redone.

Perioperative HBOT

All of these patients benefit from HBOT. Our protocol calls for at least 15 perioperative dives with 1-5 before surgery and the remainder done afterwards, beginning the same or next day. Patients with the extent of scarring shown in Figure 15 are recommended for up to 30 dives, ideally with 5-10 preop. All patients with multiple complications have decreased vascularity and impaired wound healing and need more than a reoperation to start making things right.

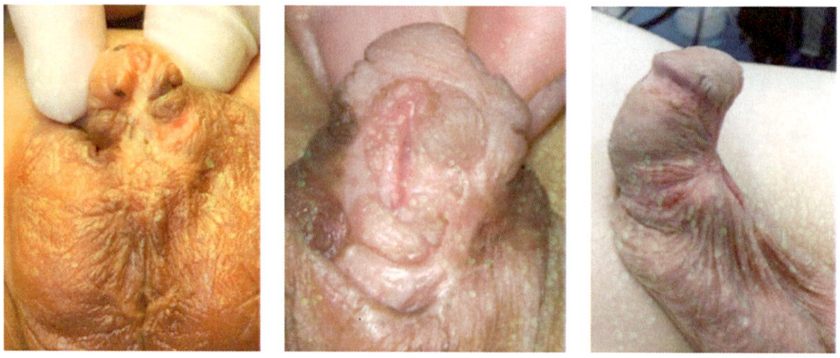

Figure 16. Multiple complications requiring STAC reoperations.
A,B, extensive scarring of the ventral shaft skin, neourethra and glans. C, ventral curvature and scarred, deficient ventral skin.

Decision-Making

A mentioned, patients presenting with multiple complications and/or VC ≥ 30° are best managed by STAC. Once the penis is made straight and the skin healthier, placing a neourethra within it is both easier and more likely successful. The first STAC was done in a patient who presented after multiple failed repairs, and the STAG that we did also failed with both penile shaft skin and oral graft contracture. Both we and the parents were amazed at the obvious improvement gained by excising the scarred graft and then simply closing the shaft skin and treating with additional HBOT. For the first time in his life that boy had a straight penis with symmetric and supple penile shaft skin. All that remained was to complete a staged graft urethroplasty to the tip of his glans under these improved circumstances.

Surgical Technique: Reoperative STAC 1

Skin incision

The key steps in reoperative STAC 1 repair are shown in Figures 17 and 18. An incision is made down the median raphe, usually continuing to at least the mid-scrotum. The skin is dissected away from the neourethra and corpora, preserving the underlying dartos with it. Subcutaneous scar tissue is also released, particularly across the ventral glans which is often tethered downwards.

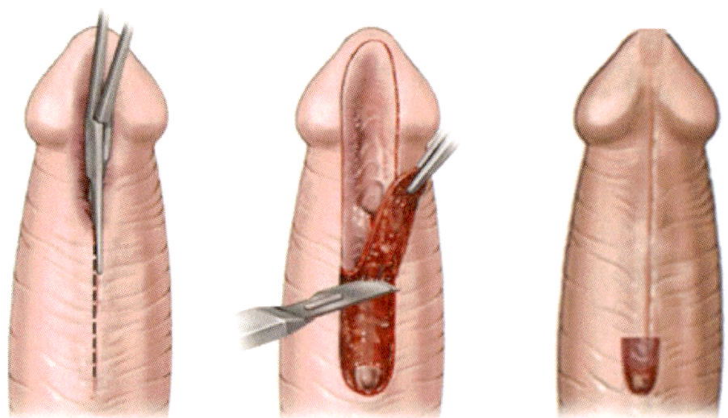

Figure 17. Reoperative STAC 1 repair.
A, ventral midline incision is made. It is rarely necessary to completely deglove the penis in reoperations, and best *not* to release the dorsal skin since overall skin deficiency can make it difficult to suture it back. B, the scarred neourethra is removed, and corporotomies made when there is ventral curvature (not shown). C, the proximal urethrostomy has been created and the shaft skin and glans edges approximated to close the wound without urethroplasty grafting.

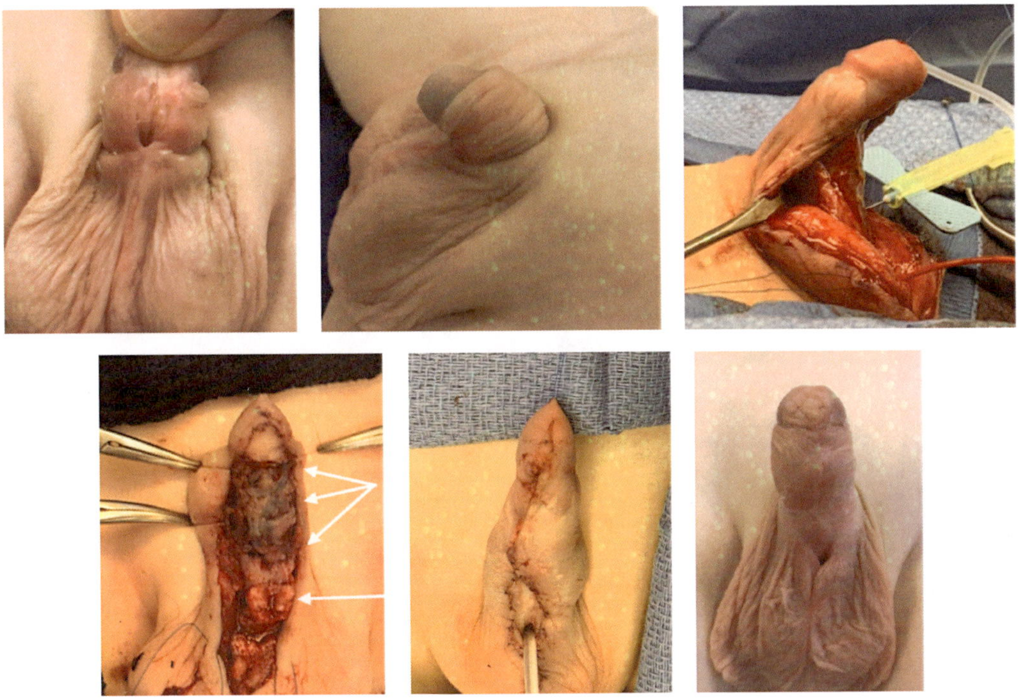

Figure 18. Reoperative STAC 1 repair.
A, wound dehiscence and short ventral skin following Byars flap repair. B, preoperative indication that there is recurrent ventral curvature. C, artificial erection confirms recurrent curvature, measuring 70° by goniometer. D, 3 corporotomies have been made. The lower arrow shows the urethrostomy below the corporotomies. The upper 3 arrows indicate where the corporal incisions were made. These have been covered by a dartos flap to contain any bleeding and prevent the skin from adhering to the incisions. E, the shaft skin is closed without urethroplasty grafting. Perioperative HBOT was done to improve skin vascularity. F, appearance 6 months later, showing the penis is straight, longer than before, and has healthier ventral shaft skin. Contrast its appearance to the photograph in A. Now attention can turn to the urethroplasty.

Artificial erection

The next step is artificial erection. Sometimes the ventral shaft skin is so short that it restricts erection and makes it difficult, or impossible, to accurately determine if the penis is straight or measure the degree of bending. In this situation the skin must first be lengthened by excision of dense scar along its edges and/or judicious cuts at angles where most the tension is localized (see Chapter 21).

Straightening ventral curvature

VC is corrected as described in Chapter 2. When there is < 30° bending, and the Adson test shows a plication will straighten it without tension, a Heinicke-Mikulicz dorsal plication is done, exposing the dorsal midline by lifting the shaft skin.

When VC is ≥ 30° the urethra is transected at the corona and dissected proximally into the scrotum. Then 3 corporotomies are made across the region of greatest curvature. Next, a dartos flap is created from adjacent shaft skin to cover the incisions, suturing it to the corpora around the area of the incisions and to the isthmuses between them to contain blood that might ooze from the corporotomies when the tourniquet is released.

Proximal urethrostomy

The urethra is advanced back distally while the penis is maximally stretched and sutured at intervals to the corpora using 6-0 PDS. The proximal urethrostomy is secured with Vicryl suture where the urethra easily reaches without tension, either on the corpora below the most proximal corporotomy or on an isthmus between corporotomies.

Glans closure

If it was opened, the glans is sewn back together in the midline after excising the distal neourethra and scar tissue. 7-0 Vicryl subepithelial sutures are used to avoid visible glans scars. Any severe glans scars/divots are addressed at this stage by excision of the scar and subepithelial anastomosis to smooth the appearance as much as possible. As in primary STAC, it is otherwise not necessary to open the glans at the first operation.

Suturing the penoscrotal junction

Similar to primary proximal STAC repairs, it is important to tack the ventral penile skin to the corpora at the penoscrotal junction on both sides of the urethra using 5-0 PDS in prepubertal patients, or 3-0 PDS in adults. This provides a fixed point against which the skin can stretch during natural postoperative erections. It does not matter that this fixation will have to be redone during the final stage. A key goal of reoperative STAC is to optimize the remaining penile skin and increase the likelihood that final skin closure can be done without tension using only penis skin. In this way Cecil maneuvers, scrotal flaps and skin grafts are almost never required. To achieve this, the penoscrotal junction needs to be secured with suture so that the foreshortened shaft skin can have a fixed point to stretch agains when erections occur. Otherwise, if not affixed, the scrotum will lift up during erections and leave the skin short.

Shaft skin closure

Skin closure can be quite difficult, depending on the extent of scarring and loss. The first priority is to use penile skin to cover the penile shaft, rather than scrotal flaps. Scar excision from along the skin edge usually lengthens the skin, as do oblique cuts into the skin as discussed in Chapter 21.

Because the skin nearly always improves after reoperative STAC plus HBOT, every effort is made to utilize all available penile skin to close the shaft. On occasion this skin will contract despite not stressing it with a urethroplasty graft and providing HBOT. In those uncommon cases it may be necessary to skin graft the ventral penis at the second operation and allow that to heal before proceeding with urethroplasty.

Urinary diversion and bandage

An 8Fr catheter into the bladder provides urinary diversion for 1 week. Adaptic and Coban™ make a gentle compression bandage around the penis.

Postoperative management

This is described in Chapter 8. We emphasize here the benefit of using Aquaphor to coat the ventral skin with each diaper change, or 4 times daily in older boys, once the bandage falls off. Beginning 1 month after surgery, betamethasone 0.1% cream is used morning and evening for 12 weeks, replacing 2 of the daily Aquaphor applications.

HBOT also helps skin to heal and rejuvenate and so deficient and scarred ventral skin is a key indication for this therapy, which begins the afternoon of surgery, or the following day.

Results

We published that 3 corporotomies achieve durable straightening in over 98% of patients with persistent or recurrent ventral curvature ≥ 30° after initial attempts at straightening by chordee excision, dorsal plication or single ventral corporotomy with corporal grafting (Snodgrass and Bush, 2017).

Patients with short, scarred penile skin have had significant, often dramatic, improvement in the length and health of their skin following STAC plus HBOT (Figures 17,18). As a result, their next stage oral mucosa grafts successfully take more than 90% of the time (Ahmed et al, 2024).

Reoperative STAC 2

2nd stage oral mucosa grafting is the same as described for primary STAC repairs as described in Chapter 8 and is shown in Figures 20 and 21.

A ventral midline incision is made from coronal to, or around, the meatus. The skin is opened laterally, preserving its dartos, and then artificial erection is done to verify that the penis remains straight. Then the glans wings are opened flat and a lip graft harvested from either upper or lower lip depending on the length needed, as described in Chapter 11. The graft is secured first at the corona, and then circumferentially. The proximal end is buttonholed around

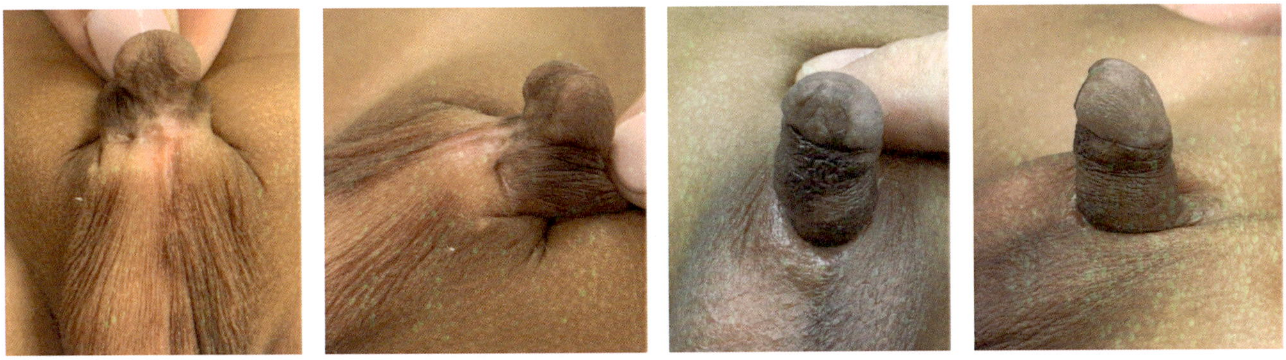

Figure 19. Dramatic, yet typical, shaft skin recovery after STAC plus HBOT.
A,B, wound dehiscence and scarring with almost no ventral shaft skin. C,D, normal appearing shaft skin after STAC plus HBOT. Staged graft urethroplasty can now be done with primary shaft skin closure at the final stage, avoiding a skin graft, scrotal flap or Cecil maneuver.

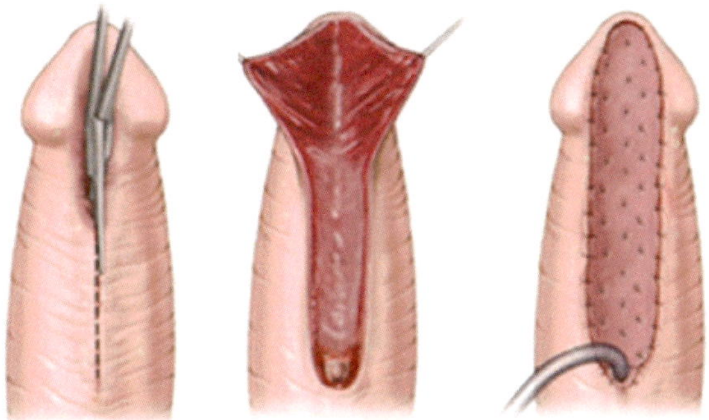

Figure 20. Reoperative STAC 2 repair.
A, ventral midline incision is made. It is rarely necessary to completely deglove the penis in reoperations, and most often best to leave the dorsal skin undisturbed. B, after confirming that the penis is straight by artificial erection, the glans wings are developed laterally to open the glans widely, like the middle of a book. C, lip graft is sewn around the perimeter using interrupted 7-0 Vicryl, and quilted to the underlying corpora with 6-0 Vicryl on a RB1 needle.

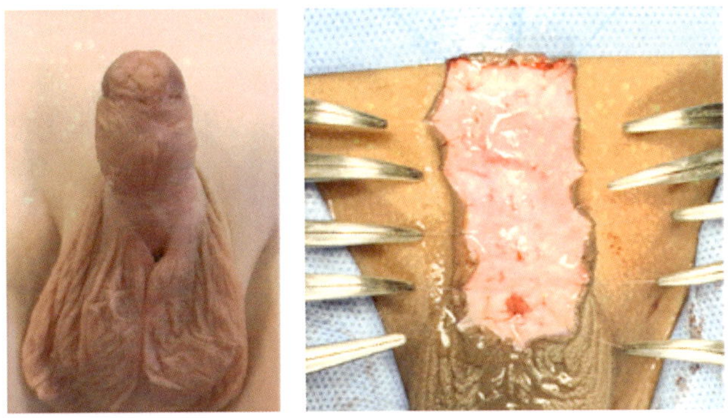

Figure 21. Reoperative STAC 2.
A, straight penis with well-healed skin after reoperative 1st stage STAC plus adjuvant HBOT shown above in Figure 17. B, the glans and shaft skin have been opened and a lower lip graft placed, buttonholing it around the meatus. The patient will next receive additional HBOT.

the meatus when it is on the penile shaft or penoscrotal junction, or tapered and advanced within the meatus in the scrotum after it is spatulated dorsally. The graft is quilted to the corpora and then a catheter and tie-over bandage placed.

Patients additionally receive 20 perioperative HBOT to help with graft healing.

Results

Paired graft measurements (taken when the graft was placed and then again before tubularization) proved that HBOT benefits these reoperative oral grafts. We found the percent of graft contracture was the same in reoperative oral grafts receiving HBOT as in primary prepucial grafts, even though the redo patients averaged 3 prior failed repairs. In contrast, reoperative oral grafts in patients who had an average of only 1.5 failed operations and so were not initially recommended for HBOT had double the rate of graft contraction (Ahmed et al, 2024). Once we recognized

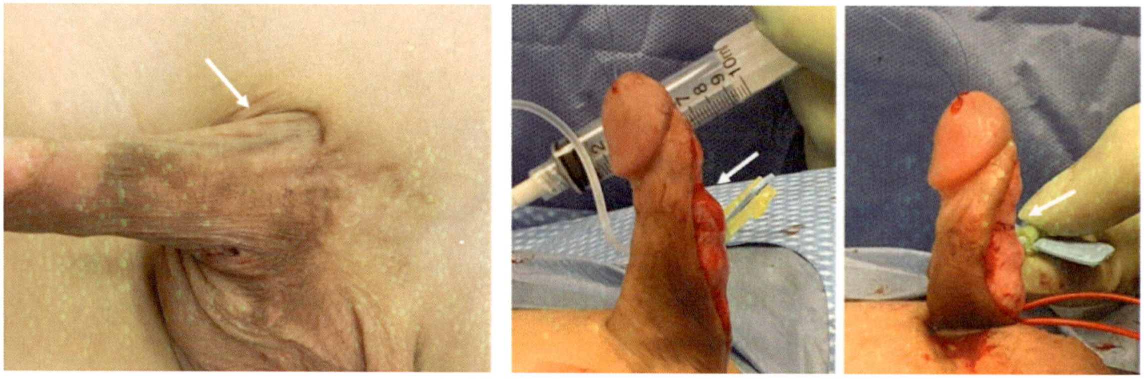

Figure 22. Dorsal curvature after corporotomies in a patient with short dorsal shaft skin.
A, deficient, scarred dorsal shaft skin with arrow indicating band of tension that pulled on the corporotomy incisions as they were healing. B, arrow points to the over-stretched corporotomy creating the dorsal bend. C, Adson test indicated straightening would be best achieved by Nesbit plication, incising through the center of the tunica albuginea over the prior corporotomy and then suturing the defect closed with interrupted subepithelial 4-0 Prolene sutures.

---

this, we changed our protocol to include perioperative HBOT in all reoperative graft procedures.

Lip distortion

As discussed in Chapter 11, oral mucosa donor sites, whether lip or cheek, can heal with scar contracture. Parents and patients are informed of this before 2nd stage grafting, and reassured that the scar can be released with transverse incisions as needed at the next operation, which also resolves any lip irregularity. We also recommend mouth exercises such as pretending to blow up a balloon, blowing a pinwheel, or even blowing a large wooden train whistle for younger children. Massage to the healing lip to help with wound contracture can also help, although this can be difficult in the toddler age group.

Dorsal penile curvature

Sometimes artificial erection at the second stage finds dorsal curvature developed after VC was corrected by the 3 corporotomies. This problem is uncommon after primary STAC repairs, but can occur in reoperations associated with short dorsal skin that can stretch a corporotomy during postoperative erections while it is healing.

Dorsal curvature less than 30° occurs normally and has not been reported to cause sexual dysfunction. Greater curvature should be corrected before the graft is placed. An Adson test is done to test how much force is needed to overcome the bend and then either a Heineke-Mikulicz plication or a Nesbit elliptical incision (Figure 22) is done ventrally for lesser or greater dorsal tension, respectively.

Reoperative STAC 3

We schedule the final operation 6 months or longer after grafting. While some surgeons routinely wait a year, we have not seen a perceptible change in graft health after 6 months. Certainly, waiting indefinitely will not improve poor graft take due to insufficient revascularization.

The key steps in the procedure are shown in Figures 23 and 24.

Measuring the graft

First, we place a 5-0 Prolene stay suture transversely in the glans and then measure the graft dimensions in the same way as when it was placed, i.e. its length and the widths at the corona, mid-graft and at the urethrostomy. There should be little change in the dimensions, and a decrease of more than a few millimeters in any of these measurements should prompt closer inspection of the graft visually and by stretching it to detect tension from scarring.

Marking skin incisions

Most often, the lines for incision are along the junction of the shaft skin and graft below the glans. However,

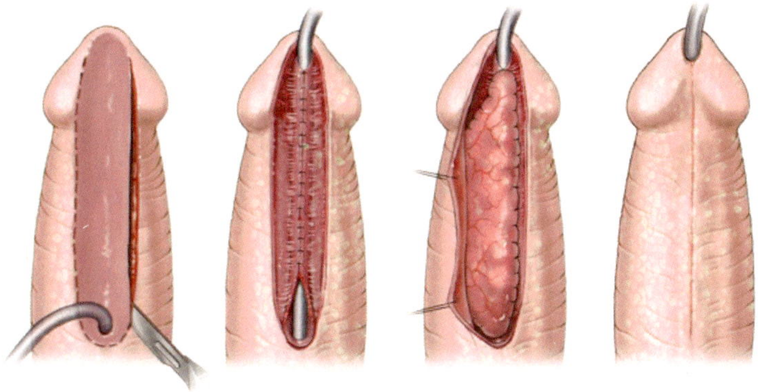

Figure 23. Reoperative STAC 3: Tubularizing the neo-urethral plate.
A, incision is made alongside the graft through its junction to the skin. Although the diagram shows that beginning within the glans wings and then continuing down, we first start at the level of the corona and do not disturb the glans until we have verified that the penis is straight and the graft will easily tubularize. B, tubularization begins distally and moves proximally. The first stitch is placed at the midglans level, the same as during TIP repair. The first layer is sutured using *interrupted* subepithelial 6-0 Vicryl. The closure is then checked for water-tightness, and a second layer is run subepithelially back proximally to distally using 6-0 or 7-0 PDS. C, a tunica vaginalis flap covers the entire neourethra and is sutured to the corpora around its perimeter. D, glansplasty is done using 3 interrupted subepithelial 6-0 Vicryl stitches to secure glans wing to glans wing, as in TIP repairs. The glans is not directly sewn to the urethral opening. Then the mucosal collar and shaft skin are closed in the median raphe using interrupted subepithelial 7-0 Vicryl.

as discussed in Chapter 8 regarding primary STAC, if there is an area of focal graft narrowing with some excess adjacent skin the incision can extend more laterally to include that skin - after determining there will still be enough to close the penile shaft without tension, and that the skin is in a non-hair-bearing region.

Similarly, if there is an area of deficient skin with extra adjacent graft, the line for incision can be moved medially to include the excess graft with the skin to facilitate shaft closure. That will leave a red line in the median raphe which can be excised after healing.

If there is induration at the junction of graft to skin without graft narrowing but which decreases mobility of the graft needed for tubularization, the incision can be moved slightly wider to make skin the lateral edge of the neourethra.

Once this inspection is completed, planned skin incisions are marked along the visible junction of the glans wings to the graft, and then down the penile shaft. Proximally, marks go just inside the urethrostomy so that shaft or scrotal skin sewn there at the prior operation can be excluded from the neourethra. Then the mark continues down the midline to the mid-scrotum to facilitate later tunica vaginalis harvest.

There is no reason to completely deglove the penis.

Initial dissection

Next, we inject the glans wings with 1:100,000 epinephrine to set up while the ventral penis is degloved. We do not incise the glans wings until we have verified that the penis is straight and the graft is satisfactory for tubularization.

Incision extends down the marks, and then the skin is dissected away from the graft and the corpora taking down any scars that may have developed. We have observed that HBOT greatly reduces scar tissues.

Releasing scar along the graft edges

Next, the graft is stretched looking for scars along the sides. Sometimes thickened dartos exerts tension on the graft and this is excised or incised transversely. Thin bands of scar can also be found running under the epithelial edge, which similarly are either excised or cut transversely. These maneuvers slightly

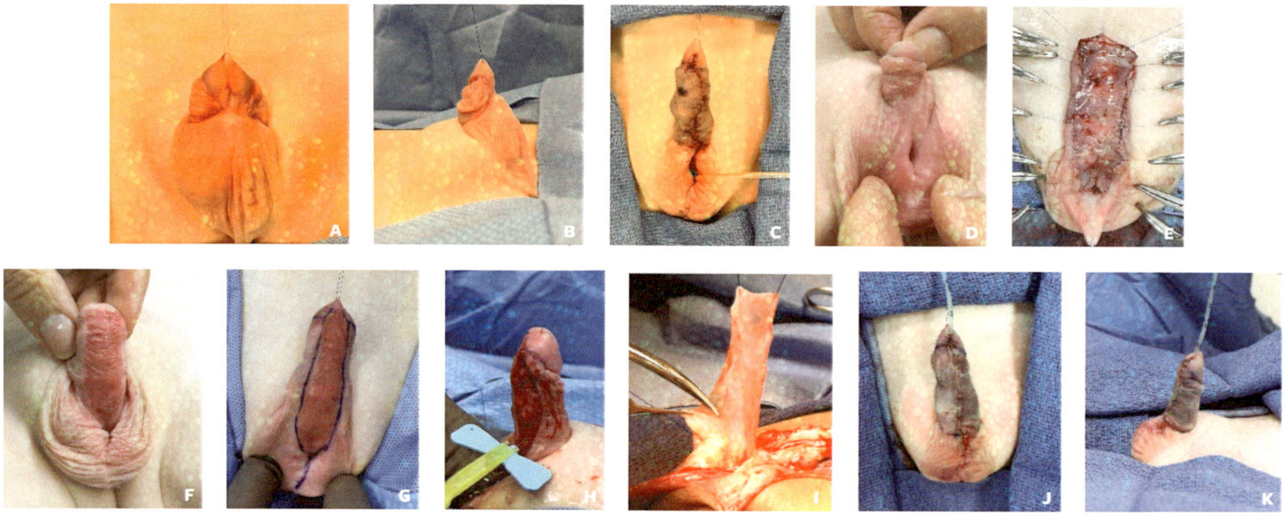

Figure 24. Reoperative STAC 3.
A,B, Preop appearance after failed TIP, with glans dehiscence, persistent curvature, and severe ventral skin deficiency. C, appearance at the end of STAC 1, after 3 corporotomies and skin revision. D,E, at the beginning and end of STAC 2, where lower lip graft was placed. F,G, lines of incision marked along the glans wings, down on either side of the graft, inside the urethrostomy to exclude hair follicles, and then down the midline of the scrotum to access tunica vaginalis. H, after mobilizing the skin, artificial erection confirms the penis is straight. Then the glans wings are developed with extended dissection to minimize risk for glans dehiscence. 2-layer tubularization of the neo-urethral plate is done, the first layer is sewn with interrupted subepithelial 6-0 Vicryl, beginning at the midglans so as not to create iatrogenic meatal stenosis by placing the first stitch too far distally. The closure is tested by infusing saline to confirm it is watertight. Then a second layer is sewn using subepithelial running 6-0 PDS. I, a tunica vaginalis flap is developed up to the external ring, and covers the entire neourethra. Glansplasty is done as described for TIP repairs, with 3 interrupted subepthelial 6-0 Vicryl stitches, with no stitches through the epithelium. J,K, completed appearance intraoperatively after tacking the penoscrotal junction and subepithelial skin closure. Note the normal glans fusion enclosing the neomeatus.

lengthen that region of the graft. This process continues up and down the entire graft. Releasing tension not only makes tubularization easier, but also decreases risk for postoperative fistulas or dehiscence.

There is usually some scarring of scrotal fat and dartos to the native urethra in the distal scrotum, and this is also taken down to relieve tension on the urethra.

Artificial erection

Artificial erection should *always* be done at this point to be certain the penis remains straight. It is a serious technical error to tubularize the graft when the penis is bent. The operative reports we review show that most surgeons assume the prior straightening remains successful, when that is often not the case when chordee excision, dorsal plication, or single ventral corporotomy rather than 3 corporotomies were done originally. Even if straightening maneuvers were not needed originally, artificial erection should still be done. We have been surprised in a few cases by new curvature that is difficult to explain, unless the prior artificial erection was falsely negative from leakage preventing firm distention of the corpora.

Recurrent VC found at this stage when straightening was done by 3 corporotomies almost always results from lengthwise graft contraction. When release of tethering dartos tissues and small subepithelial scars is not sufficient, additional interventions such as notching the graft edge, patch grafting, or complete graft replacement are needed and are described in Chapter 11.

Artificial erection sometimes reveals dorsal penile curvature at this stage. In contrast to dorsal curvature found before the graft is placed, which is corrected by Nesbit plication as described above, straightening at the final stage is achieved by Heineke-Mikulicz plication on each side of the graft opposite the point of maximum bending. It is much easier to correct dorsal curvature at the time of graft placement than at the time of tubularization, so carefully checking at STAC 2 is critical.

Glans wings dissection

A superficial incision into the marked lines along the junction of glans wings to graft is made with a sharp knife. Deeper dissection is done using tenotomy scissors, freeing the glans laterally to 3 and 9 o'clock and then superiorly another few millimeters off the corpora as needed to relieve tension. It is very important that there be no tension on the glans wings when they are closed later. Sometimes there are small bands of scar on the underside of the wings, which are released by lightly cutting across them with a knife.

Tubularizing the neourethral plate

A 6Fr stent is passed into the bladder and sewn to the glans stay suture. If the glans is < 14mm, we use a 5Fr feeding tube for urinary diversion to avoid the catheter exerting pressure on the edematous urethroplasty and glansplasty early postoperatively.

The first stitch of the neourethra is placed in the mid-glans as was previously described for TIP repair (Chapter 6). We use interrupted subepithelial 6-0 Vicryl for the first layer, moving distally to proximally. Grafts almost always heal with some asymmetry, especially in reoperations, and interrupted stitches best adjust for those minor differences from side to side. This closure also reduces the likelihood for postoperative fistulas, or for urinary extravasation if the stent comes out prematurely.

Next, an angiocatheter is inserted into the end of the neourethra and fluid is infused to test for leaks. Those are oversewn. Then, a second layer is run subepithelially from proximally to distally using 6-0 PDS.

Tunica vaginalis flap

Next, one testicle is exposed through the scrotal incision and the tunica vaginalis is opened transversely near the inferior pole. A stay stitch of 5-0 absorbable suture is then placed superficially at the inferior pole, and an additional 2 traction sutures hold the corners of the flap. With the scrub tech keeping the testicular stitch taut and an assistant lifting the other 2 stays cephalad, a rectangle of tunica vaginalis is dissected off the spermatic cord to the external ring. An army/navy retractor provides exposure superiorly to release bands tethering the flap. Medially and inferiorly a sheet of scrotal fat connects to the flap and this is also released, taking care to maintain sufficient length for the flap to easily cover the entire neourethra suture line without exerting tension.

If the flap is not adequately freed it can pull the penis laterally during erections. If the blood supply is not protected the flap can contract postoperatively and cause glans dehiscence, a fistula, or recurrent penile curvature.

The testicle is suture pexed back to the scrotal wall, and then the hemiscrotal compartment is sewn closed. These are important steps, and we have seen testicles that adhered to the urethra in the midline during healing when both these maneuvers were not done, causing discomfort when sitting.

The tunica vaginalis flap is spread out and first secured to the neourethra distally on either side of the suture line just below the meatus using 6-0 or 7-0 PDS. Additional sutures attach the flap to the corpora at intervals proximally. The assistant should hold the penis taut as these stitches are placed as another precaution to avoid tension from the flap.

Sometimes dartos muscular contractions are noted in the flap as it is manipulated. We incise transversely through the muscle avoiding damage to the pedicle, as otherwise these contractions postoperatively can cause the penis to intermittently torse.

Glansplasty

Next, the glans wings are lifted and stretched again to be certain there is no tension. This is a critical final check to reduce glans dehiscence. Then they are approximated as described for TIP repair. They are first aligned with a 9-0 Vicryl epithelial suture in the midglans. Then 3 interrupted 6-0 Vicryls are placed subepithelially from under that alignment stitch to the corona, the second also catching a bite of the tunica vaginalis to hold it in place. Glans fusion should be 3-5mm, even in small glans with a preoperative width < 14 mm.

We *never* suture close the glans epithelium, since stitches placed through the skin can leave visible marks or divots and are not needed.

Approximating the mucosal collar

Next, the mucosal collar is checked for scar or tension. After those are released the edges of the collar are sewn together in the midline with interrupted subepithelial 7-0 Vicryl. The collar should not exert any tension onto the glansplasty, but rather serves as an important buffer to help reduce tension from the shaft skin on the glans wings. We try to line up the incisions from the prior circumcision in redo cases for visual symmetry.

Shaft skin closure and scrotoplasty

Skin closure is often difficult in reoperations because of scarring and loss from prior surgeries. We emphasize again that surgeons should have a very low threshold to begin reoperations with STAC repair plus HBOT to give the skin an opportunity to rejuvenate and stretch. Otherwise, even if a urethroplasty graft heals satisfactorily, a lack of skin can lead to complications from tension or the need for a Cecil maneuver to be able to close the shaft - meaning there will be an additional operation done anyway to repair the urethra or take down the scrotum and repair the skin.

As in primary repairs, it is important that the skin be arranged so that it is symmetric in length from the base of the penis to the corona circumferentially, and does not exert tension on the urethroplasty or glansplasty. Scar excision or Heinecke-Mikulicz incisions across scars can lengthen the skin, as do oblique cuts as discussed in more detail in Chapter 21.

Scrotal skin is also scarred in many cases from prior surgery, especially when it was used to fill penile skin deficiencies. These scars are excised as much as possible, and, as with penis skin, surprising length can be gained by removing scar along the edge of the incision and/or by cutting obliquely into the skin.

Establishing the penoscrotal junction; Shaft skin closure

Next, the optimal location for the penoscrotal junction is determined. Although it is preferable to place it as low as possible to make the penis appear longer, sometimes shaft skin deficiency dictates the junction be raised up to 5mm higher to make the skin closure easier with less tension.

5-0 PDS tacks the penile skin at the penoscrotal junction to the tunica albuginea of the corpora on either side of the urethra. We then also sew the skin together temporarily with the same suture and leave a hemostat on a long tail to give counter-traction as shaft skin sizing and closure is done. Otherwise, it is easy to inadvertently pull the skin distally and further shorten it.

The scrotum is closed with continuous subepithelial 6-0 PDS. Penile shaft skin is approximated with interrupted subepithelial 7-0 Vicryl.

Bandage

A small Tegaderm™ is wrapped around the penis. Gauze is placed to hold the penis upwards against the abdomen and then large Tegaderms™ are placed over them to provide gentle compression. The bandage falls off spontaneously and is not replaced.

Postoperative Care

The stent diverts urine for 2 weeks to allow for some of the edema that develops within the neourethra to subside. The earlier the stent is removed, the greater the possibility that voiding against edema will cause urine extravasation and require the stent to be replaced. Analgesics, antibiotics and anticholinergics are prescribed as discussed for TIP repair in Chapter 6.

When the bandage comes off, Aquaphor is coated on the wounds with every diaper change, or 4 times daily in boys who are toilet trained. Beginning 1 month after surgery, betamethasone 0.1% cream is applied to the incisions if there was concern intraoperatively that they might contract, or if contraction is seen postoperatively, especially at the penoscrotal junction.

Results

The addition of HBOT has improved oral graft take in reoperations, such that most can be successfully tubularized. HBOT also helps revascularize native penile tissues, to the extent that results in these reoperations are similar to those from primary repairs. Fistulas or glans dehiscence develop in 20%. Other complications including meatal stenosis, urethral stricture, or diverticulum are unusual after reoperative STAC.

When there is extensive glans scarring and/or volume loss it might only be possible to approximate the glans wings with a single 6-0 Vicryl stitch at the corona. Naturally, glans dehiscence is more likely in this circumstance.

These outcomes are significantly improved over the nearly 40% complication rate WS previously reported after 2-stage graft reoperations (Snodgrass and Bush et al, 2009). This reflects changing to STAC and the addition of HBOT. In addition, in the earlier series WS joined segments of grafts, taking pieces of both lip and cheek before realizing that the lower lip graft properly harvested is sufficient for most urethroplasties, as shown in Figure 24. He did not measure the grafts to confirm healing without contracture, and he did not repeat an artificial erection at the second stage. Glans wings dissection was less extensive, and skin management did not reliably provide sufficient penile shaft coverage to avoid tension on the glansplasty.

The technical methods described in this chapter represent more than a decade of continued improvements made based on reviews of our outcomes.

Impact of Failed Repairs on Families

The patient, his parents, and even his siblings are all potentially impacted by failed hypospadias repair. We used the validated Impact of a Child with Congenital Anomalies on Parents survey to better understand the emotional effects of hypospadias on caregivers (Snodgrass et al, 2021). Of 260 participants, 64% responded they "worry a great deal about my son's health" which increased to 88% when repair was not successful. In fact, three-quarters of these wondered if their son would *ever* be healthy. For many these fears were compounded when the surgeon told them the complication rarely happened in his practice.

In our survey, a third of parents whose sons had failed surgery complained their surgeon did not explain things clearly, writing in free-text responses that they wanted more information about expected results and the potential for complications. Knowing this, we matter-of-factly inform parents the percentage likelihood of a fistula, glans dehiscence, or obstruction the proposed repair has in our hands, and then refer back to that conversation if one of those occurs.

This information does not relieve the disappointment that their son was one of the minority of patients who has a complication, but it provides perspective that says this is a known problem that happens in a known percentage of patients despite our efforts to prevent it. In fact, we emphasize before surgery that all parents hear there is, for example, a 5% risk of a fistula and reassure themselves it will not happen to their son - yet someone's boy is going to be a 5 percenter. For those parents it is reassuring to hear that we have seen the complication many times before and know how to correct it.

Older boys who develop a complication will naturally be apprehensive about having another operation. Those who have had several can become distraught. Accordingly, surgeons discussing reoperations should ask parents how their son is coping and recommend counselling if appropriate.

Siblings are also impacted, having previously seen their brother come home in pain with a catheter and bandages. Beyond that stress, some become jealous at the attention their brother is receiving, or angry when other family plans such as vacations are interrupted by the need for more surgery. Acknowledging these concerns can provide support to parents trying to cope with unsuccessful surgery.

Key Points

Management of complications and the results of reoperations are primarily determined by the extent of VC and the availability and health of penile skin. Accordingly, decision-making for reoperative TIP and STAC follows the same algorithm used in primary repairs.

However, the surgeon also has to consider the general health of penile tissues after failed operations. Decreased vascularity and scarring complicate wound healing and require attention beyond the technical details of surgical procedures. HBOT is currently the best adjunctive therapy to both increase vascularity and decrease tissue scarring. Accordingly, we have found it significantly improves graft and skin healing and so consider HBOT a necessary adjunctive treatment in essentially all reoperations.

The goal of reoperations is the same as for primary repairs, to make abnormal anatomy into a normal penis. This can usually be accomplished, although some damage to the glans cannot be repaired and lost glanular tissues cannot be replaced. Similarly, scarred penile skin that does not respond to revision plus HBOT may require skin grafts, which never have the same characteristics as penis skin. Furthermore, scars in the penile skin serve as a lifelong reminder of the birth defect for both the patient and his lovers.

In contrast, making a new neourethra is relatively easier. When the penis is straight, reoperative TIP or inlay grafting can be done when the urethral plate has minimal scarring. Otherwise, excision of the plate and replacement with a lip graft is best when scarring is more extensive, and as part of a reoperative STAC repair when the penis is bent 30 degrees or more.

It is important to emphasize again that the best source of urethroplasty grafts when the foreskin is no longer available is lip, and not cheek.

Failed hypospadias repair also exacts a toll on the parents, who often already feel guilt for their son having hypospadias now made even worse when surgery results in complications. But in the end it is the child who suffers from unsuccessful surgery, sometimes for his lifetime. There is no stronger way to say again that surgeons have an obligation to do everything possible to get the first repair right.

References

Ahmed H, Bush N and Snodgrass W: An objective analysis of over 600 paired graft measurements: prepucial vs oral results. Abstract presented to ESPU, Naples, 2024.

Bush N and Snodgrass W: Hyperbaric oxygen therapy improves oral graft take in hypospadias staged tubularized autograft reoperations. *J Urol* 202: 1, 2019

Husmann DA and Rathbun SR: Long-term followup of visual internal urethrotomy for management of short (less than 1cm) penile urethral strictures following hypospadias repair. *J Urol* 176: 1738, 2006

Husmann DA: Erectile dysfunction in patients undergoing multiple attempts at hypospadias repair: Etiologies and concerns. J Pediatr Urol 17(2): 166, 2021.

Jayanthi VR, McLorie GA, Khoury AE and Churchill BM: Can previously relocated penile skin be successfully used for salvage hypospadias repair? *J Urol* 152: 740, 1994

Snodgrass W and Bush NC: Re-operative urethroplasty after failed hypospadias repair: how prior surgery impacts risk for additional complications. *J Pediatr Urol* 13: 289, 2017

Snodgrass W and Bush NC: Staged tubularized autograft for primary proximal hypospadias repair with 30-degree or more curvature. *J Urol* 198: 680, 2017

Snodgrass WT, Bush N and Cost N: Algorithm for comprehensive approach to hypospadias reoperation using 3 techniques. *J Urol* 182: 2885, 2009

Snodgrass W, Grimsby G and Bush NC: Coronal fistula repair under the glans without reoperative glansplasty or urinary diversion. *J Pediatr Urol* 11: 39, 2015

Snyder CL, Evangelidis A, Snyder RP, Ostlie DJ, Gatti JM and Murphy JP: Management of urethral diverticulum complicating hypospadias repair. *J Pediatr Urol* 1: 81, 2005

Van der Toorn F, De Mooij K, Nijman R, Van der Horst E, Callewaert P, Steffens M, Hoebeke P, Van der Heijkant M, Froeling F, Wildhagen M, Willemsem S, Bryan S, and de Gier R: The Dutch hypospadias study: complications and prognostic factors after distal- and mid- type hypospadias repair. Abstract presented to the ESPU, Prague, 2015

Vallasciani S, Berrettini A, Nanni L, Manzoni G and Marrocco G: Observational retrospective study on acquired megalourethra after primary proximal hypospadias repair and its recurrence after tapering. *J Pediatr Urol* 9: 364, 2013

Ye WJ, Ping P, Liu YD, Li Z and Huang YR: Single stage dorsal inlay buccal mucosa graft with tubularized incised urethral plate technique for hypospadias reoperations. *Asian J Androl* 10: 682, 2008

Chapter 18

Hyperbaric Oxygen Therapy

Surgeons cannot only focus on technical performance and routine perioperative care to achieve the best outcomes in hypospadias repair. Although most complications result from surgical errors, poor wound healing also contributes. This is especially true in reoperations, with authors consistently reporting higher complications despite using the same operations and perioperative care they do for primary cases. We found that the first reoperative urethroplasty has double the risk for additional complications as did the initial repair, increasing to near 50% as the number of prior failures increases (Snodgrass & Bush, 2017).

This is largely due to decreased vascularity, which is not surprising given that the penis is an end organ and the tissues of most interest near and on the glans are furthest away from the main blood supply entering at the base.

This message was driven home to us by a 40-year old who presented after 10 failed repairs. WS successfully repaired his glans dehiscence, but a 4mm distal shaft fistula developed. His notes from the fistula closure stated the tissues looked ischemic, and the fistula soon recurred. That prompted a search for treatments to improve tissue vascularity before attempting another repair.

Testosterone has been advocated for this purpose in prepubertal hypospadias reoperations as discussed in Chapter 12, but seemed less likely to benefit a healthy adult. We could not find an available stem cell therapy. Then NB recalled a colleague who became a hyperbaric physician and began researching that option.

Our patient received perioperative HBOT. The tissues appeared healthier intraoperatively, and his second fistula closure was successful, with follow up to 6 years. This anecdotal case did not prove a benefit to HBOT, but it encouraged us to try it in other difficult situations, including patients with urethroplasty graft failures.

One criticism of HBOT is that the level of evidence for treatment is low. This relates to the difficulty in defining objective outcomes, as well as controlling confounding factors that impact wound healing and the results of reoperations. For example, a trial randomizing HBOT in patients undergoing hypospadias reoperation to determine if it decreases complications would have to control for many variables - including the number of prior operations, the original location of the meatus, the extent of VC and need for straightening procedures, the surgical techniques and variations in key steps as done by the participating surgeons, and the definition of outcomes and how they are assessed.

Paired graft measurements provided an objective way to test HBOT. Given the high complication rate in patients undergoing their 3rd or more reoperation, we created a protocol in consultation with hyperbaric medical experts for 20 preoperative dives to improve vascularity and prepare the graft bed, followed by 10 postoperative dives to support graft take. These patients were compared to controls who had fewer failed surgeries and so did not receive HBOT. Graft lengths and widths were recorded when they were placed and again at the next stage tubularization.

We found that patients receiving HBOT had significantly better oral graft healing, with less graft contracture and fewer graft failures – even though they were at higher risk due to having significantly more failed operations (Bush and Snodgrass, 2019).

After that study, we tweaked the protocol for 2 reasons. First, was the difficulty, and sometimes the impossibility, to obtain insurance authorization for preoperative treatment. Second, there was subjectively more bothersome bleeding during surgery from revascularization. Our current regimen is explained below. Nevertheless, we re-evaluated graft outcomes in a much larger cohort of over 600 patients and again found that HBOT improves oral graft healing in reoperations, in fact with a risk of contracture the same as in primary grafts. Furthermore, this translated into fewer skin and urethroplasty complications (Ahmed et al, 2024).

We also changed indications for treatment, nearly always recommending HBOT to patients undergoing any reoperative hypospadias repair. We are also exploring its use in primary perineal repairs with little ventral penile skin.

Effects of HBOT

Tissue hypoxia is an underlying factor contributing to poor graft take and skin flap loss. HBOT has several positive effects on wound healing. It decreases hypoxia and edema, releases stem cells, and stimulates angiogenesis (Gill and Bell, 2004; Thom, 2011; Francis and Baynosa, 2017).

We reported that oral grafts objectively benefited from perioperative HBOT. This improvement was so obvious in terms of robust appearance and reduced scarring along the junction to skin that a blinded trial would be difficult. In addition, we observed diminished scarring under the penile skin despite many failed surgeries in those who received HBOT. After multiple failed operations dartos tissues can be so thick and indurated that it is difficult to cut through them with scissors. Soon after beginning HBOT we realized there was usually much less reaction, to the extent that some had tissues which seemed nearly virginal.

We also observed that penile skin healing improved with HBOT. Adding treatment to reoperative STAC repair made the skin more supple and elastic, reducing need for scrotal flaps, Cecil maneuvers, and skin grafts despite the skin deficiency most patients with failed surgery have when they present.

However, these benefits are not universally realized and HBOT is not a panacea to prevent complications. Furthermore, decreased scarring and increased vascularity are difficult to quantify objectively. But, like the importance of choosing the best operation and using good surgical technique, HBOT helps improve outcomes, especially in reoperations – where the need and the benefit are most obvious.

Most parents also comment that they see less swelling and bruising when their son received HBOT compared to their recollections of prior operations done without it. They often report that overall healing seemed faster and less uncomfortable. Plastic surgeons have recognized similar benefits and some now incorporate HBOT in their postop management of face lifts, for example, as do athletes hoping for improved healing after an injury.

Indications for HBOT

HBOT is approved for the treatment of "compromised skin flaps or grafts", and for "chronic nonhealing wounds" both of which describe findings in some primary and most reoperative hypospadias surgeries.

How Many Dives Are Needed?

Available data suggest that approximately 20 dives are needed to stimulate angiogenesis. Fewer dives are still useful to increase available tissue oxygen, but effects are longer lasting when accompanied by revascularization (Wright, 2001).

Generally, treatment for other non-hypospadias conditions with impaired wound healing has averaged approximately 30 dives. We have recommended 30 dives for patients with severe skin deficiency and scarring, and in those who contract their urethroplasty grafts despite receiving 20 postoperative dives. Otherwise, a maximum of 20 dives seems sufficient for hypospadias wound healing in otherwise healthy patients.

HBOT Protocol

As mentioned above, we changed the protocol after our publication regarding graft healing. We currently recommend 1-5 dives before a reoperation. The purpose of preoperative treatment is to prepare the tissues for the stress of additional surgery and start stem cell induction. However, if preop treatment cannot be done for a variety of reasons, postoperative treatment is still beneficial.

Following a reoperative STAC 1 we recommend 15 perioperative dives. Similarly, 20 perioperative dives are done to support reoperative STAC 2 graft revascularization. A total of 15 perioperative dives are then recommended again with reoperative STAC 3. Additional dives to a total of 30 are sometimes advised if scarring is subjectively judged to warrant further treatment, such as in those patients with tendency for keloiding or severe hypertrophic scarring.

Treatment Parameters

Hypospadias patients are exposed to 2 ATM pressure for 1 hour, breathing 100% oxygen. An additional 15 minutes is usually needed to reach that depth, and another 15 minutes to surface afterwards, meaning that each session lasts 1.5 hours. This is the recommended treatment for compromised grafts and flaps (Francis and Baynosa, 2017).

Air "breaks" are thought to stimulate stem cell release by simulating relative tissue hypoxia after breathing 100% oxygen. Older patients who will tolerate putting on a mask to provide room air for 5 minutes during treatment have 2 or 3 such breaks.

Surgeons should be aware that many "spa" hyperbaric facilities dive patients to only 1.3 or 1.5 ATM. While reviewing treatment in patients who had graft contraction despite HBOT, we found that some had less than the 2 ATM recommended, and/or a total treatment duration of 1 hour, meaning they spent less time at depth.

Multichamber Versus Monochamber

HBOT can be administered simultaneously to multiple patients seated in a large chamber, or to 1 patient at a time in a monochamber. To safely treat more than 1 patient in a multichamber, 100% oxygen is delivered through a helmet to each individual rather than filling the entire chamber. This arrangement makes air breaks easier, since the helmet is simply removed for 5 minutes. It also allows a parent to sit with the child during treatment.

Monochambers are more prevalent in the US. Patients are usually treated alone in these, which are filled with 100% oxygen so that helmets are not needed. However, the youngest children (< 2 years of age) will fit in the chamber with a parent and often are more comfortable that way. Most other children aged 2 years and up tolerate treatment in monochambers, since parents are visible and they are distracted by a television screen placed just outside (Figure 1). A disadvantage is that air breaks in monochambers require a mask be worn for the 5 minutes to deliver room air, which young children cannot manage alone and so are typically not performed until children are able to follow instructions regarding this.

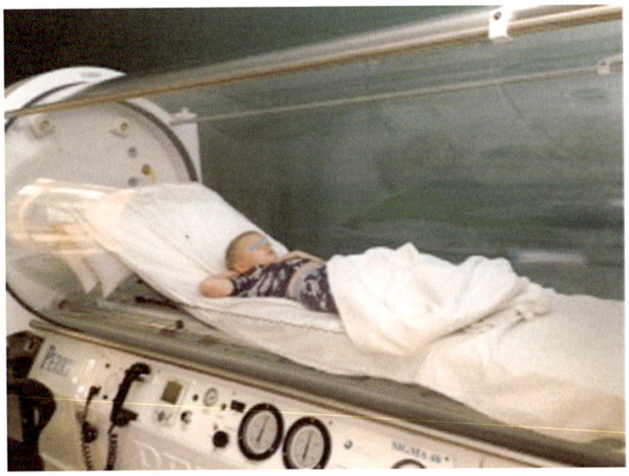

Figure 1. Young boy in a monochamber.
This young patient is comfortably laying in a monochamber watching TV as he receives HBOT. His mother is nearby, just outside the picture. She told him he was riding in a spaceship.

Although we originally thought that young boys would require treatment with a parent in multichambers, HBOT facilities informed us that a parent can accompany them in a monochamber. Furthermore, most toddlers accept therapy alone after acclimation by the initial dive. Accordingly, we have referred infants and toddlers for treatment in monochambers.

Myringotomy

Increasing pressure requires equilibration of the gradient between the middle ear and the external environment. Older boys and men can readily "pop" their ears, but that can be more difficult for younger patients. In part, this depends on the treatment facility and the speed at which compression is done. If a boy appears uncomfortable during this phase, slowing the rate of pressurization can help him acclimate.

Some patients are not able to tolerate compression and develop ear pain. Myringotomy allows the pressure to rapidly equilibrate, making routine treatment possible. Initially, we recommended myringotomy for boys less than 3 years of age, but local hyperbaric facilities found that most patients do not require ear tubes if taken to depth more slowly during the initial dives.

We have also learned that pre-treatment with Afrin nose spray and Zyrtec before each dive can help avoid myringotomy, as can instructions to make "shark jaws", opening and closing the mouth to equilibrate pressure.

Effects of HBOT on grafts

As mentioned above, we found that patients who received perioperative HBOT had better graft outcomes than patients who did not (Bush and Snodgrass, 2019). All these had reoperations using oral mucosa grafts. Treated patients had significantly more failed operations than did those not treated (mean 3.5 vs 2.5, p=0.001). Despite the worse baseline features, there was significantly less graft contracture (9% vs 26%, p=0.04) and significantly less graft failure defined as graft contracture > 50% (6% vs 28%, p=0.03) in patients who received HBOT. A comparison of treated and untreated grafts is shown in Figure 2.

While partially contracted grafts can sometimes still be tubularized, scarring and loss of length and/or width increase the difficulty of the procedure and the potential risks for complications. In fact, we reported that graft contracture > 10% increases skin and urethroplasty complications by more than 60% (Ahmed et al, 2024).

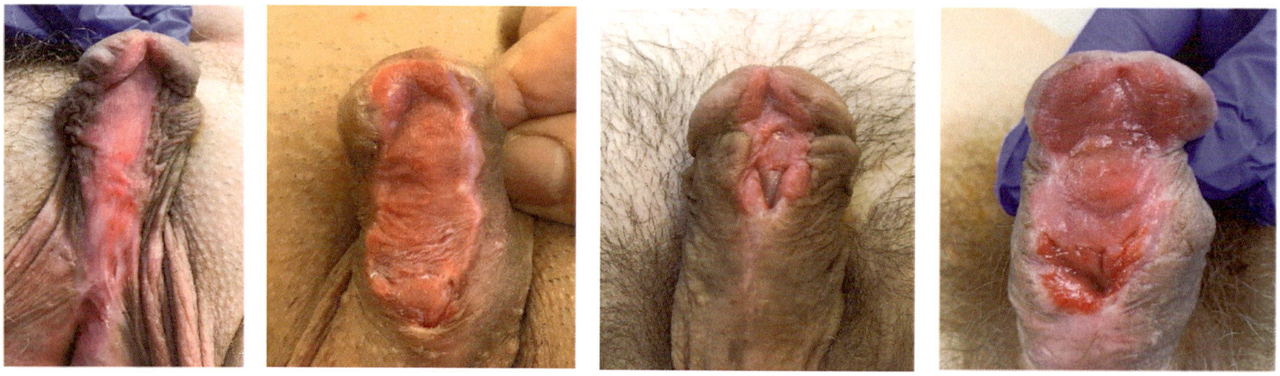

Figure 2. Impact of HBOT on oral mucosa grafts in reoperations.
A, no HBOT. There is graft contracture with loss of width, particularly on the left side extending from near the proximal urethrostomy to within the glans. The junction to skin is also difusely irregular from graft loss along the edges. B, no HBOT. Graft contracture and visible scarring are seen along the left junction of the graft to shaft skin extending into the glans. Scars within the glans make graft tubularization and glansplasty particularly difficult, and usually require distal patch re-grafting. C, no HBOT. This patient had graft failure with > 50% contracture. Note the visible graft scarring and also the thickened junction of graft to skin bilaterally. D, another graft treated with HBOT. The graft is smooth and symmetrical with no visible scarring or thickening within the graft or at its junction to shaft skin and glans wings.

Side Effects

We reported that one 7-year-old out of 21 prepubertal boys developed ear pain and required myringotomy to continue treatment (Bush and Snodgrass, 2019). That was the only side effect observed in that series of 32 treated patients. Our use has steadily increased but no other ill-effects besides the occasional ear pain have occurred. Temporary change in vision (myopia) has been reported in a small number of patients undergoing HBOT, but is reported to be reversible usually within a few weeks after treatment is completed.

Disadvantages of HBOT

There are several disadvantages to HBOT. First, treatment is expensive, and not affordable for many patients without insurance coverage. The cash price is at least $400 per dive, although many facilities charge substantially more. Second, treatment is time-consuming. Added to the 1.5 hour dive is the additional time needed to change in 100% cotton clothing before entering and again upon leaving the chamber, and the commute to and from the facility. Third, although 2 dives can be made daily, some insurances will only pay for 1 a day, meaning a course of 20 dives takes a month since most facilities do not treat on weekends. In addition, many facilities are not accustomed to treating children, and some have policy restrictions forbidding it. However, after the initial dives most facilities rapidly adjust to pediatric treatment and even enjoy the opportunity to dive a young and otherwise healthy patient. Another challenge is insurance authorization can be difficult to obtain.

Despite these disadvantages, parents readily accept HBOT for their sons. In fact, many inquire about it for primary repairs even though that is not part of our routine management. Parents of boys with unsuccessful hypospadias surgery tolerate the inconveniences of treatment for the hope of a better outcome and the feeling of contributing to the process. And many parents have commented on how much better the tissues have looked after HBOT when compared to surgeries their son had without it.

Insurance Authorization

Although a urologist may recommend HBOT, insurance authorization has to be obtained by the treating facility. Justification in hypospadias surgery is based on "compromised skin flaps or grafts" and "chronic nonhealing wounds".

Approval for preoperative therapy can be challenging, in part because Medicare will not pay for it and so other insurances may also refuse it. However, in cases of severe vascular compromise, such as those with high-risk skin grafts, preop therapy to improve the vascular bed is considered a standard of care by many treating facilities.

Postoperative therapy most often is approved. A picture taken intraoperatively at the conclusion of surgery and forwarded to the HBOT facility with an operative note mentioning concerns regarding vascularity helps obtain authorization. We have found that waiting to start HBOT until actual skin flap necrosis develops, typically between 7-10 days postoperatively, is less effective in helping to salvage at-risk penile skin.

Starting HBOT Therapy

Some US surgeons practice in areas that either lack an HBOT facility or one which will treat boys. This was more common when we first incorporated treatment into our hypospadias reoperation protocol, and today fewer facilities refuse to treat children. Families that do not have nearby access to HBOT have arranged to stay near a facility for the duration of treatment needed for each operation.

Colleagues outside the US commonly say that HBOT is not available. However, facilities generally exist in developed countries, and usually can be persuaded to dive boys with hypospadias. Published data showing improved results and decreased complications have also convinced some national health services to approve treatment.

Probably the greatest obstacle to date has been a lack of enthusiasm by surgeons to persuade facilities and insurances to treat hypospadias patients when they are not yet convinced HBOT is necessary.

Key Points

Reports summarizing hypospadias reoperations consistently find increased complications compared to primary repairs, which relates to decreased tissue vascularity and impaired wound healing. HBOT improves vascularity and tissue oxygen and therefore deserves consideration as adjunctive treatment to proper surgical technique. We published objective evidence that HBOT improves oral graft healing in reoperations. Furthermore, we have shown that less graft contracture decreases skin and urethroplasty complications. The protocol we recommend is based on expert opinion, and so it may be that some patients would have satisfactory results with fewer dives while others might require more. Regardless, the evidence is clear that HBOT improves graft and skin healing in reoperations and that is sufficient reason for hypospadias surgeons to begin using it routinely.

References

Ahmed H, Bush N and Snodgrass W: An objective analysis of over 600 paired graft measurements: prepucial vs oral results. Abstract presented to ESPU, Naples, 2024.

Bush N and Snodgrass W: Hyperbaric oxygen therapy improves oral graft take in hypospadias staged autograft reoperations. *J Urol* 202: 1, 2019

Francis A and Baynosa RC: Hyperbaric oxygen therapy for the compromised graft or flap. *Adv Wound Care* 6: 23, 2017

Gill AL and Bell CN: Hyperbaric oxygen: its uses, mechanisms of action and outcomes. *QJM* 97: 385, 2004

Snodgrass W and Bush N: Re-operative urethroplasty after failed hypospadias repair: how prior surgery impacts risk for additional complications. *J Pediatri Urol* 13: 289e, 2017a

Thom SR: Hyperbaric oxygen–its mechanisms and efficacy. *Plast Reconstr Surg* 127: 131, 2011

Wright J: Hyperbaric oxygen therapy for wound healing. Available at http://www.worldwidewounds.com/2001/april/Wright/HyperbaricOxygen.html, 2001

Managing Penile Skin

Chapter 19

Prepucioplasty

The goal of hypospadias surgery is to make the abnormal anatomy of this birth defect into a normal penis. That includes managing the incomplete foreskin that most boys with hypospadias have, repairing it into either a normal prepuce or removing it by circumcision.

This is not a minor consideration. Boys who live in communities in which few are circumcised who have their foreskin removed during hypospadias surgery still look different from "normal" even if their repair is otherwise aesthetically perfect. Looking different is a major concern for teens and adults, who worry about the questions friends and lovers may ask when they see their circumcision.

Nevertheless, many surgeons will not offer prepucioplasty, some erroneously informing parents that there are too many complications when it is done, or that the foreskin does not look or function normally, or that it will not retract after puberty. Few recommend that interested parents seek another surgeon willing to reconstruct the foreskin.

This chapter explains the steps in prepucioplasty and discusses outcomes.

Surgical Technique

Patient Selection

We simply ask parents if they planned on circumcision or leaving the foreskin natural before their son was born, and then manage the skin accordingly. Nearly all boys can have hypospadias repair with prepucioplasty. This includes most of those with proximal hypospadias, if the family agrees to harvesting oral mucosa for the graft urethroplasty.

However, we advise circumcision when a urethroplasty graft is needed and the glans width is less than 10mm, simply because foreskin heals more thin than does graft taken from any other location, including the lip. Using foreskin grafts in this uncommon situation reduces the likelihood for glans dehiscence. On the other hand, glans dehiscence is less obvious when the glans is covered by foreskin, so we discuss that option as well.

Rarely, the partial foreskin does not extend ventrally beyond 3 and 9 o'clock, or it is relatively small in comparison to a larger than usual glans, which potentially make foreskin reconstruction without tension on the skin closure difficult. These can be anticipated preoperatively and the family informed that circumcision could be necessary if prepucioplasty cannot be done without tension.

We have also realized that a single dorsal midshaft skin hump decreases the likelihood for a successful prepucioplasty, because efforts to smooth the hump devascularize the foreskin distally. Similarly, patients with distal hypospadias plus penile torsion heal better from circumcision than prepucioplasty because the necessary manipulations to reduce twisting and then reconstruct the foreskin can devascularize the prepucial skin.

Small foreskins, midshaft dorsal humps and hypospadias plus penile torsion are all uncommon, meaning

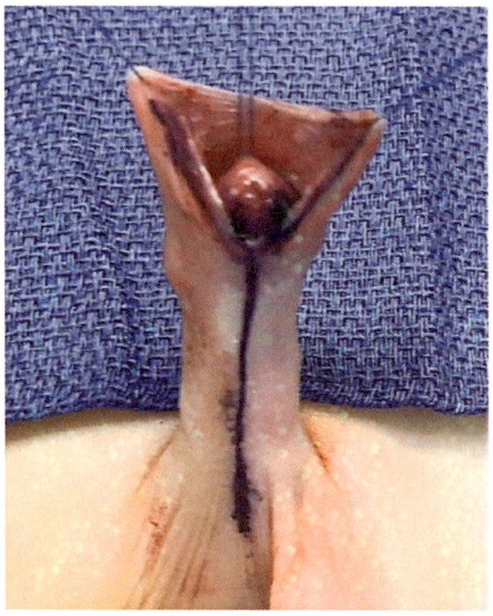

Figure 1. Ventral skin incision for distal TIP with prepucioplasty.
This incision provides excellent exposure for hypospadias repair and then closes into a normal median raphe. The penis should not be degloved dorsally when prepucioplasty will be done.

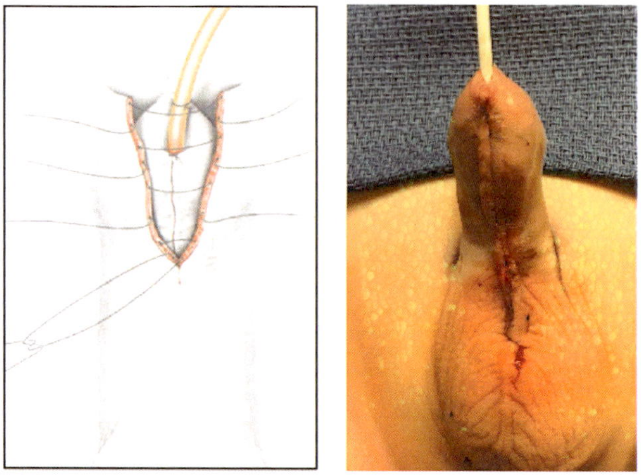

Figure 2. Completing prepucioplasty and the final result. The inner prepuce, dartos, and outer skin are each closed separately using interrupted subepithelial Vicryl stitches. The outer skin is closed to give a normal, circular tip as shown here, even if it will not then retract intraoperatively.

there are few relative contraindications to prepucioplasty when that is the family's preference.

Operative Technique

The major difference in distal TIP with prepucioplasty versus circumcision is that the penile skin is not degloved dorsally when the foreskin will be reconstructed (Figure 1). Instead, the corners of the dorsal hood are identified and stays placed, from which the lines of incision are made ventrally to beneath the meatus and down the midline of the shaft towards the scrotum.

Dissection on the ventral shaft is done directly under the skin to preserve dartos for a flap to cover the neourethra.

Once the ventral penis is degloved, the operation proceeds as usual, as described in Chapter 6, except that the suture securing the stent is tied with a longer loop. That makes it easier to cut and then remove the stent postoperatively when the foreskin is swollen. After urethroplasty, ventral dartos preserved during the initial dissection is made into a flap to cover the neourethra.

Skin closure is done in 3 layers. First the inner prepuce is approximated with interrupted subepithelial 7-0 Vicryl stitches. That closure is reinforced with a few additional interrupted stitches approximating the dartos. Finally, the outer skin is closed, also with interrupted subepithelial 7-0 Vicryl (Figure 2).

Sometimes closure of the outer skin to give a normal appearance with a circular opening at the tip prevents the foreskin from retracting intraoperatively. Originally we then stopped the closure lower so that the foreskin would retract. However, that leaves the abnormal appearance of a partial foreskin. Today we suture to make a normal-appearing foreskin and do not worry if it does not initially retract – knowing that it will with time, like a normal foreskin gradually does. However, it is often possible to retract the reconfigured foreskin intraoperatively, albeit with a narrowed waist until it stretches with time (Figure 3). Alternatively, some surgeons prefer to make a dorsal Heineke-Mikulicz incision at the 6 o'clock position, closing it transversely to allow easier retraction of the foreskin without compromising the aesthetics of the ventral foreskin reconstruction. This maneuver is not recommended during foreskin reconstruction at a STAC repair, since it leaves a scar in the tissue which will later be used for grafting. But it is a helpful maneuver during distal TIP with foreskin reconstruction or at STAC 3 with foreskin reconstruction if the foreskin reconstruction subjectively feels too tight.

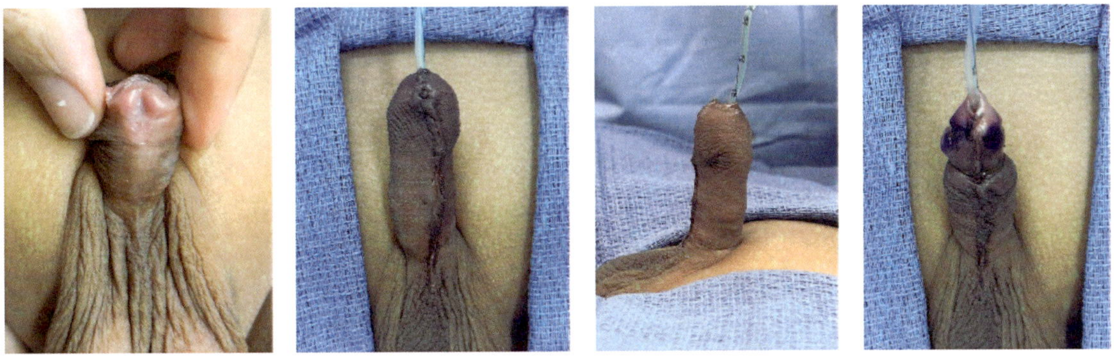

Figure 3. Distal TIP with prepucioplasty.
A, preop appearance in a patient with subcoronal hypospadias. B,C, typical results of prepucioplasty. The outer skin is closed to give a normal, circular tip as shown here. D, in most patients with distal hypospadias, the reconstructed foreskin will retract, simply leaving a slightly narrowed waist as is typical in boys whose foreskin has only recently begun to retract. However, parents are instructed to avoid retracting the skin for several months postoperatively in order to avoid tension on the healing skin.

We inform all parents that postoperative swelling of the foreskin may prevent retraction of the foreskin for several months, meaning that the hypospadias repair cannot be immediately inspected.

Prepucioplasty During Proximal Hypospadias Repair

The procedure is the same for prepucioplasty during proximal TIP repair, except the initial plan of dissection. Degloving is done ventrally, which gives excellent exposure for artificial erection. But for proximal TIP, the urethroplasty is covered by a tunica vaginalis flap (Figure 4). Accordingly, the plane of dissection should leave the dartos tissue with the shaft skin, just as described for STAC repair, in case significant penile curvature is encountered that will need to be straightened with corporotomies and covered with a dartos flap from the skin.

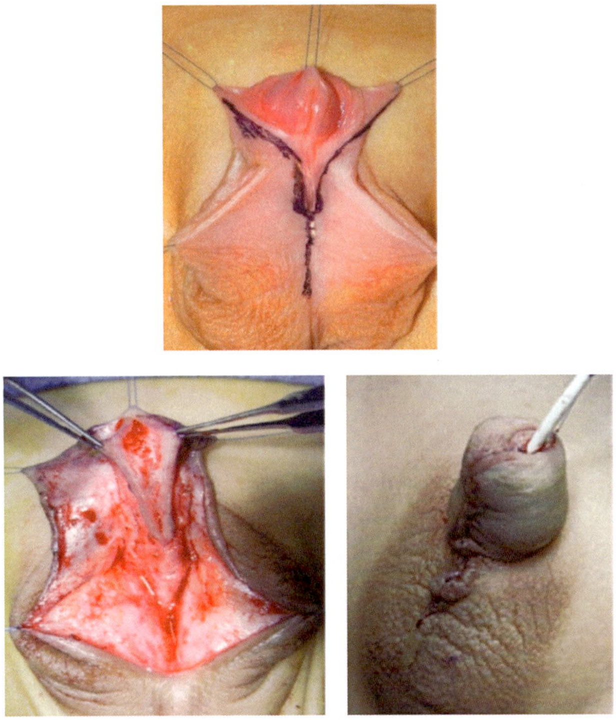

Figure 4. Proximal TIP with prepucioplasty.
A, incision lines are similar to those made for distal TIP with prepucioplasty, but extend lower to beneath the proximal meatus. B, after release of penile and scrotal dartos there is excellent exposure for hypospadias repair. C, completed repair.

If there is curvature that measures less than 30°, dissection can extend completely around the penile shaft *under* the dorsal skin without complete degloving up to the level of the corona dorsally. A vessel loop is used to retract the skin out of the way during dorsal plication.

As mentioned in Chapter 6, we use a tunica vaginalis flap to cover the neourethra in all proximal repairs, which is easy to access through the ventral incision. After urethroplasty and glansplasty, the shaft skin at the penoscrotal junction should be sutured to the

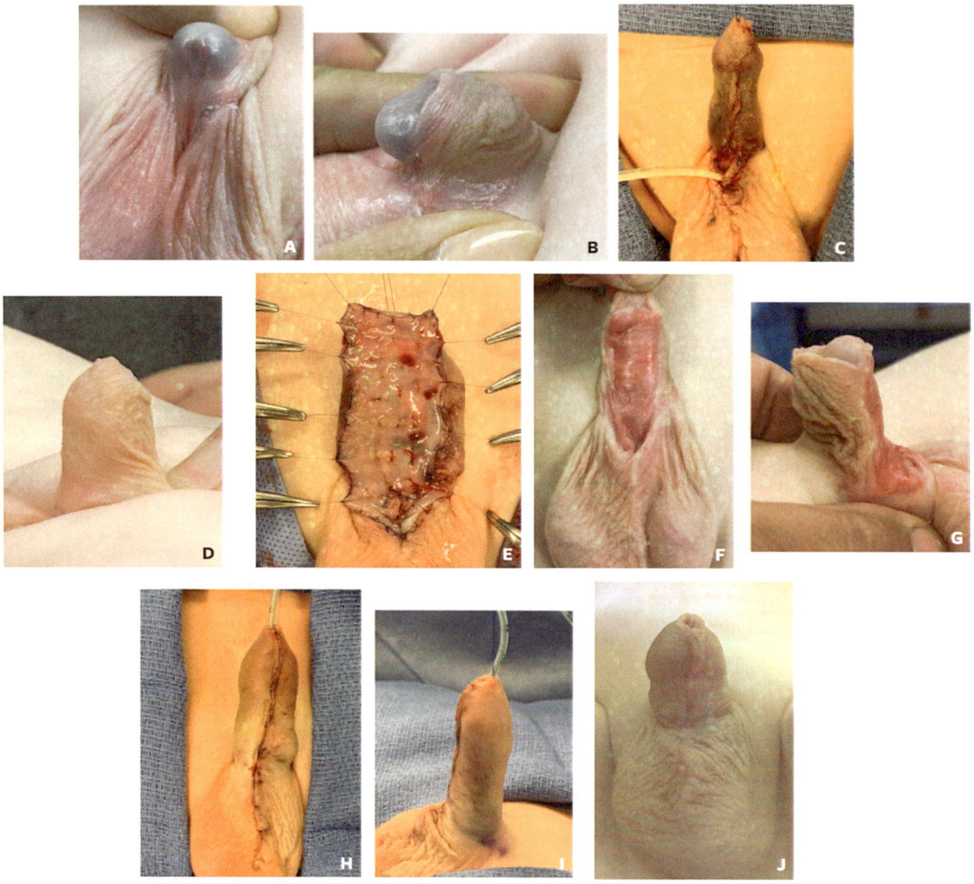

Figure 5. STAC repair with prepucioplasty.
A,B, scrotal hypospadias with 95° ventral curvature and essentially no ventral penile shaft skin. C, appearance after STAC 1 with 3 corporotomies, ventral skin rearrangement, urethrostomy and prepucioplasty. D, straight penis with symmetric shaft skin and foreskin 6 months later. E, lower lip urethroplasty graft has been placed at STAC 2, extending from the urethrostomy to the tip of the opened glans. F,G, healed lip graft 6 months later at STAC 3. Note the available foreskin for prepucioplasty. H,I, completed foreskin reconstruction. J, normal uncircumcised appearance several months postop.

corpora on either side of the urethra to better define the penile shaft. This junction can be moved a few millimeters distally if needed to assure adequate skin for prepucioplasty.

Prepucioplasty is a standard step in all primary STAC 1 repairs. That foreskin is then removed during STAC 2 to make the urethroplasty graft when the family prefers the final outcome to be a circumcised penis. When a natural penile appearance is preferred, the reconstructed foreskin is opened in the ventral midline during STAC 2 and lip mucosa is used for the urethroplasty graft. An example is shown in Figure 5.

Postoperative Care

The reconstructed foreskin needs no special care. We specifically instruct caregivers *not* to manipulate the skin, especially in the initial weeks during healing when the foreskin is edematous. It is better for the surgeon to first test retractability before parents do. We also inform them it is not necessary to retract the foreskin for hygiene until the foreskin retracts on its own, in keeping with the American Academy of Pediatrics guidelines for care of the uncircumcised penis.

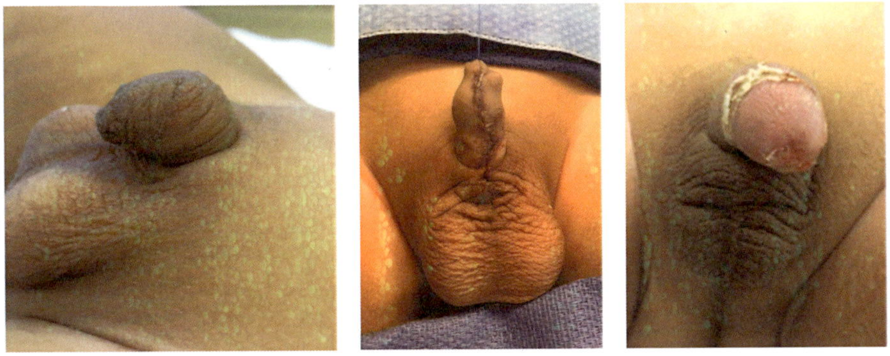

Figure 6. Skin slough after prepucioplasty with midshaft dorsal skin hump.
A, single dorsal midpenile skin hump. B, immediate postoperative appearance after distal TIP with prepucioplasty. C, the foreskin sloughed early postoperatively, leaving a circumcised appearance that did not require skin revision.

The main "disadvantage" of prepucioplasty is that the associated hypospadias repair may not be seen postoperatively for some time to confirm healing without glans dehiscence. However, glans dehiscence should not occur in more than 5% of distal cases, and there is no urgency to identify it when it happens.

Topical Steroids

Physiologic phimosis responds to topical betamethasone for the skin to retract, and can be applied to the reconstructed prepuce to induce its retraction and expose the repaired glans after hypospadias repair. However, there is rarely a clinical need for treatment before the skin retracts naturally.

Betamethasone can also be used on the suture line twice daily for 6-12 weeks beginning 1 month postoperatively if it appears to contract, similar to its benefit after hypospadias repair with circumcision when skin contraction is noted around the penoscrotal junction.

Results

We did prepucioplasty in 91 consecutive patients whose parents preferred that option, which comprised 17% of our distal repairs. No conversion to circumcision was done intraoperatively. The foreskin retracted by 6 months in all but 5 boys, who were successfully treated with topical betamethasone. A single late circumcision was done for BXO 5 years later.

Our series compared these patients to others operated during the same study period who had distal TIP with circumcision. There was no difference in either urethroplasty complications or skin problems resulting in reoperation, the latter occurring in 2% of cases. Those were a persistent dorsal skin hump in 1 and BXO mentioned above in another. There were no foreskin fistulas or dehiscences (Snodgrass and Bush et al, 2013), although we have seen each of these infrequently since that time.

We also reported prepucioplasty in 20% of consecutive proximal TIP repairs, finding that none had either a urethroplasty or skin complication (Snodgrass and Bush, 2011). Similarly, prepucioplasty was done in 10% of STAC patients, with 1 developing a fistula.

As mentioned above, skin abnormalities including a single dorsal midline hump or penile torsion can impact healing after prepucioplasty, presumedly because of the altered vascularity of the affected penile skin. Skin reactions, sloughing and foreskin dehiscence can develop around 10 days postoperatively.

We have not found a reliable way to manage single dorsal midline humps without unwanted skin reactions. For example, we attempted to smooth the hump by removing underlying dartos, but that caused the foreskin to slough (Figure 6). Varying degrees of ventral skin reactions have occurred despite less manipulation such that we recommend HBOT in these patients to try to improve their vascularity.

Similarly, we have not found a means to avoid skin complications related to hypospadias with penile torsion, either. Figure 7 shows a distal hypospadias managed by TIP repair with prepucioplasty in which

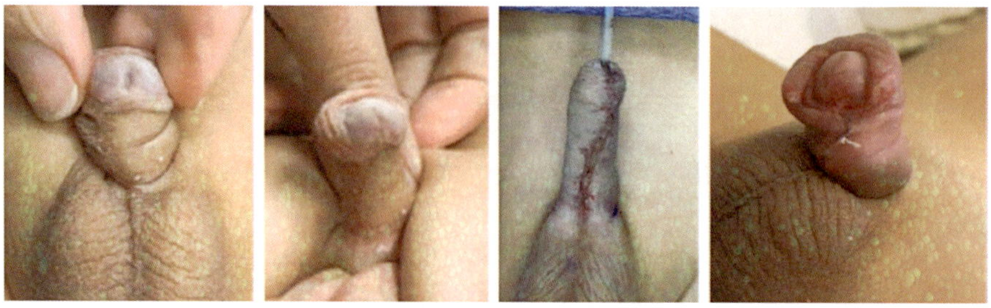

Figure 7. Foreskin dehiscence related to penile torsion.
A, B, coronal hypospadias with penile torsion. Note the median raphe extends to the right of midline and that there is left lateral skin deficiency. C, skin closure showing the median raphe now deviating to the left because of the need to rotate skin from the right to address the relative skin deficiency. D, foreskin dehiscence occurred on postoperative day 10.

the foreskin dehisced. When circumcision is done instead, varying degrees of ventral skin reaction and loss can still develop.

When the entire prepucioplasty dehisces, either circumcision or repeat foreskin repair can be done (Figure 8).

A foreskin fistula can also occur after prepucioplasty, with urine exiting the urethral meatus and then escaping through the hole in the ventral foreskin (Figure 9). We have encountered that complication, and found it was straightforward to repair the foreskin fistula after ensuring there was no simultaneous urethral fistula by pressurizing the repair with an angiocath just as we do in STAC 3 repairs.

Most other authors describing hypospadias repair with prepucioplasty had similar findings to ours, with urethroplasty and skin complications comparable to repairs done with circumcision. However, Klijn et al (2001) said that foreskin reconstruction led to complications in 33% of their patients, with 21% isolated

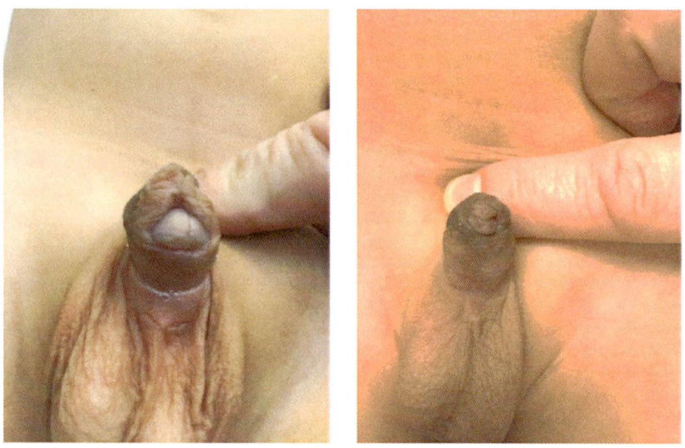

Figure 8. Foreskin dehiscence and redo prepucioplasty.
A, the foreskin repair completely dehisced. B, the parents preferred repeat prepucioplasty, which was successful

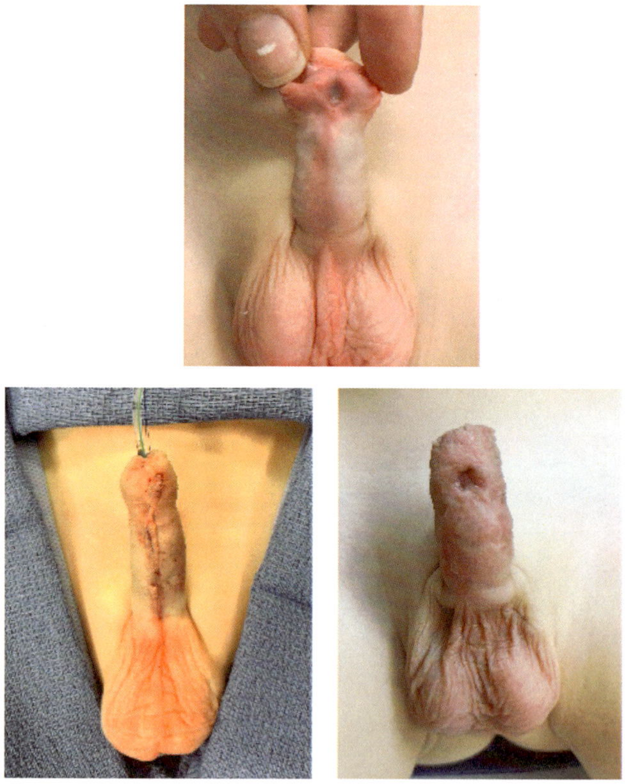

Figure 9. Foreskin fistula.
A, preop appearance. B, intraop appearance after distal TIP and foreskin reconstruction. C, the patient healed with an isolated foreskin fistula, which was repaired.

to the prepucioplasty. These included foreskin fistulas and partial or complete dehiscence.

It is important to note that most of these were Mathieu repairs, which uses ventral shaft skin in the urethroplasty. Antoa et al (2006) similarly found that Mathieu and the related Barcat procedure performed with concomitant prepucioplasty had significantly greater foreskin complications than did prepucioplasty with MAGPI and TIP. This increased risk for foreskin fistulas or dehiscences when flap urethroplasties were done likely relates to a tighter skin closure.

Klijn also instructed parents to begin retracting the foreskin 10 days postoperatively, well before edema resolves. Most likely this added more stress to the suture line and accounted for the increased complications they reported in contrast to other authors.

Outcome at Puberty

Critics claim that successful prepucioplasties in childhood develop secondary phimosis during puberty. To our knowledge that has not been documented, and we have not encountered it in our practice. Rather, the tendency is for improved retraction of the reconstructed foreskin as time passes, mimicking the natural history of unoperated foreskin (Figure 10).

Even if a few patients develop problems related to a reconstructed foreskin during puberty, surgeons should still perform prepucioplasty when parents request it. Phimosis can be treated with steroid creams, or with a minor Heineke-Mikulicz release as needed. If the teen or adult requests circumcision instead, that can be done.

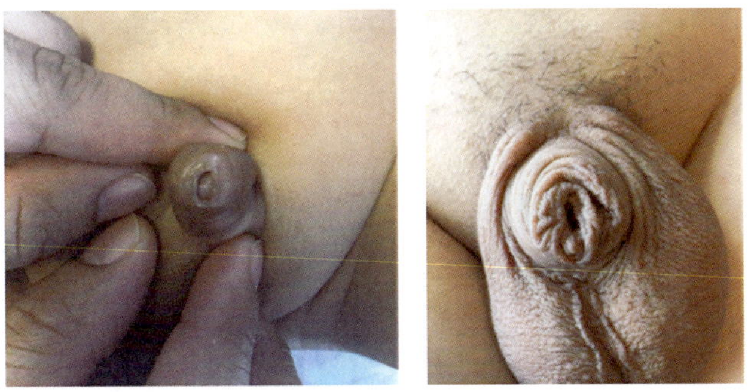

Figure 10. Pubertal follow up after childhood prepucioplasty.
A, the reconstructed foreskin partially retracts to expose only part of the glans prepubertally. B, natural appearance of the same patient at puberty. The foreskin retracted freely and normally.

However, when circumcision is done during childhood repair because the surgeon prefers it, there is no way to restore a complete foreskin if the child grown into a man wants it back.

Learning Curve for Prepucioplasty

Our study also asked if there was a difference in complications following the first 50 prepucioplasties versus those done later (Snodgrass and Bush et al, 2013). We found results were the same, meaning there was no learning curve to this procedure, which WS learned from watching a single operation during a visiting professorship to Sweden. Consequently, there is no reason that others capable of performing hypospadias repair cannot similarly repair the foreskin.

As stated above, we initially tailored the foreskin repair to ensure that the skin retracted. Today we emphasize reconstruction to achieve a normal-appearing foreskin, even if that results in temporary phimosis.

Key Points

Prepucioplasty does not increase either urethroplasty or skin complication after TIP or STAC hypospadias repairs and can be done in nearly all patients who request it. Foreskin repairs done with flap-based distal repairs such at Mathieu or Barcat are associated with a higher rate of prepucial complications.

The main contraindications are a disproportionately small foreskin relative to the glans size that results in tension on the skin approximation, or glans width less than 10mm during STAC repair since a prepucial graft is less likely than a relatively thicker lip graft to result in glans dehiscence. Both these are rarely encountered.

Hypospadias repair when there is also penile torsion or a single dorsal midline hump has increased likelihood for postoperative skin complications whether prepucioplasty or circumcision is done. Nevertheless, if the reconstructed foreskin dehisces it can often be sewn back together once the skin has healed.

Prepucioplasty is important to many families, especially those living in societies in which a circumcised penis is not the norm. A hypospadias repair that heals without complication with a normal meatus still cannot be considered a success if the patient believes his penis to be different than that of others.

Any surgeon with the skills to repair hypospadias can reconstruct the foreskin, too. Those who choose not to do so should not mislead parents about the results of this procedure, but rather simply recommend them to a willing surgeon.

References

Antao B, Lansdale N, Roberts J, and Mackinnon E: Factors affecting the outcome of foreskin reconstruction in hypospadias surgery. *J Pediatr Urol* 3: 127, 2007

Klijn A, Dik P, and de Jong, TPVM: Results of preputial reconstruction in 77 boys with distal hypospadias. *J Urol* 165: 1255, 2001.

Snodgrass W and Bush N: Tubularized incised plate proximal hypospadias repair: continued evolution and extended applications. *J Pediatr Urol* 7: 2, 2011

Snodgrass W, DaJusta D, Villanueva C, and Bush N: Foreskin reconstruction does not increase urethroplasty or skin complications after distal TIP hypospadias repair. *J Pediatr Urol* 9:401, 2013

Chapter 20

Correcting Penoscrotal Transposition

Transposition of the scrotum up onto the penile shaft is commonly associated with hypospadias. The higher location blurs the distinction between penis and scrotum, creates a deficiency of ventral penile shaft skin, and also makes the penis appear shorter than it is.

Correcting transposition is done for aesthetic reasons, to give the penis as much visible length as possible. But there can also be functional concerns associated with hair-bearing, rugated skin on the penile shaft after puberty, where it can cause irritation/discomfort to sexual partners.

As with all aspects of hypospadias, penoscrotal transposition presents a spectrum of abnormal anatomy requiring varying extents of correction (Figure 1).

Cause of Transposition

Transposition results from scrotal dartos tethering the scrotum to the penile shaft and, in more severe cases, also to the pubis on either side of the penis. Release of these tissues drops the scrotum to a normal anatomic position.

Surgical Correction

Incision through the median raphe

Midline incision down the median raphe of the penis into the scrotum provides optimal access to release the dartos tethering the scrotum to the penile shaft and pubis. It also facilitates creating the new

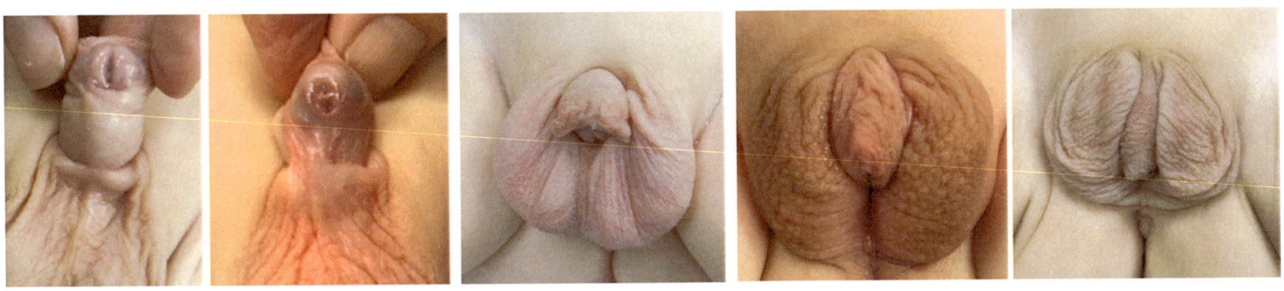

Figure 1. Varying extents of penoscrotal transposition.
A, scrotal encroachment on the proximal shaft just above the penoscrotal junction in a boy with distal hypospadias. B, scrotal encroachment extends to the midshaft in another boy with distal hypospadias, creating a ventral penile skin deficiency which will have to be corrected during repair. C,D,E, more severe transposition with the scrotum extending above the penis in boys with proximal shaft to perineal hypospadias.

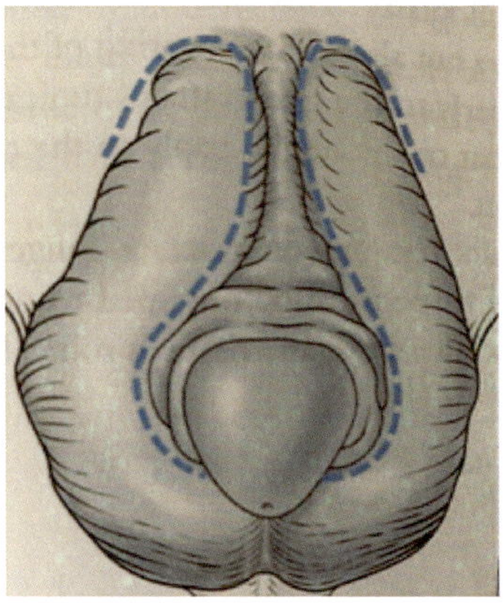

Figure 2. Traditional scrotal flaps.
This diagram shows the incision releasing the scrotum from the penis extending alongside their visible junction on the shaft and continuing above the penis and around the uppermost scrotum, creating 2 scrotal flaps to rotate down. While effective, this method leaves scars that can remain visible after puberty. We have not used this method in more than 20 years to correct transposition.

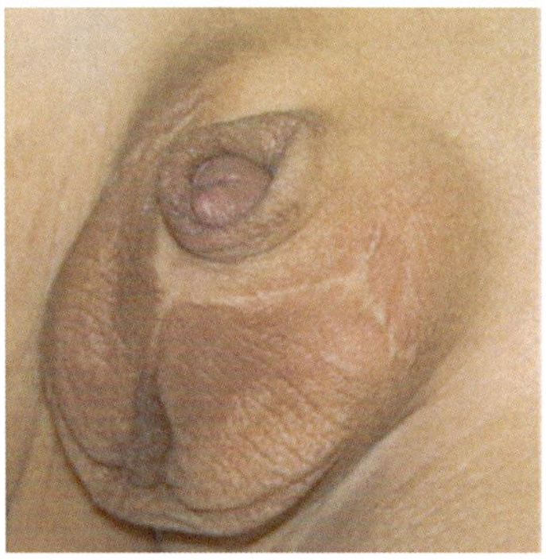

Figure 3. Visible scars left by scrotal skin flaps.

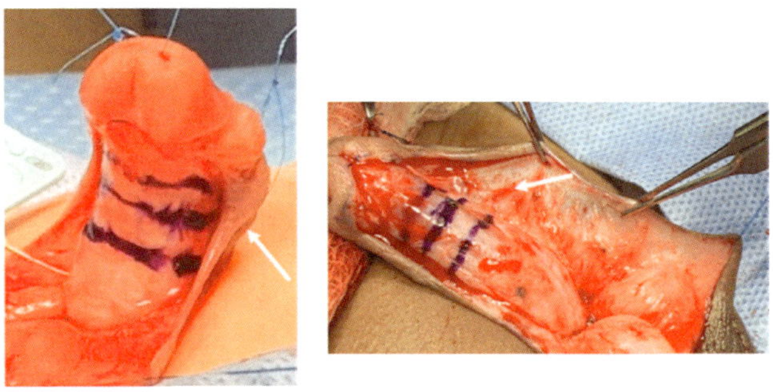

Figure 4. Lengthening ventral skin from skin humps. A, short ventral skin is apparent after dropping down the scrotum. The arrow indicates an ipsilateral dorsal skin hump with excess penile skin. B, oblique incision towards the skin hump will lengthen the ventral shaft skin to help correct the skin deficiency.

penoscrotal junction and lengthening the ventral penile skin to fill any resulting deficiency on the shaft.

If circumferential degloving is done, additionally splitting the ventral skin and scrotum through the median raphe assists in correcting transposition.

Release of scrotal dartos

Degloving ventrally releases both penile and scrotal dartos, reducing transposition off the shaft. When transposition extends around the penis, scrotal dartos running alongside the shaft and inserting into the pubis is identified and transected so that the scrotum can move down to its normal position.

The traditional approach creating scrotal skin flaps illustrated in Figure 2 is *not* needed to move the scrotum down to a normal location, and the incisions creating flaps can leave visible scars (Figure 3).

Lengthening the ventral penile shaft skin

As the scrotum drops lower, any ventral skin deficiency becomes greater. Consequently, the penile skin needs to be lengthened to provide symmetric shaft coverage circumferentially. This is best accomplished with oblique cuts extending towards any available skin humps (Figure 4), usually in the midshaft region.

Creating the penoscrotal junction

Once the scrotum is moved down and the ventral skin is lengthened, it is important to establish and secure a new penoscrotal junction. The location can be adjusted up to 5mm distally if needed to accommodate remaining penile skin deficiency, but is otherwise placed at the visual junction of the penis to the scrotum. The penile shaft skin at approximately 3 and 9 o'clock is then sutured to the tunica albuginea of the corpora on either side of the urethra using 5-0 PDS to maintain the junction (Figure 5). In staged procedures, this step also helps the shaft skin to stretch during postoperative erections.

Put together, these steps correct penoscrotal transposition without the risk for visible scars that can result from making scrotal skin flaps in a primary repair (Figure 6), and in a reoperation (Figure 7).

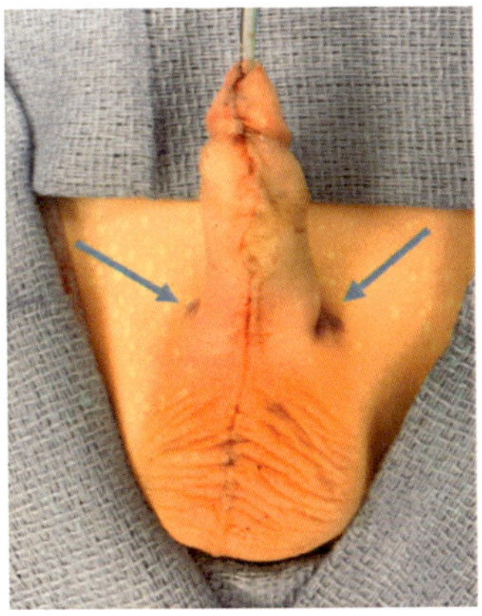

Figure 5. Pexing the penoscrotal junction.
After moving the scrotum down and lengthening the ventral penile shaft skin, a new penoscrotal junction is established. The penile skin at 3 and 9 o'clock is sewn to the tunica albuginea of the corpora to either side of the urethra using an interrupted subepithelial 5-0 PDS suture, as indicated by the arrows.

Timing of Correction

When most proximal hypospadias repairs were done using skin flaps, there was concern that simultaneous correction of scrotal transposition could impair the blood supply to the urethroplasty flap. Consequently, some surgeons postponed this step to a later operation (for example, see Stanasel et al, 2015).

However, the different embryonic origins of the scrotal folds and genital tubercle make it possible to separate the penis and scrotum without devascularizing either. Scrotal transposition repair can safely be done during proximal TIP. Similarly, we perform all or most of a transposition correction at the first operation of STAC repair, completing any remaining encroachment during STAC 3.

There is no reason to plan a separate operation to correct penoscrotal transposition.

Key Points

Penoscrotal transposition commonly occurs with hypospadias, often shortening the ventral penile skin. Correction involves release of underlying scrotal dartos attaching to the penile shaft and the pubis on either side of the penis.

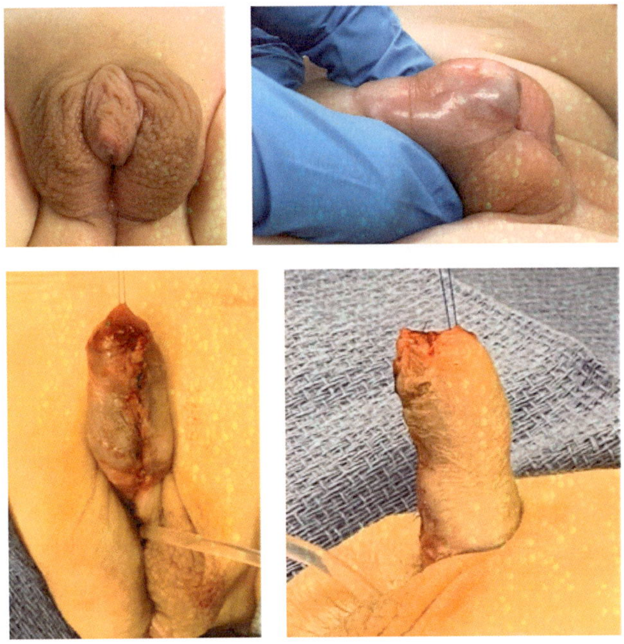

Figure 6. Reducing extensive penoscrotal transposition without scrotal flaps, primary repair.
A, scrotal hypospadias with scrotal transposition above the penile shaft. B, side view showing the absence of ventral penile skin with scrotal skin fusion to the penile shaft. C, D, appearance after reduction of transposition by releasing scrotal dartos attachments to the penile shaft and pubis without making inverted U incisions or scrotal flaps.

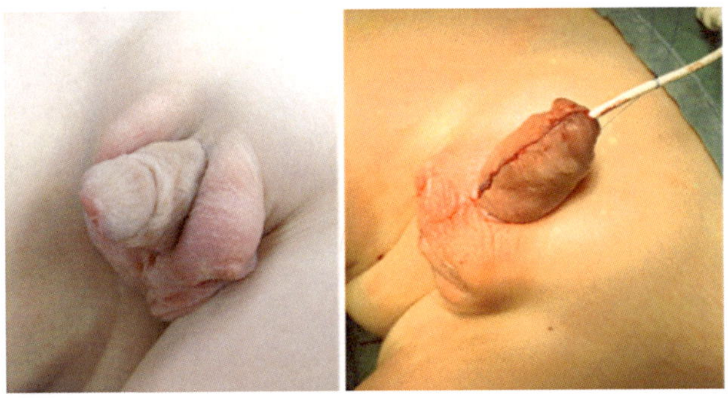

Figure 7. Reducing extensive penoscrotal transposition without scrotal flaps, reoperation.
A, another patient with proximal hypospadias and transposition extending above the shaft which was not corrected by the original surgeon. B, completed hypospadias repair with correction of the transposition by releasing dartos extending towards the pubis without making scrotal skin flaps, then pexing the penoscrotal junction to the penis with 5-0 PDS.

The aesthetic concerns which prompt correction of penoscrotal transposition should also prompt repair without leaving visible scars. While surgeons might consider this aspect of hypospadias repair a minor consideration, boys grow into teens and adults who do not want scrotum extending above their penis or scars near their penis.

References

Stanasel I, Le HK, Bilgutay A, Roth DA, Gonzales ET, JR, Janzen N, Koh CJ, Gargollo P and Seth A: Complications following staged hypospadias repair using transposed prepucial skin flaps. *J Urol* 194: 512, 2015

Chapter 21

Managing Penile Skin in Hypospadias

Even though the ventral shaft and foreskin are most often deficient and likely have altered vascularity in patients with hypospadias, management of the skin and its outcomes receive far less attention than urethroplasty and orthoplasty. Yet the goal of changing the abnormal anatomy of the condition into a normal penis requires the penile skin to be re-distributed so that it has symmetric length circumferentially and shows no scars except for the circumcision and median raphe incisions.

The decreased attention to skin correction may historically relate to the challenge of producing a normal-appearing penis. WS recalls how his mentor often left the OR while the urology resident and fellow did their best to close the skin, probably because the Mathieu and tubularized flap repairs then in vogue usually created an abnormal meatus. Perfectly tailored shaft skin could not overcome the otherwise disappointing results.

Today many surgeons likely consider skin management one of the easiest steps in hypospadias surgery, which they accomplish by some variation of splitting the dorsal foreskin to move skin flaps ventrally. However, that skin can be mis-sized, or approximated leaving scars outside the median raphe, and in any event is not available in many reoperations because it was either already utilized or removed by circumcision previously.

Furthermore, there are no objective criteria to define outcomes of skin management, much less means to measure them. The best we have devised are paired measurements of the stretched length of dorsal and ventral skin from the penopubic or penoscrotal junctions to the coronal of the glans to document changes after repair.

Meanwhile, we have learned the critical role that healthy penile shaft skin plays in healing after hypospadias repair. One major impetus for STAC was the observation that skin relocated ventrally could not reliably provide needed nourishment to the urethroplasty graft along their junction until the skin first had an opportunity to heal. We have also seen fistulas and wound dehiscences develop from tension generated by a tight skin closure. Similarly, dorsal curvature can occur when the dorsal shaft skin is cut too short. Finally, there are extreme situations in which there simply is not sufficient penis skin to cover the shaft and so scrotal flaps or skin grafts are necessary – which have a different color and texture than penis skin and are likely to sprout unsightly hair at puberty.

There is no equivalent substitute for penis skin to cover the penile shaft. Therefore, it should be handled carefully, with greater priority given to using it to enclose the penis rather than making the neourethra when there is not enough to accomplish both.

It is another improvement in this textbook over the first edition that we devote an entire chapter to the challenges of penis skin management during hypospadias repair.

General Principles

Despite the seemingly endless variations in the shape and configuration of hypospadias penile skin, we have learned some general guidelines for management.

1. *The penis skin will nearly always stretch longer, even when it is markedly deficient ventrally in a severe primary hypospadias or shortened and scarred by prior surgery.*

   There is almost always sufficient penis skin to symmetrically cover the shaft and provide tissue for the urethroplasty, even in perineal cases – if the skin is utilized as we describe during the first operation of a STAC repair. Similarly, we have learned that shortened and damaged skin after failed operations can rejuvenate and stretch longer in STAC reoperations combined with perioperative HBOT. In most of these situations there is also ventral curvature, and straightening the penis with ventral corporotomies while tacking the shaft skin at the penoscrotal junction provides the means for skin to lengthen during natural postoperative erections. Prepucioplasty during the first operation similarly facilitates stretching by postoperative erections to provide more foreskin for the urethroplasty graft.

2. *Dorsal whorls are repositories supplying additional penile skin.*

   The humps commonly found on each side of the hooded foreskin are comprised of excess skin that can be used to cover the penis shaft or make the neourethra. These are generally best accessed by short oblique cuts from the ventral skin edge angled into the whorls.

3. *Mirror image incisions along the ventral skin edges should be avoided.*

   The most common example of this is cutting the penoscrotal junction towards 3 and 9 o'clock. While it may appear this is a natural line for incision, incising the skin in opposite directions and then re-approximating the new edges narrows the overall width, often resulting in a visible waist. It is usually better to offset similar incisions, whether at the penoscrotal junction or more distally, or angle one up and the other down to mimic Z-plasties.

4. *Excising scar from the skin edge lengthens it.*

   It is counterintuitive to cut off skin to make the skin longer, but removing the scarred edge usually accomplishes that, sometimes to a surprising extent. Incising a notch across a band of scar along the skin edge can also provide length, although less.

5. *Exaggerating stretch will reveal tension bands in the skin to be released.*

   Both the congenitally short skin of proximal hypospadias and the scarred skin after failed repairs often reveal bands of tension when they are stretched. Unless these are released their pull can result in urethroplasty complications, including fistulas and glans dehiscence. It can be surprising to find such bands extending from within the scrotum to the glans. Some can be released by incision across the underlying dartos, while others require incision through the tight skin. When the band is located within an expanse of skin rather than along its edge, a Heineke-Mikulicz transverse incision across the tension line releases it and subsequent closure longitudinally lengthens the skin. We have found this maneuver to be useful to lengthen short dorsal shaft skin in reoperations, concealing the incision within the penopubic junction.

6. *Placing a urethroplasty graft against relocated penile skin at the first stage of a proximal hypospadias repair can stress the skin and cause scarring of both the skin and graft.*

   Grafts derive their vascularity from both the underlying surface of the corpora cavernosa and the shaft skin sewn along their edges. Newly relocated skin needs time to recover before it can reliably provide neovascularity to a graft, and skin scarred from prior operations similarly needs the rejuvenation gained from HBOT before it can support graft take. While these grafts will sometimes heal, when they do not the resulting scarring impacts not only the graft, but also the adjacent penile skin – adding to the overall skin deficiency and damage. STAC repair and perioperative HBOT decrease these risks.

7. *Penile skin in hypospadias has altered vascularity.*

   This clinical observation derives from superficial skin necrosis seen after hypospadias surgery, whether primary or reoperative, distal or proximal, which rarely occurs after circumcision of a normal penis. The likelihood for this abnormal wound healing is further increased when there is also penile torsion or a solitary dorsal hump. This skin reaction becomes apparent approximately 10-14 days postoperatively, and is sometimes confused for a wound infection.

Skin Considerations in Distal Hypospadias

There is a range of skin anomalies associated with distal hypospadias. For example, MIP variants by definition have normally formed penile shaft skin with a complete foreskin. At the opposite end of the spectrum are otherwise typical distal cases with such ventral skin deficiency that the shaft skin retracts to the penoscrotal junction after it is released by the initial skin incision, creating a large deficit comprising the entire ventral side to be covered. The occasional addition of penile torsion also complicates skin management by creating a skin deficit on the side to which it turns.

MIP hypospadias

These often present after hypospadias is found during circumcision. Stopping the procedure often leaves excess ventral skin which has to be revised during the hypospadias repair.

Those with an intact foreskin can be managed according to the preference of the parents for either circumcision or foreskin preservation. Because any patient, even one with MIP, can have VC greater than 30°, we no longer begin repairs with the traditional circumferential incision. Instead, we make a midline incision down the median raphe and deglove ventrally until artificial erection is done and confirms the penis is straight or has less than 30° of curvature. Then routine sleeve circumcision is completed without need for skin flaps since there should be no ventral skin deficiency (Figure 1).

Circumcision is not required if the parents wish to maintain the foreskin intact. TIP repair can be easily done with the foreskin retracted as shown in Figure 1 B, marking incisions along the glanular wings that

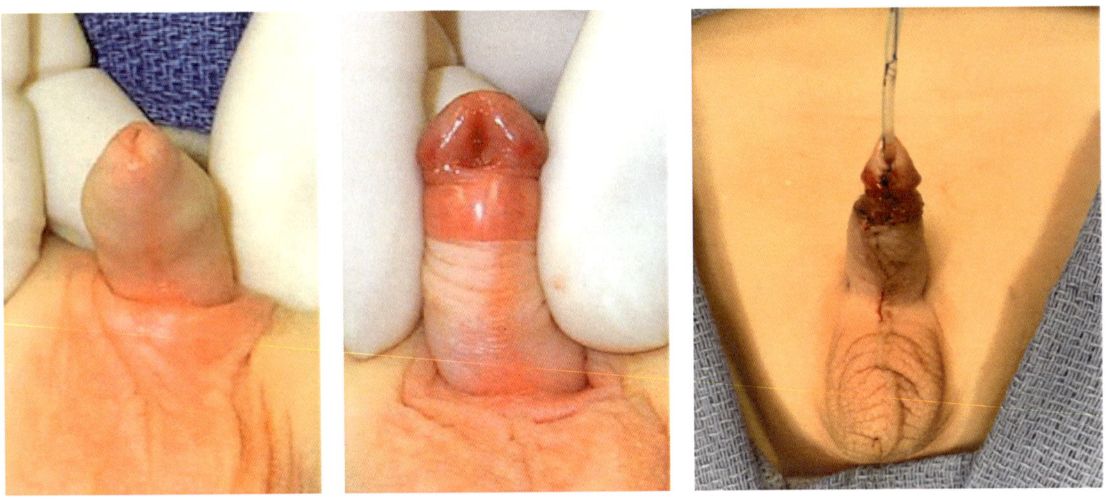

Figure 1. MIP hypospadias.
A, normal-appearing penis with a complete foreskin, concealing a coronal hypospadias seen in B when the skin is retracted. A midline incision down the median raphe is done and dissection confined to the ventral shaft until artificial erection demonstrates there is either no or less than 30° VC. C, the parents wanted the final result to be a circumcision and so that was done along with distal TIP repair. There should be no ventral skin deficiency in these patients since the shaft skin and foreskin are normally developed.

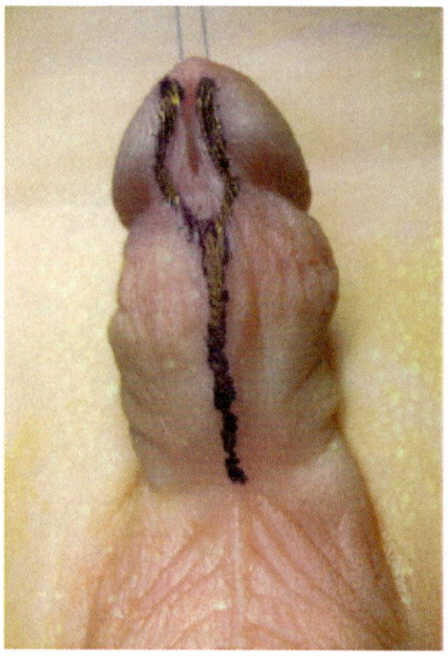

Figure 2. Ventral incision to repair MIP found after circumcision.
The incision can be carried down the median raphe as far as necessary to excise any excess skin remaining after the circumcision. It is rarely necessary to completely deglove the penis in this circumstance.

meet below the corona in the midline and continue through the inner prepuce. After urethroplasty, glansplasty, and coverage of the neourethra by a ventral dartos flap, the incision in the inner prepuce is sutured and the still-intact foreskin reduced.

When hypospadias is discovered after circumcision was completed, repair is also done using a ventral degloving incision as shown in Figure 2. This approach provides ample exposure for the urethroplasty, glansplasty, and ventral dartos flap coverage over the neourethra, as well as excision of any residual excess skin without degloving dorsally.

If circumcision was stopped after the dorsal slit revealed hypospadias, the choice between ventral versus circumferential degloving depends on the extent of excess dorsal skin that remains. In many cases the dorsal slit extends to near the corona and the excess skin is mostly ventral, where it can be revised by a medial raphe incision.

Distal hypospadias with a partial "hooded" foreskin

The extent of ventral skin deficiency varies among patients with distal hypospadias and a partial foreskin. In some the distal edge of the ventral skin comes to lie at or only a few millimeters below the glans, while in others the skin retracts to the penoscrotal junction.

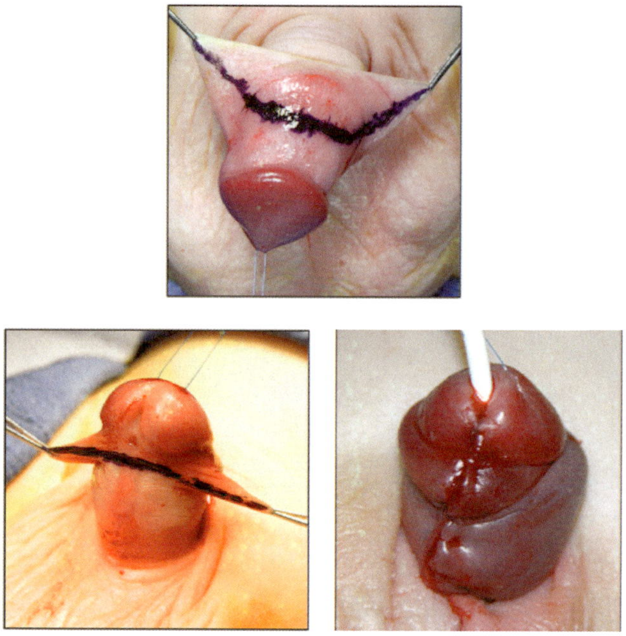

Figure 3. Traditional Firlit skirts.
A, dorsal incision is made approximately 1cm below the corona, extending towards the corners of the hooded prepuce. This incision can be made closer to the corona to create a less wide collar. B, ventral aspect showing the lack of inner prepuce near the meatus. The "skirts" made by this incision rotate ventrally to make a circumferentially symmetric collar, as seen in C.

The size of the defect to be filled is also influenced by the length of the mucosal collar that the surgeon creates.

The end result of distal hypospadias repair can be either a circumcised penis or a natural penis with reconstructed foreskin, done according to the preferences of the parents. Both should create a median raphe where the ventral skin deficiency was corrected.

Mucosal Collar

The mucosal collar is not only important for the aesthetic outcome, but also to buffer tension from the ventral shaft skin which might cause a fistula or glans dehiscence. In addition, the collar can be used to address lateral shaft skin deficiency resulting from penile torsion or lateral curvature.

North American surgeons generally create Firlit skirts to redistribute the inner prepuce ventrally and provide a symmetric collar circumferentially (Figure 3).

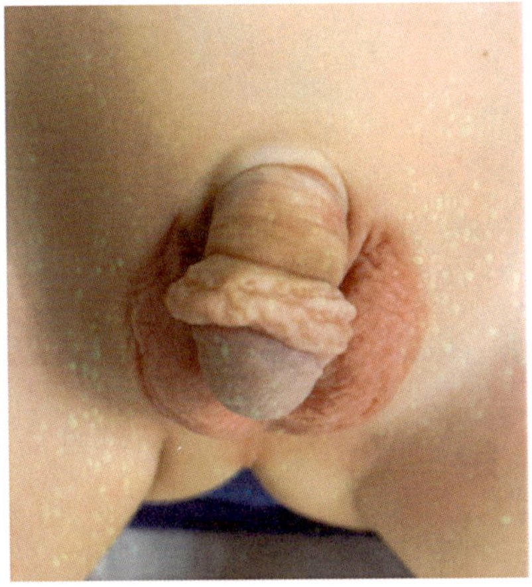

Figure 4. Unsightly mucosal collar.
Postoperative edema in the thin inner prepuce sometimes leaves an unsightly distinction with the shaft skin. This is more likely to occur when a long mucosal collar is created.

The length can be adjusted and is commonly made approximately 1cm to mimic the result of newborn circumcisions done with Gomcos or plastibells.

However, this long collar is prone to postoperative edema in the thinner inner prepucial skin which can leave it visibly more thick that the shaft skin when healing is complete (Figure 4).

When an Italian mother complained about the mucosal collar after her son's hypospadias repair, we learned that Europeans, who generally do not practice clamp-based newborn circumcision, prefer a much shorter collar. We were already making a smaller collar in boys undergoing proximal staged graft repairs to conserve as much prepuce as possible for the urethroplasty graft, and so we subsequently applied this to distal hypospadias circumcisions.

Now the distance from the corona to the transverse incision line dorsally is made closer to the glans, which then adjusts the remaining incision lines and creates a shorter collar to the length the surgeon decides (Figure 5).

However, when there is penile torsion or lateral penile curvature the shaft skin is shorter on one side, usually the left. In these cases, a longer mucosal collar helps resolve the needed shaft skin deficiency.

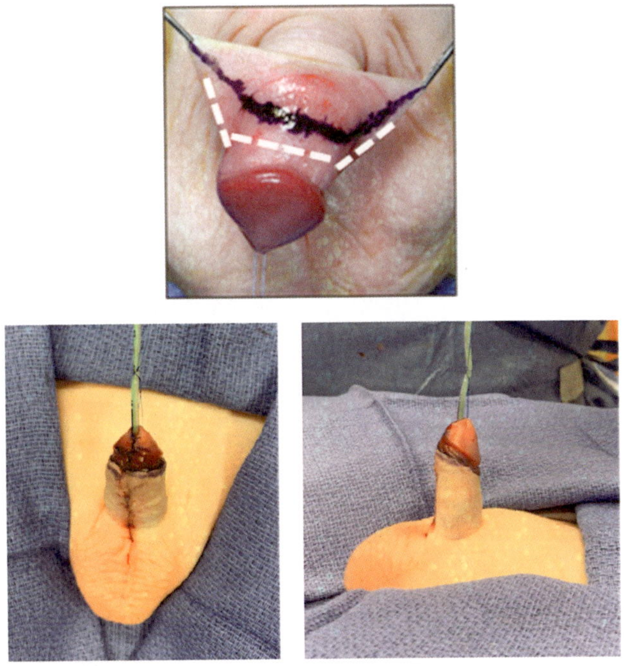

Figure 5. Circumcision creating a less prominent mucosal collar.
A, the dotted line shows the dorsal incision made to create a narrow mucosal collar. The less prominent collar is still symmetric and buffers against shaft skin tension on the hypospadias repair. This is the preferred appearance after circumcision for many Europeans. A similar short collar is made during circumcision in STAC repairs to save more of the foreskin for the urethroplasty graft.

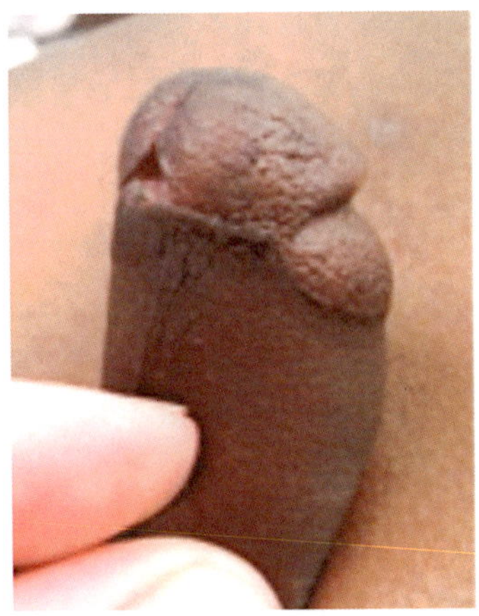

Figure 6. Absent ventral collar contributing to glans dehiscence.
It is obvious that the inner prepuce is absent from 3 to 9 o'clock in this patient after distal hypospadias repair, creating an abnormal appearance compared to circumcised boys. In addition, the ventral shaft skin is tight, and that tension contributed to glans dehiscence.

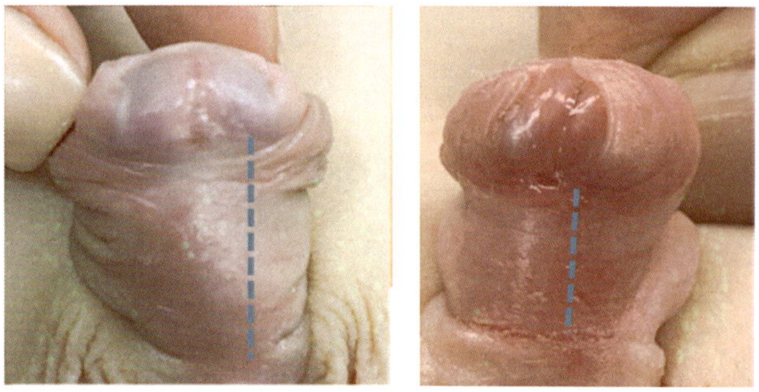

Figure 7. Varying ventral skin length in 2 boys with coronal hypospadias.
Although both patients have coronal hypospadias, the boy in A has longer ventral skin than does the one in B.

Failing to create the ventral aspect of the mucosal collar leaves an unsightly appearance to the penis. It also increases the risk for urethroplasty complications, including fistulas and glans dehiscence, from tension generated by the shaft skin (Figure 6). Therefore, steps to preserve sufficient inner prepuce to cover the ventral deficiency and provide a symmetric collar must be taken at the outset of the operation when the skin incision is made. Then care must be exercised throughout the surgery to avoid inadvertant damage to this ring of skin.

Byars Flaps

The differences in ventral skin length in boys with otherwise similar meatal location is shown in Figure 7. It is well-recognized that release of the skin reveals a variable ventral deficiency. In addition, tethering from short ventral skin explains the "chordee" that resolves when the penis is degloved.

The gap from the skin edge to the corona is filled using either the dorsal foreskin moved ventrally by Byars flaps, or ventral shaft skin lengthened by small oblique incisions.

Byars flaps are the natural choice when circumcision is preferred by the parents. Historically, the bilateral flap wings created by splitting the dorsal foreskin were often wrapped around the penis and sewed crisscrossed one above the other ventrally, making unsightly Z-shaped ventral scars. Today this tissue transfer is fashioned into a median raphe (Figure 8).

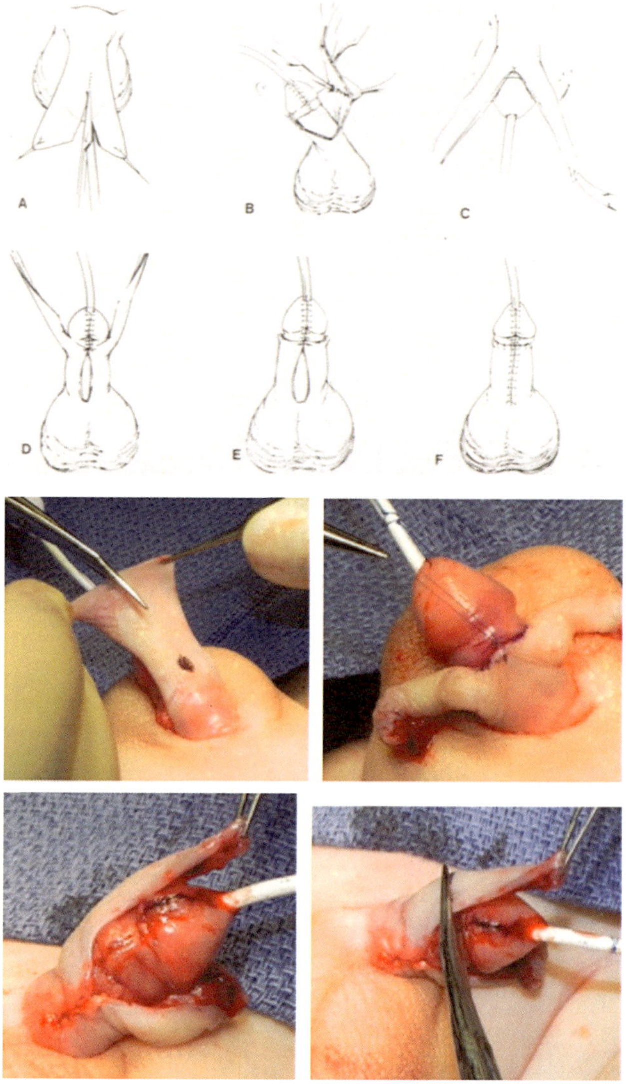

Figure 8. Byars flap skin closure.
As the diagram and pictures show, the hooded dorsal foreskin is first incised down the midline to the corona, marked with a blue dot in the photo. Underlying dartos is released from under the flap on each side as shown in B in the diagram. Then the dorsal skin is sewn to the mucosal collar at 12 o'clock. The 2 flap wings rotate laterally, providing the skin needed to correct the ventral deficiency. These edges are approximated into a median raphe as indicated by the arrow. Then the remaining excess skin is excised to complete the circumcision. Skin should be approximated subepithelially to avoid a "ruffled" appearance and/or suture tracks.

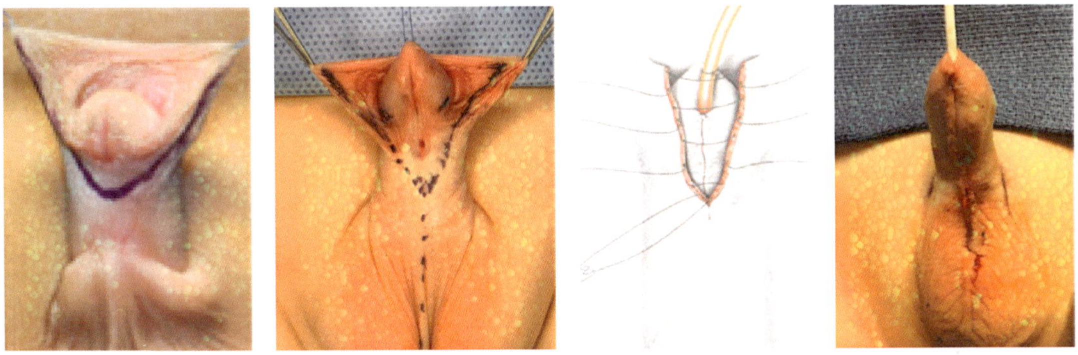

Figure 9. Foreskin reconstruction.
A, incision lines are marked from the lateral edges of the foreskin extending approximately 3mm below the meatus. Care is taken to ensure there is at least 3mm of ventral skin below the glans so that the inner prepuce can be reconstructed. Note that the scrotum is encroaching up the base of the penis in this patient. This is corrected by next incising down the ventral midline through this scrotal tissue, as shown in another patient in B. When the hypospadias repair and scrotoplasty are completed, the inner and outer layers of the foreskin, and the intervening dartos between them, are separately approximated in a 3-layer closure shown in C that creates the median raphe seen in D.

Prepucioplasty

When the parents do not want their son to be circumcised, the skin on the dorsal side of the penis is left untouched. Ventral degloving is performed through a Y-shaped incision that extends from near the corners of the foreskin to below the meatus and down the ventral midline as needed. After urethroplasty and glansplasty, limited dissection is done to separate the inner and outer layers of the prepuce sufficiently for tension-free closure. As discussed in Chapter 19, the inner layer is approximated, dartos under it is then sewn in a second layer to reinforce it, and finally the outer skin is closed into a median raphe (Figure 9).

Heineke-Mikulicz Lengthening

Newborn circumcision of a penis with torsion or lateral curvature can result in ipsilateral shaft skin deficiency when straightening is done. One option for managing this situation is to lengthen the shorter skin by a Heineke-Mikulicz maneuver at the base of the penis. The tension line of the shorter skin is identified by stretching it, and then a transverse incision is made through that line until the tension is released. Longitudinal closure of the skin adds the needed length and leaves a proximal scar that is hardly noticeable (Figure 10).

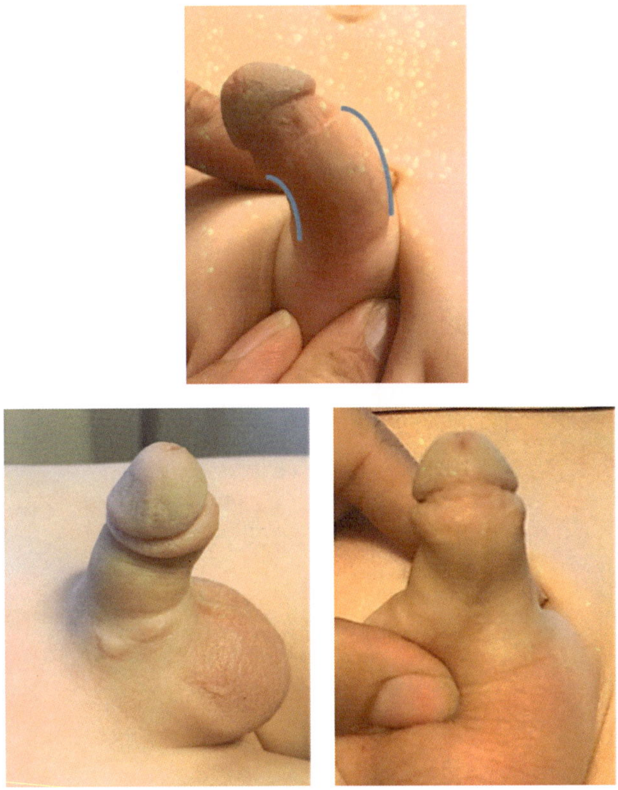

Figure 10. Heineke-Mikulicz skin lengthening.
A, right lateral curvature with visible skin deficiency. Heineke-Mikulicz straightening was done via a transverse incision made at the base of the penis across the area with greatest tension and then closed longitudinally. B,C after healing the penis is straight with symmetric skin length circumferentially. Only a small scar is visible.

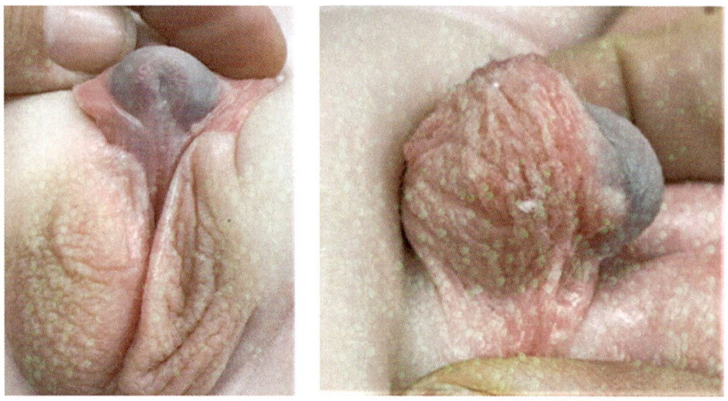

Figure 11. Ventral penile skin deficiency in proximal hypospadias.
A, B, there is no ventral penile shaft skin - only the urethral plate, a narrow strip of inner prepuce and scrotum, covering the shaft.

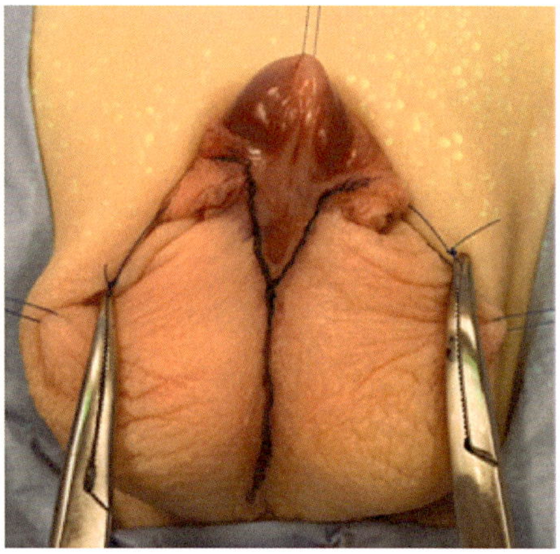

Figure 12. Skin incision for hypospadias repair. Complete degloving is not done for proximal repairs. Instead, a ventral incision is made as shown, extended a short distance along the inner prepuce on each side, along side the urethral plate to below the meatus, and then through the scrotum to near the perineum.

Skin Management in Proximal Hypospadias

Everything involved with repairing proximal hypospadias - straightening the penis, urethroplasty, and skin closure - is much more complex than in distal hypospadias. Of these, skin management receives the least attention yet is vital both to achieve a normal appearance and to avoid urethroplasty complications.

The challenge is that most patients have ventral skin deficiency that is much greater than in distal hypospadias (Figure 11), and which increases when the penis is straightened. The penile skin which is available has to be re-allocated to provide symmetric coverage around the shaft.

Initial skin incision

Proximal repairs begin through a ventral skin incision as shown in Figure 12. This gives excellent exposure to complete the major steps in STAC 1: straightening VC, creating the urethrostomy, and lengthening the ventral penile skin.

Lengthening the penile skin

The default method used by surgeons to address ventral skin deficiency is to split the dorsal foreskin hood into 2 Byars flaps rotated to the underside. However, that limits options for proximal urethroplasty. Tubularization of Byars flaps into the neourethra has at least double the complications as creating the neourethra from grafts (Snodgrass and Bush, 2017). If foreskin flaps are used to cover the penile shaft, then urethroplasty grafts have to be taken from the mouth. Those heal more thick than do prepucial grafts, making glansplasty more difficult in patients with a small glans.

Consequently, we lengthen the lateral skin edges created by the ventral degloving incision to cover the shaft skin deficiency. That involves short oblique incisions through the skin edges towards nearby humps of skin. These should be made in opposite directions on each side to resemble Z-plasties and avoid creating narrow waists in the skin that form when straight mirror-image incisions are made at right angles to the skin (Figure 13).

Tacking the penoscrotal junction

Postoperative erections will further lengthen the shaft skin, if the surgeon tacks it to the tunica albuginea on each side at the penoscrotal junction (Figure 14). We use 5-0 PDS in prepubertal patients, increasing the size to 4-0 or 3-0 PDS in post-pubertal patients.

Prepucioplasty

Reconstructing the foreskin during the first STAC operation similarly allows that skin to stretch during postoperative erections. This helps provide enough foreskin to create the urethroplasty graft at Stage 2. By pexing the penoscrotal junction and closing the foreskin around the glans, we have been able to

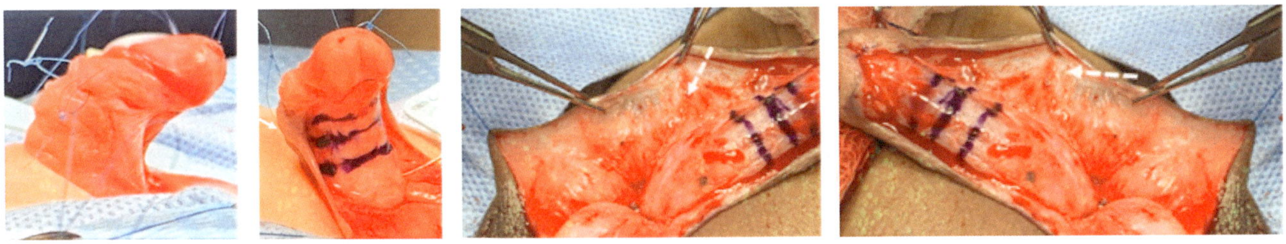

Figure 13. Lengthening the penile skin.
A, skin edges created by the ventral degloving incisions. These will be lengthened to release tension and provide needed shaft coverage. B, the tight skin seen from a different angle. The arrow points to a small skin hump which will provide additional skin. B,C, short oblique cuts at roughly 45 degree angles are made into the humps which lengthens the skin. The cuts are offset in differing directions on the right and on the left so that skin defects can be filled in with the resulting "Z" of skin edges. Mirror-image, perpendicular horizontal cuts are that could create a narrow waist are avoided.

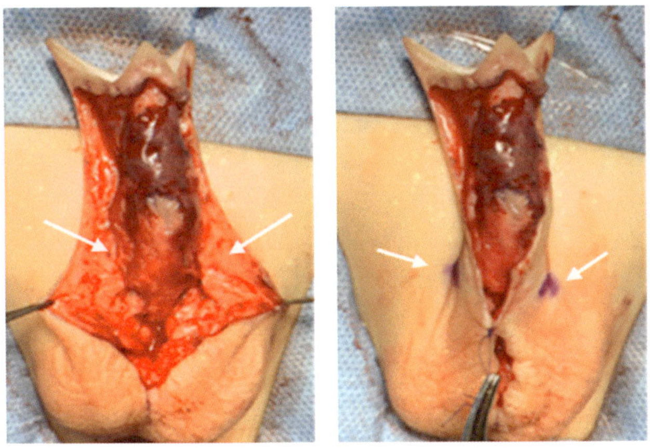

Figure 14. Fixing the penoscrotal junction to facilitate stretching of the shaft skin.
Suture-pexing the penile skin to the corpora on either side of the urethra at the penoscrotal junction provides 2 fixed points against which erections will stretch the skin postoperatively. This is a key maneuver performed at each step of the STAC repair.

correct even the most severe cases of proximal hypospadias without the need to take oral mucosa grafts for the neourethra or use scrotal flaps, skin grafts, or Cecil maneuvers to close the skin during the final stage (Snodgrass and Bush, 2024).

Prepucial grafts are preferred because they heal more thin than do grafts taken from the mouth. This is an important consideration since many boys with proximal hypospadias have a smaller glans that is more prone to dehiscence. There is also greater morbidity associated with the donor site when grafts are harvested from the mouth.

The skin incisions are extended towards the corners of the dorsal foreskin hood. Then the inner and outer surfaces are separated sufficiently that each can be approximated to the other side without tension in a layered reconstruction – inner skin, dartos, and outer skin (Figure 9 above).

Results

Lengthening the skin without Byars flaps, pexing the penoscrotal junction, and doing prepucioplasty without simultaneously placing a urethroplasty graft has essentially resolved the problem of ventral skin deficiency in severe hypospadias. We compared outcomes from 3-stage STAC versus 2-stage STAG and found that nearly 1 of every 10 STAG patients required a scrotal flap, Cecil maneuver, or skin graft to close the skin, versus needing none of these at the final STAC (Snodgrass and Bush, 2024). The skin lengthening achieved by STAC is remarkable, as shown in Figure 15.

As explained in Chapter 11, delaying urethroplasty grafting from the first stage to a second significantly improves graft health. This is in part due to allowing the relocated shaft skin to better vascularize before stressing it with demands from the graft. Less graft scarring and contracture in turn benefits the skin, since grafts that scar and contract cause the adjacent skin to also scar and contract.

Healthy, symmetric penile skin covering the shaft is one of the three pillars of a successful hypospadias repair, along with a straight penis and a terminal meatus correctly positioned in the glans.

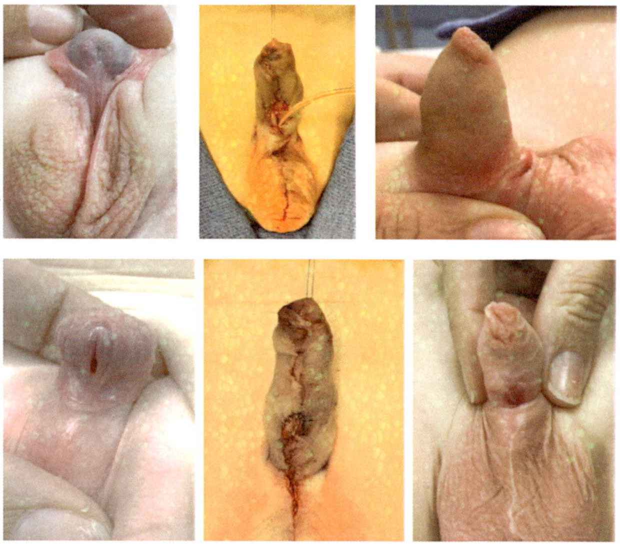

Figure 15. Successful STAC skin lengthening. Both of these patients had near absence of ventral penile skin and underwent the first stage of STAC repair with the results shown at the end of that procedure and 6 months later. The shaft skin was symmetric circumferentially and the foreskin provided the urethroplasty graft extending from the penoscrotal junction to the tip of the glans. These are the nearly universal results achieved by lengthening the ventral skin, pexing the penoscrotal junction, and prepucioplasty during the first STAC operation.

Skin complications

As stated above, the abnormal penile skin in hypospadias has altered vascularity. Consequently, the lengthened ventral skin can partially contract, or even necrose after surgical manipulation– problems that are unusual when a normal penis is degloved for circumcision or other non-hypospadias surgery.

Partial Skin Contracture

Typical circumcised penile skin length from the penoscrotal junction to the coronal is approximately 30mm. Boys undergoing proximal hypospadias repair may have less than 5mm. Ventral lengthening of that skin by oblique incisions towards skin humps should result in symmetric skin circumferentially. However, it is not uncommon for some of the gained length to be lost postoperatively from skin contraction, for example decreasing the measured length that changed from 5 preop to 32mm at the end of STAC 1, down to 25mm at the beginning of STAC 2. We inform parents why this happens and explain that it does not indicate failure of the corporotomies.

Emollients applied to the skin after the bandage falls off keep it moist, which helps reduce contracture. So does 0.1% betamethasone applied twice daily beginning a month after surgery and continuing for 6-12 weeks.

Skin contracture that persists most often is due to underlying thickened dartos and bands of scar tethering it. STAC 2 always begins with a ventral midline incision followed by excision of tethering dartos and transverse release of scars which usually restore the diminished length. Skin that remains tight after these maneuvers is lengthened again by short oblique incisions.

Necrosis

The ventral skin can also necrose after STAC 1, which occurs between 7-14 days postoperatively (Figure 16). This should not be confused with wound infection, which rarely occurs and is diagnosed by the accompanying fever, erythema and purulent discharge.

We review skin healing 2 weeks after surgery either in-person or by emailed photographs looking for signs of ischemic necrosis. When found, we change the emollient from Aquaphor to Manuka honey, which helps debride the skin and provides antimicrobial benefits. Progress is monitored weekly until healing is completed.

Rarely, ischemic necrosis is more extensive, as seen in Figure 17. In these situations, HBOT is begun to help revascularize the skin. Most often the skin will recover without gross scarring.

Skin Contracture Requiring Redo Stac

7% of our primary STAC patients had skin contracture that was more extensive and required an unplanned additional operation to revise it. Nearly all of them had a preexisting skin anomaly in addition to their hypospadias, specifically either penile torsion or a single large midline hump "gnome hat" deformity (Snodgrass and Bush, 2024) shown in Figure 18.

We have not yet found a reliable way to address these gnome hat skin anomalies. Initially we removed their underlying dartos to smooth them but that resulted in autoamputation of the foreskin. Next we tried minimally manipulating that skin while lengthening the ventral skin, but necrosis with scarring still occurred.

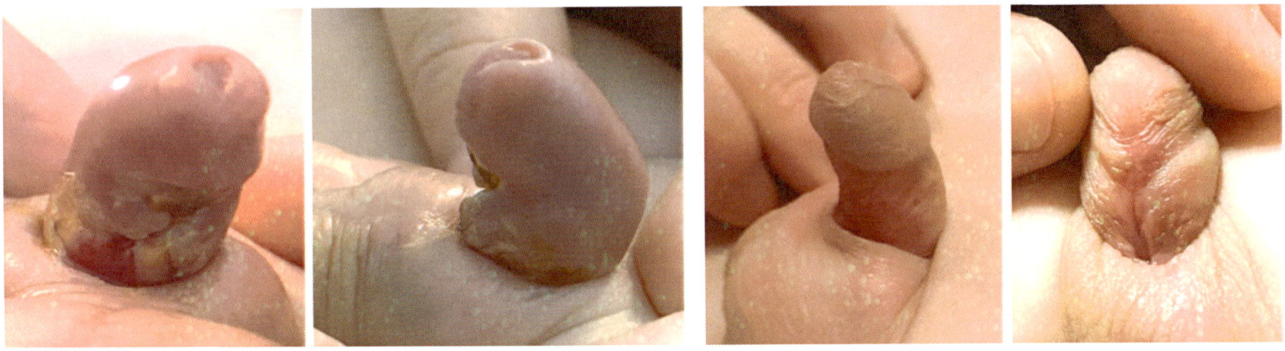

Figure 16. Skin necrosis after STAC.
A,B 2-week postoperative photos showing intact reconstructed foreskin with ventral right shaft skin necrosis. Note the absence of surrounding erythema or purulent discharge, indicating this is ischemic necrosis. The skin reaction is also causing ventral curvature during erection. The wound was treated with Manuka. C,D appearance 3 months later showing the penis is nearly straight again and the ventral shaft skin is healed and appears supple.

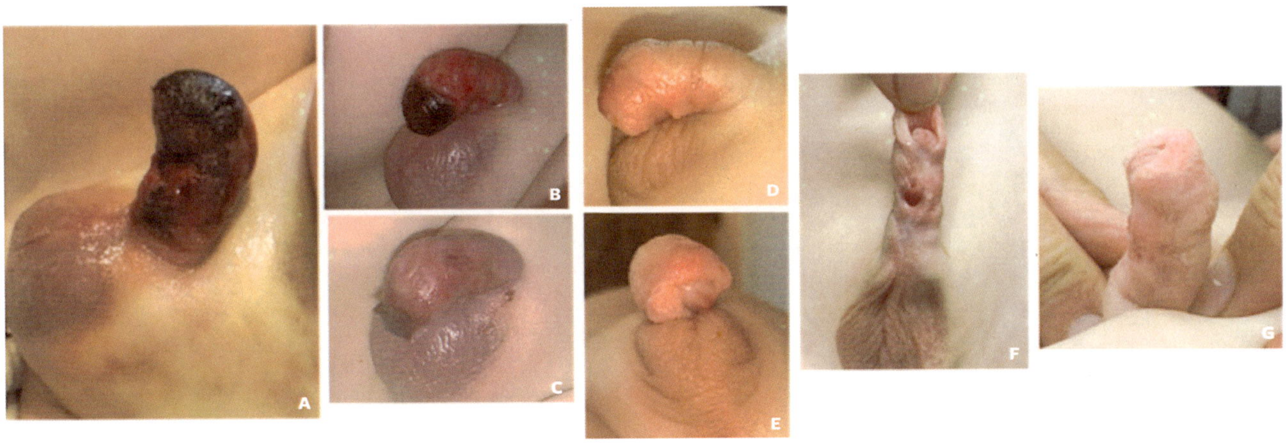

Figure 17. Skin necrosis after STAC treated with HBOT.
A, appearance 1 week after surgery. HBOT began immediately, with rapid improvement noted a week later in B and another 3 days later in C. D, appearance at 1 month after 20 HBOT dives showing progressively healthier skin, although with ventral skin contraction seen in E. Betamethasone 0.1% was next applied twice daily for 12 weeks. F,G pictures taken intraoperatively before Stage 2, 6 months after the initial operation, showing the penis was straight with supple shaft skin and sufficient remaining foreskin to make the urethroplasty graft.

Fortunately, redoing the skin lengthening in a second STAC 1 skin revision with adjuvant HBOT has successfully restored vascularity and avoided need to place an external penile skin graft (Figure 18). Unfortunately, oral grafting has been necessary in many of these patients since the penile skin that remains after severe contracture/necrosis is used preferentially to cover the penis in a symmetric fashion.

Ironically, this complication illustrates another advantage of STAC over STAG, as this skin contracture is identified and corrected before proceding with urethroplasty grafting and final skin closure. Now, we start HBOT immediately postoperatively in boys with a "gnome hat" configuration, and that has alleviated the need for redo skin surgery and/or oral grafts in many of these patients.

Skin management in reoperations

Short penile skin is a common feature after unsuccessful surgery, especially in patients with proximal hypospadias. The general principles guiding skin management in primary cases apply in these cases too. Oblique cuts into the skin will lengthen it, although mirror image incisions should be avoided so that a

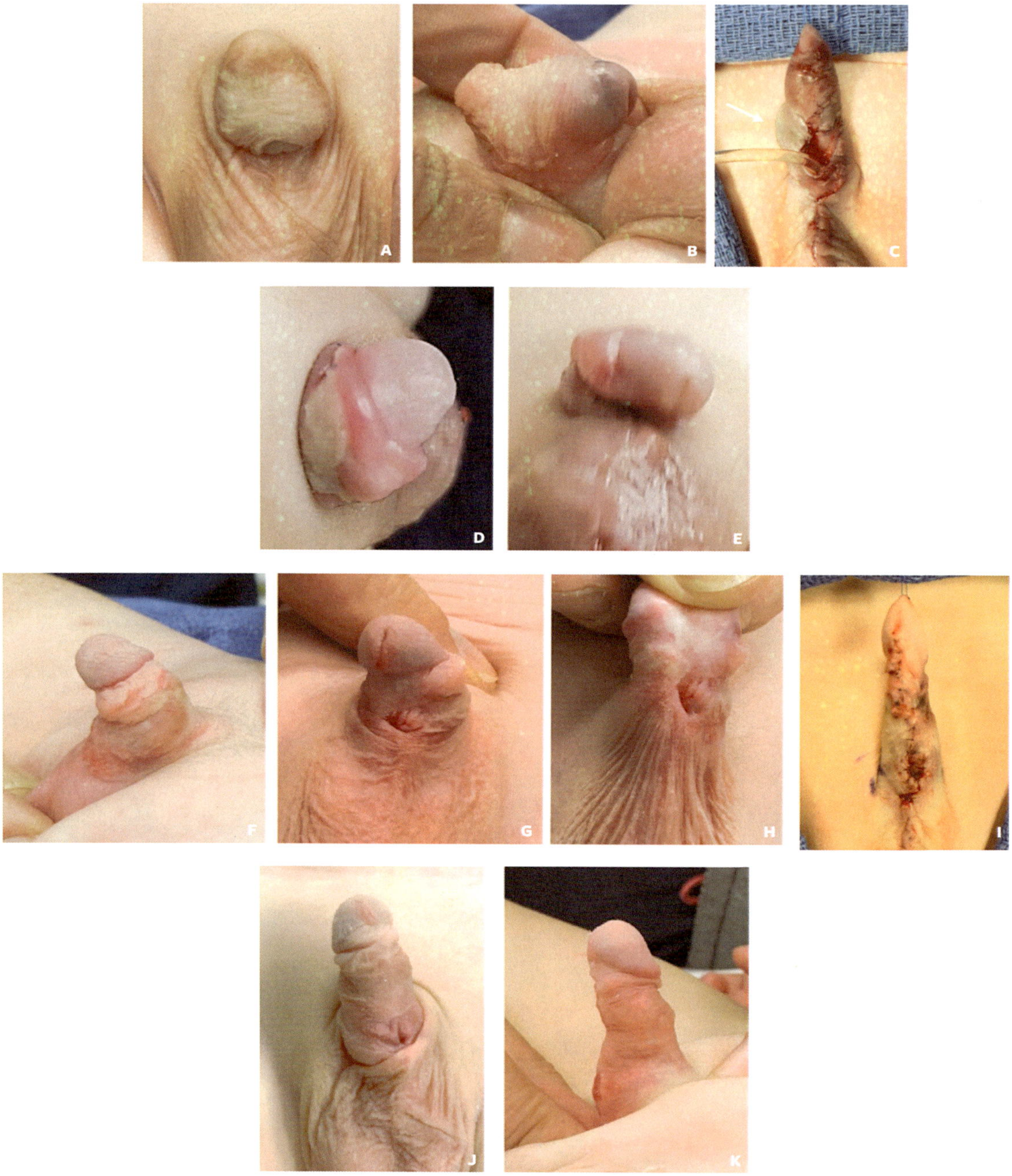

Figure 18. Gnome hat skin deformity requiring redo STAC skin revision.
A,B, single dorsal midline hump resembling a "gnome hat". C, Intraoperative appearance after STAC 1. Arrow shows the residual hump now deviated towards the right side after skin lengthening with minimal manipulation of the gnome hat. D,E 2-week postoperative photos sent by the parents showing necrosis extending from the hump around to the underside. F, appearance 6 months later showing loss of the foreskin and recurrent ventral curvature from skin contracture. G,H shaft skin loss and visible scarring on the right side. STAC skin revision was done removing as much scar as possible and lengthening the skin again. I, completion of the redo STAC. Adjuvant HBOT with 20 dives was also given. J,K, restored skin length and suppleness apparent 6 months later. 2-stage oral graft urethroplasty was next done to complete the repair, meaning his 3-stage STAC required 4 operations for success.

narrow waist is not created. Then postoperative erections will stretch the skin more, especially when VC was also straightened. With adjuvant HBOT, which is nearly always beneficial in reoperations, even short, scarred skin can recover and revascularize so that scrotal flaps, Cecils and skin grafts are rarely needed.

As in primary repairs, the penis should be straightened and the skin lengthened and allowed to heal before urethroplasty grafting is done. Reoperative STAC is preferable to redo STAG or skin flap urethroplasties. In fact, reoperative skin flap urethroplasties are best avoided since the previously operated skin has diminished vascularity (Jayanthi et al, 1994) prone to contracture, and harvesting flaps exacerbates the skin deficiency for covering the penile shaft.

Nevertheless, skin management in reoperations is more complex than in primary repairs for several reasons. One is that the skin deficiency affects not only the ventral shaft, but often the dorsal or lateral sides of the penis, too. The skin that remains is commonly grossly scarred, and there is less shaft skin and usually no foreskin available. Consequently, there is little margin for error in designing skin coverage, and even the best executed repair may not heal properly without HBOT.

Contracted skin leads to several complications. Short skin can restrict erections, creating ventral, dorsal or lateral curvature. Tension that a tight skin closure exerts can pull open fistulas or dehisce the glans and neourethra. Older patients can also have pain with erections when skin is very short and/or tight.

In addition, scars on the glans and penile shaft skin outside of natural lines create anxiety in teens and adults, who worry that a lover will ask why his penis is scarred and be unhappy that it is ugly. Consequently, surgeons also must remove as much scarring as possible and strive to make the penis look normal, or as close to normal as possible.

Figure 19 demonstrates a reoperative STAC repair to correct persistent 65° ventral curvature, short scarred skin and a nonterminal meatus with stenosis after a Byars flap repair.

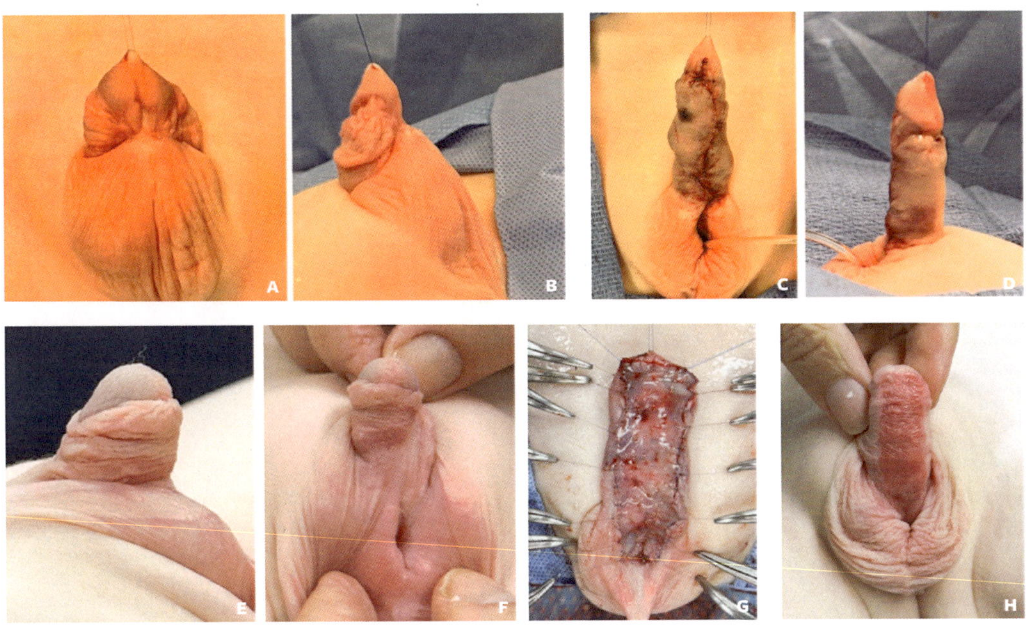

Figure 19. Reoperative STAC.
A,B, short, scarred and contracted ventral skin pulling the glans down and the scrotum up. C,D intraoperative appearance after scar excision, penile straightening, skin lengthening, and scrotoplasty. E,F, appearance 6 months later following adjuvant HBOT showing symmetric and supple shaft skin. G, after artificial erection confirmed the penis was straight from 3 corporotomies done at the last stage, the glans was opened along with the ventral penile skin and a lower lip graft was placed reaching from the tip of the glans to the scrotal meatus. With additional HBOT this graft has a 95% likelihood to heal healthy for final stage tubularization as shown in H, 6 months later.

Subepithelial skin closures

Regardless if the hypospadias is distal or proximal, or undergoing a primary versus a reoperative repair, skin stitches should be placed subepithelially. Skin marks and suture tracts are both more likely when stitches traverse the epithelium. A smooth scar within the median raphe or circumcision line calls less attention to prior surgery than do irregular scars and suture tunnels.

Adjuvant HBOT

Chapter 18 discusses the use and benefits of HBOT in hypospadias surgery. We have published how it improves urethroplasty graft healing in reoperations, using paired graft measurement to objectively assess results. It is also clear to us that HBOT is required to optimally repair skin damaged by prior operations. Accordingly, we recommend 15 perioperative dives with the first reoperation, generally with up to 5 given immediately preoperatively and the remainer postoperatively starting either the same day or day after surgery. This treatment makes it more likely the contracted skin will lengthen and better vascularize. Occasionally 15 dives is not sufficient and the patient returns with skin that is still thickened and inelastic. In these cases we double the recommended dives, which usually achieves the goal.

We cannot overemphasize the importance of adjuvant HBOT. Even a technically perfect operation may not be successful if the tissues are scarred and poorly vascularized.

While we do not plan HBOT for primary repairs, the severely deficient and nearly transparent ventral skin in perineo-scrotal hypospadias may also benefit from treatment, as might less severe cases associated with penile torsion or gnome hat deformities. Except for the time commitment required, HBOT rarely has complications and so the threshold to recommend it is low.

KEY POINTS

Healthy skin is one of the pillars for successful hypospadias repair, required along with a straight penis and a terminal meatus. All boys except those with MIP have some extent of ventral skin deficiency. Lengthening the skin and reallocating it symmetrically around the penile shaft is therefore a fundamental skill required of all hypospadias surgeons. Failure to accomplish this leads to urethroplasty graft contractions, difficulties closing the skin, and complications including fistulas and glans dehiscence pulled open by tension exerted by short and/or scarred skin.

The ventral skin also has abnormal vascularity and is prone to ischemic necrosis after hypospadias surgery. This occurs between 7 and 15 days postoperatively and is often confused for wound infection. Coating the skin with Manuka honey helps its healing when this occurs. Risk for this complication is increased when there is also penile torsion or a gnome hat dorsal skin hump.

Surgical manipulation of the skin affects its ability to nourish the edges of urethroplasty grafts when placed at the initial stage of a repair, resulting in increased graft and skin contracture. Delaying grafting to a second operation after the skin has healed largely avoids these complications and is one of the reasons for STAC repair.

HBOT also helps skin healing. Adjuvant therapy is mandatory for optimal skin lengthening and revascularization after unsuccessful surgery causes it to contract. We have additionally used it for extensive skin necrosis after primary proximal repairs, and as prophylaxis against skin complications in perineo-scrotal hypospadias and hypospadias with penile torsion or gnome hat skin deformities.

Hypospadias skin incisions should be confined to the ventral median raphe and the circumcision line. These are natural or common lines and conceal scars that would otherwise call unwanted attention to the prior surgery. Closure of skin incisions should use subepithelial stitches to reduce visible scars.

References

Jayanthi VR, McLorie GA, Khoury AE and Churchill BM: Can previously relocated penile skin be successfully used for salvage hypospadias repair? *J Urol* 152: 740, 1994

Snodgrass W and Bush NC: Graft and skin complications in 342 primary proximal hypospadias repairs: STAG versus STAC. ESPU abstract, 2024

Follow-Up

Chapter 22

Duration of Follow Up to Diagnose Complications

It is commonly said that patients should be followed through puberty after childhood hypospadias repair, and that the longer the follow up the greater the number of complications that are found. This may cause surgeons to disregard published results, assuming they will change with longer follow up. The possibility that new problems can develop during puberty also concerns parents, who question the rationale for doing a repair in childhood if it is only going to have to be redone during puberty.

However, we are not aware of a single published series in which a large percentage of patients were systematically assessed at specified intervals until their growth ended. In fact, it is not practical to maintain active contact for many years with every patient after repair, especially when the operation is thought to be successful.

Consequently, we evaluated teens and adults presenting with complications after childhood hypospadias repair and found that 80% had persistent problems dating back for as long as the patients could remember. Only 5% developed new complications during puberty, and the remaining 15% occurred much later at an average age of 47 years, all obstructions from meatal stenosis or strictures. Therefore, lifelong follow up would be needed to capture all complications after hypospadias repair despite the vast majority of complications occurring in childhood (Snodgrass & Bush, 2022).

Furthermore, the timing and duration of follow up needed depends on the outcome of interest. Since most urethroplasty complications can be diagnosed relatively early after surgery, follow up into puberty is not necessary to assess most results of a repair and compare it to others. In contrast, a study on sexual function after hypospadias repair would require evaluation later in puberty and early adulthood, but not periodic follow up throughout childhood.

Finally, long term periodic follow up with examination of the penis can adversely impact the patient. For example, one adult with uncorrected distal hypospadias who had no functional problems with his urinary stream or sexual performance still wanted it repaired. He explained how the primary doctor performing his back-to- school physical exams each year always hesitated for a few moments to study his penis, and then turned to his mother to say, "Now I remember. He has a minor hypospadias that we agreed doesn't need surgery." After hearing his whole life that his penis was not right, he wanted surgery to make it right.

This chapter reviews the duration of follow up needed to diagnose most urethroplasty complications after hypospadias repair.

Diagnosis of urethroplasty complications

Before surgeons can determine the optimal duration of follow up to diagnose urethroplasty complications, those complications must be universally defined. No consensus definitions exist, and so we have provided the following:

Persistent or recurrent curvature is any degree of postoperative penile bending.

A fistula is a leak of urine from the neourethra anywhere below the meatus.

Glans dehiscence is separation of the glans wings leaving fusion < 2mm.

Meatal stenosis is a meatus < 8Fr with obstructive urinary symptoms (stranguria, retention) and/or UTI.

A stricture is narrowing of the neourethra to < 8Fr proximal to the meatus.

A diverticulum is visible ballooning of the neourethra during voiding.

When complications occur

To decide the needed duration of follow up, it is important to determine when complications occur, which may be different than when they are diagnosed or when reoperations are done. A patient might develop a fistula soon after the initial postoperative evaluation, but not return for follow up and have the diagnosis made until a year later. Then there may be an additional wait before closure is scheduled.

Similarly, it is important to know if a patient presenting with a complication several years after surgery was seen earlier postoperatively *without* that problem. Otherwise, delayed follow up or reintervention can give the false perception that the complication occurred later than it actually did and that longer follow up is needed than actually is required to detect most problems.

Within the First Year

We reported that 87% of complications after primary and reoperative distal and proximal TIP repairs occurred within the first year after surgery (Figure 1).

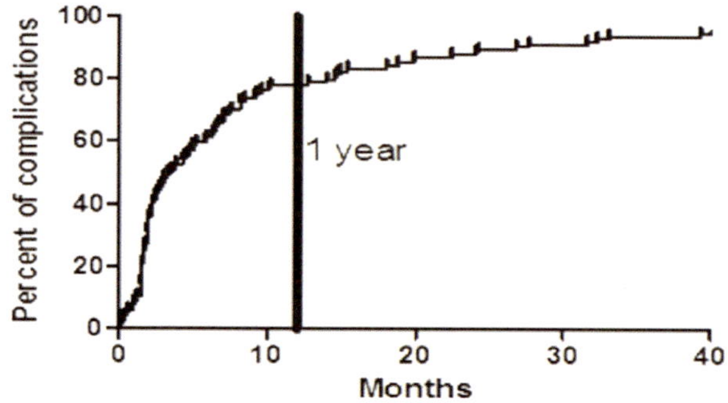

Figure 1. Kaplan-Meier curve showing detection of complications after TIP repairs in 887 patients. 88% of complications occurred within the first year or at the first postoperative visit. Only 2% of patients with follow up during the first year developed a complication later.

The median time was 6 months for fistulas, meatal stenoses, strictures and diverticula, and 2 months for glans dehiscence. At the time of that review our initial postoperative assessment was done at 6 weeks, and the second 6 months later (8 months postoperatively).

New complications that were not present during follow up within the first year occurred in only 2% of the 887 patients (Snodgrass and Bush et al, 2014).

Today we review pictures of the repair sent by parents 2 weeks after surgery and have learned that glans dehiscence has nearly always occurred by then. Many fistulas also become apparent soon after the catheter is removed. Rather than having to wait longer to diagnose complications, we have learned they can be identified even sooner than we realized.

Similarly, Castagnetti et al (2013) reviewed patients after primary proximal repairs using TIP, onlay preputial flaps, or staged grafts and found that all complications were diagnosed within the first 12 months despite follow up ranging from 4-7 years. This is noteworthy, since their overall follow up was in the "intermediate range" that some have recommended should be the standard, yet complications were only found during the first year.

After the First Postoperative Year

Long et al (2017) reported complications after primary proximal repairs using 1-stage and 2-stage flaps.

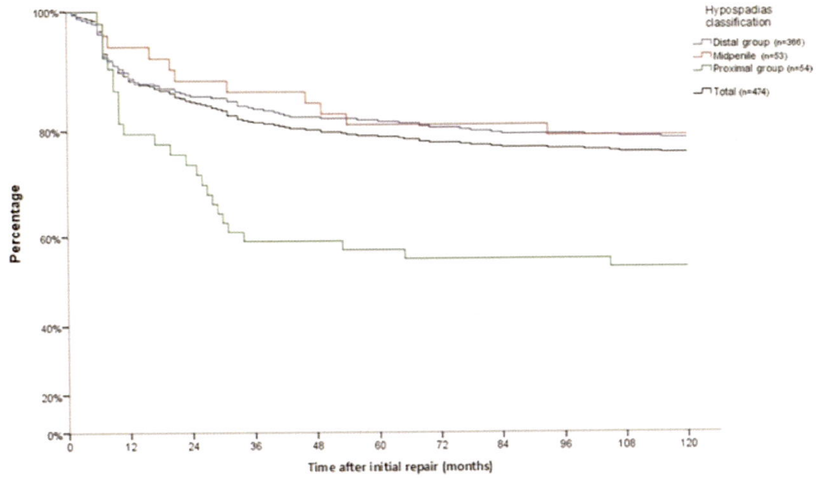

Figure 2. Time to reoperation for complications.
Spinoit et al reported follow up to reoperation, which will be longer than the time to diagnosis because of factors impacting surgery scheduling. They also did not state how many of these complications were diagnosed after an assessment with normal findings during the first postoperative year.

The median time to diagnosis was 9.7 months (IQR 3-21), but it is noteworthy that the time to occurrence was based on the *first* operation in the 50% of patients who had a 2-stage repair, meaning those complications developed within 2 months of the procedure that created the neourethra. They did not describe the timing and duration of their protocol for postoperative assessments, or state if those patients found to have complications later than a year postoperatively had negative assessments earlier.

Spinoit et al (2013) also reviewed complications after primary hypospadias repair, but with the specific aim to determine the duration of follow up needed for their diagnosis. Their standard recommendation comprised postoperative consultations at 6 weeks, 6 months, after toilet-training, and during puberty. There was a total of 474 patients, whose mean follow up was 34 months. Only 63% returned for assessment more than a year after surgery, which emphasizes the difficulty in maintaining longer routine follow up, even in national health care systems with ready access to care.

The authors did not report when complications occurred but rather when reoperations were done, which can be delayed due various factors such as waiting lists, or insurance considerations in the US. They reported nearly half of these reoperations were within 1 year of surgery, with a mean time of 25 months (Figure 2).

Both Long et al and Spinoit et al concluded longer follow up was needed to identify complications, although neither reported how many patients developed a complication which was not present within the first year after surgery. They also did not mention how many patients did not have a postoperative assessment during the first year, as happened with a third of our patients whose complications were diagnosed later.

While Spinoit et al recommended follow up twice during the first year and then another evaluation after toilet-training and in puberty, they did not say how many patients followed that protocol, and if later complications were diagnosed because of scheduled follow up, or at other times outside their protocol when parents recognized a problem.

Another reason to recommend long term follow up is concern that a complication will be overlooked or ignored by the patient or caregivers, but how often that occurs is not well-documented in prepubertal boys.

Consequently, the importance of scheduled follow up beyond 1 year when most complications occur with the goal of identifying new problems cannot be determined from these studies.

During Puberty

To our knowledge, the study with the highest percentage of patients following up during puberty after childhood repair was reported by Ekmark et al (2013). Of 147 patients eligible for follow up at age 16, 114 (77%) returned for that final assessment. The authors stated a new complication was diagnosed during puberty in only 7 (6%) patients, comprising 1 stricture after a Byars flap repair, and 6 recurrent ventral curvatures.

The original orthoplasty in those 6 with curvature was chordee excision, which the authors described as "being done so thoroughly that artificial erection was not necessary to confirm it made the penis straight". However, since chordee excision has been proven ineffective for straightening corporal disproportion (Chapter 2), the "new" curvature they found at puberty was almost certainly bending that was never made straight and could no longer be overlooked when the penis grew larger.

We reviewed findings in 82 teens and adults, 15 of whom were Tanner 2-4, presenting with complications after childhood hypospadias repair. These included glans/repair dehiscence (75%), ventral curvature (40%), strictures or meatal stenosis (30%) and fistulas (15%). Of these, 80% were present before puberty, including all ventral curvatures and dehiscences. Only 4 (5%) were new problems that developed during puberty - 2 fistulas and 2 strictures (Snodgrass & Bush, 2022).

These data refute the idea that "rapid" pubertal growth stresses otherwise successful childhood hypospadias repairs, and challenge the assertion that follow up through puberty is necessary. They also can reassure parents that successful childhood repairs are durable.

In Adults

Barbagli, an adult stricture specialist, reported men with apparently successful childhood hypospadias repair sometimes presented 10 years or later with strictures of the neourethra (2006). However, he did not state how many of the 60 adults in his series met this description, saying only that most had persistent complications from childhood.

Similarly, 15% of the teens and adult we evaluated with complications after childhood repair presented with new obstructive voiding symptoms caused by strictures (n=9) or meatal stenosis (n=3) at a mean age of 47 years (19-66).

Together, these studies show a bimodal distribution of complications after childhood hypospadias repair. Most occur early after surgery, and certainly before puberty, while there is a second group presenting with obstruction in middle age.

These series have to be considered in context. Each year approximately 10,000 boys in the US have primary hypospadias repair. By the time the first patients reach 40 years of age, 200,000 will be adults 20 years or older. Although the adults reported with complications most likely represent only an unknown portion of those living with problems, it is clear that the 12 we described are outliers.

Who Does the Assessment?

The provider tasked with postoperative assessment was not mentioned in any of the reports cited above. Probably most surgeons evaluate their own patients in the US, which has always been our practice. However, some have criticized us saying that another qualified surgeon would provide a more objective review and accurate reporting of complications.

We are aware that trainees provide most of the postoperative follow up of hypospadias patients in some large centers, sometimes without confirmation of those assessments by a staff surgeon. Increasingly, physician extenders are being used in this same role, and we have seen patients for second opinions in whom complications, including glans dehiscence and BXO, were not recognized by them.

To our knowledge no study has compared the diagnosis of complications made by the surgeon to trainees or physician extenders.

Key Points

Few publications report when urethroplasty complications occurred in patients under systematic follow up after hypospadias repair. Those that do found between 50% and 100% were diagnosed within the first 12 months after surgery. Our experience indicates that glans dehiscence develops at approximately 2 weeks, while fistulas, meatal stenosis, strictures and diverticula are diagnosed at a median of 6 months. Therefore, careful assessment is most needed during the first year to not overlook a complication.

There is no consensus regarding the length of additional follow up after a year needed to consider postoperative evaluation for urethroplasty complications adequate, or to publish outcomes of repairs. It is often quipped that the longer the follow up, the more the complications, but available data suggest that is not true after the first postoperative year except for outliers or those patients who did not attend earlier follow up, with the exception of stricture disease.

If the goal is to capture all urethroplasty complications, the finding of strictures in middle-aged adults indicates assessments would have to continue the entire lifetime after childhood repair – a standard that would never be met.

A reliance on trainees or physician extenders to provide postoperative follow up could result in delayed diagnosis, and surgeons should verify both positive and negative examinations by them, especially during the first year after surgery when most complications will be detected.

Most importantly, unless supporting data is published, surgeons should not say that new complications are common during puberty. Some parents decide against hypospadias repair in their child because they worry the operation will have to be done all over again when puberty causes new complications. Rather, care-givers can be reassured that the risk for new complications more than a year after surgery is small, and that very few occur during puberty.

References

Barbagli G, De Angelis M, Palminteri E, and Lazzeri M: Failed hypospadias repair presenting in adults. *Eur Urol* 49: 887, 2006

Castagnetti M, Zhapa E, Rigamonti W: Primary severe hypospadias: comparison of reoperation rates and parental perception of urinary symptoms and cosmetic outcomes among 4 repairs. *J Urol* 189: 1508, 2013

Ekmark AN, Svensson H, Arnbjornsson E, and Hannsson E: Postpubertal examination after hypospadias repair is necessary to evaluate the success of primary reconstruction. *Eur J Pediar Surg* 23: 304, 2013

Long CJ, Chu DI, Tenny RW, Morris Ar, Weiss DA,Shukla AR, Srinivasan AK, Zderic SA, Kolon TF, Canning DA: Intermediate-term followup of proximal hypospadias repair reveals high complication rate. *J Urol* 197: 852-858, 2017

Snodgrass W, and Bush NC: Do new complications develop during puberty after childhood hypospadias repair? *J Urol* 208: 696, 2022

Snodgrass W, Villanueva C and Bush NC: Duration of follow-up to diagnose hypospadias urethroplasty complications. *J Pediatr Urol* 10: 208, 2014

Spinoit AF, Poelaert F, Groen LA, Van Laecke E and and Hoebeke P: Hypospadias repair at a tertiary care center: long-term followup is mandatory to determine the real complication rate. *J Urol* 189: 2276, 2013

Chapter 23

Hypospadias Repair In Teens and Adults

Teens and adults present with never-corrected, usually distal, hypospadias, or with unsuccessfully repaired, usually proximal, hypospadias. They often fall into the divide between pediatric and adult urology – too old to be operated by the pediatric urologists who perform most hypospadias surgery, and therefore left to seek advice from adult urologists who are less familiar with the condition and its best management.

Many with uncorrected hypospadias report skepticism from adult urologists, who question the need for surgery while emphasizing a poor risk / benefit ratio. Patients who persist are often recommended to have only a partial repair that leaves the neomeatus in a subterminal location not properly enclosed within the glans.

This attitude arises from a few reports suggesting that adults accommodate to their hypospadias, and sometimes do not even realize they have the condition (Fichtner et al, 1995; Dodds et al, 2007). Conversely, one study of men with untreated hypospadias found they reported worse urinary function, more penile curvature and difficulties with intercourse, worse sexual health and more dissatisfaction with their meatus compared to others without the condition (Schlomer et al, 2014).

We similarly found high rates of urine spraying, penile curvature, painful intercourse, and bother by the appearance of their penis in men with uncorrected hypospadias presenting at a mean age of 42 years (Snodgrass and Bush, 2022). Rather than accommodating to their condition, even middle-aged men sought correction. Of course, we cannot know the denominator of all men with non-operated hypospadias to determine if these were representative of them or outliers, but they nevertheless prove that distal hypospadias creates functional problems in at least some patients which persist until it is repaired.

Patients suffering from persistent complications after childhood repair also present with urine spraying, ventral penile curvature and sexual dysfunction, and dissatisfaction with the appearance of their penis. They too often encounter hesitancy from adult urologists to correct their problem or refer them to a specialist who can, telling them they need to learn to live with their situation. Some men report they were told there is nothing that can be done to help them. Accordingly, they may end their search for repair unless problems develop, such as obstruction from a neourethral stricture, that requires intervention. Even in these situations, several men were under the impression that nothing could be done about their urethral stricture other than painful periodic dilations. Definitive surgical treatment was not discussed for several of our patients until after urgent obstruction and placement of a suprapubic tube.

Concern has been expressed in recent years that successful hypospadias repairs done in childhood can develop new complications during pubertal growth, including fistulas and ventral curvature. That worry can influence parents to delay surgery, believing it will all have to be redone later anyway. However, we reported a series of Tanner 4 and 5 patients with complications after childhood repair and found that most had persistent problems never corrected after earlier surgery, while a smaller group presented in middle age with new obstructive symptoms from strictures or meatal stenosis. Only 5% developed new complications during puberty – comprising fistulas or strictures, but no ventral curvature (Snodgrass and Bush, 2022).

Those observations are similar to what Barbagli et al (2006) reported. Most the men he evaluated had persisting complications from childhood hypospadias surgery, while another group appeared to have had successful repairs until they presented many years later with strictures.

The reason for the apparently late development of complications decades after repair are not known. Barbagli et al speculated strictures occurred as a result of sexual trauma to the neourethra lacking corpus spongiosum. Most of the men in reported series likely had skin flap urethroplasties in childhood, which may have unreliable vascularity to their ends which become the meatus or the junction to the native urethra. Perhaps a marginal blood supply eventually leads to stenosis. In others, we have found strictures at the site of their persistent ventral curvature. Regardless, these patients are outliers, given their small numbers in contrast to the thousands of hypospadias repairs done annually.

None of these teens and adults we evaluated with lingering complications after childhood repair expressed the wish that surgery had been delayed until they could have given consent. Nor did any adult with uncorrected hypospadias say that he was pleased his condition was not repaired before he could participate in the decision-making. Rather, their uniform complaint was that the hypospadias was not fixed, or successfully fixed, when they were younger, before the condition caused ongoing frustration trying to void standing without splattering outside the toilet, embarrassment in the locker room, or hindered intimacy with lovers.

This is especially true in teens who are often angry to learn their hypospadias could have been repaired in childhood, sparing them the anguish of being different and having to discuss their penis with their parents. A few have attempted suicide to escape their hypospadias. Others act out during recovery, punishing their parents for their bitterness. One teen with BXO started drinking heavily because of the pain and embarrassment of his penis problem. His liver enzymes had to recover prior to proceeding with oral grafting. These raw emotions are so prevalent that we strongly advise all teens facing surgery to talk with a licensed therapist, psychologist, or psychiatrist to help manage them.

Without doubt recovery after surgery is also more taxing to these older patients than to younger boys. Their pain is greater, especially the nocturnal erections during urinary diversion which cannot be prevented, particularly when short penile skin is present as is common in most reoperations. They are also quickly impatient with the time it is taking to recover.

But most are also extremely gratified when their penis is made normal for the first time in their lives. When they can stand to urinate without worrying if the spraying stream will soil their pants. When their bent penis is finally straight. When they no longer have to conceal their condition from a new lover or worry if they will hear the dreaded question, "What's wrong with your penis?"

We did not know the extent that hypospadias can affect teens and adults when we practiced in a children's hospital. Nor did we hear men say again and again after their hypospadias was repaired that they had no idea how much it affected their sense of their own masculinity.

There are important lessons in these observations for pediatric urologists advising parents if their son would benefit from hypospadias repair, and in deciding what the final result of surgery should be.

Whatever those conclusions, we already acknowledged that some critics will question if men who seek surgical repair are really representative of the unknown denominator of men with hypospadias that was never operated, or was only partially repaired. While that question cannot be answered by either advocates for surgery or skeptics of its benefits, the experiences of these men are still useful to know what happens to at least some who have not had surgery, or had incomplete and/or unsuccessful correction.

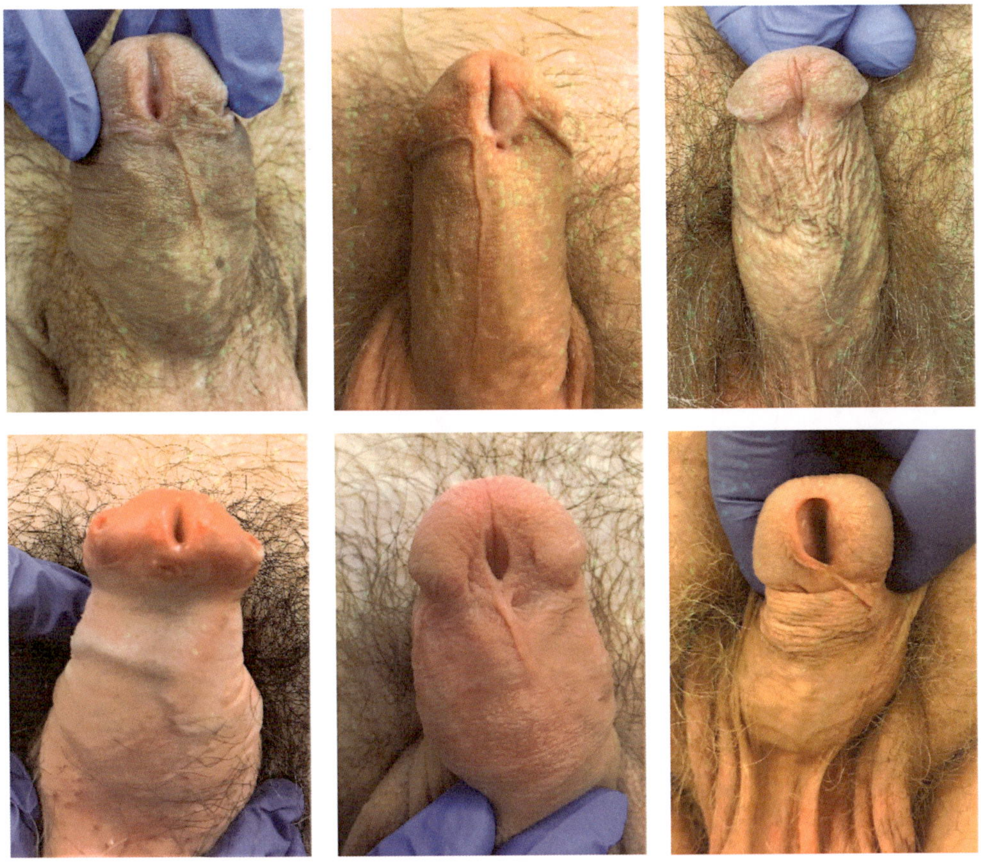

Figure 1. Meatus of men with urine spraying from uncorrected distal hypospadias.
These representative photos show that every man with urine spraying had abnormal anatomy with deficient or absent glans fusion. Boys with similar anatomy are therefore at risk for urine spraying as they grow older.

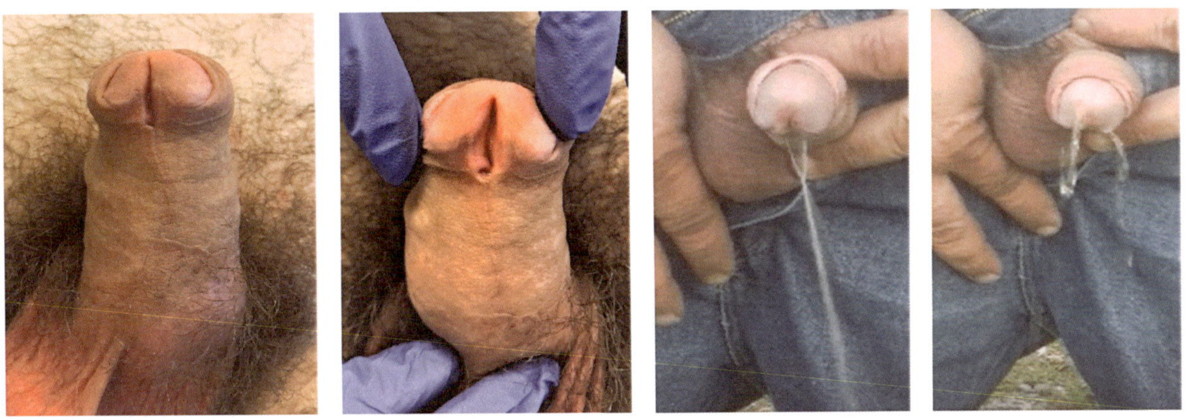

Figure 2. Urine spraying from subcoronal meatus.
A,B, man with uncorrected hypospadias and a subcoronal meatus. C and D show the stream defected down and spraying, and then splattering towards the end of voiding. This was his usual voiding pattern.

Uncorrected Hypospadias in Adults

We reported observations in 35 men with uncorrected hypospadias presenting at a mean age of 42 years (median 44, 18-63). Of these, 3 had distal shaft and the remainder had coronal or subcoronal hypospadias, including 10 with MIP (Bush and Snodgrass, 2023). Representative photos of their hypospadias are shown in Figure 1.

Urine Spraying

The most common complaint these men had was urine spraying, present in 80%. Typically, this was not predictable and many of them were able to stand to void at least some of the time. Nevertheless, their stream was a constant source of concern, proving that merely asking if a patient voids standing does not determine if he voids normally.

Splattering was most likely when the force of their stream was less, typically near the end of urination or when they voided with an incompletely filled bladder. Most chose to sit when there were others in a public bathroom, and several admitted they had to change clothes at work on a few occasions after soiling their pants.

Examination in all of them found a meatus which was not normally enclosed by the glans, as seen in Figure 1. One function of the glans is to focus the urine into a compact, straight stream, and spraying is a rare complaint from men with normal anatomy or following hypospadias repair which creates normal glans fusion. That normal anatomy has been defined in boys as glans fusion between the ventral lip of the meatus and the corona measuring > 2.3mm and averaging 4.7mm (Hutton and Babu, 2007). We have consistently measured fusion averaging 10mm in adults.

Parents of boys with similar anatomy to that seen in Figure 1 should be advised that at least some, and possibly most, will grow into men who will experience urine spraying and related concerns if the hypospadias is not successfully repaired to create normal glans fusion.

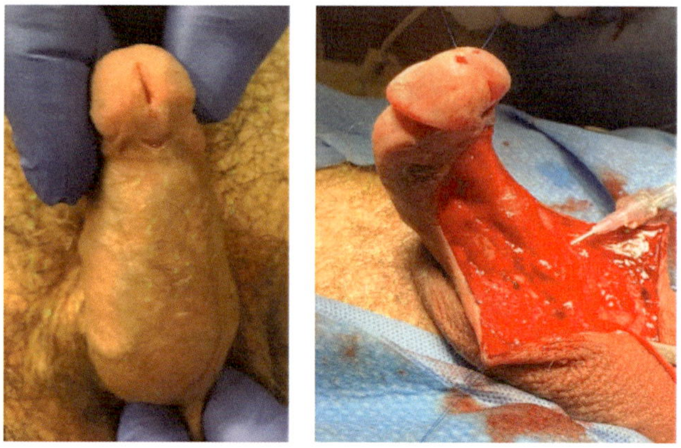

Figure 3. Ventral curvature despite a distal meatus. Uncorrected distal shaft hypospadias with 65° VC. Sexual intercourse was so uncomfortable for his wife that she threatened to divorce him unless it was repaired.

Several men sent videos of their voiding to demonstrate the spraying, shown in representative photos in Figure 2. These emphasize again that abnormal anatomy leads to abnormal function.

Ventral Curvature

Penile curvature ranging from 10° to 65° was found in 37% of these men, 11 with VC and 2 having lateral bends. This bending caused difficult penetration for 1 man, and discomfort for sexual partners in various positions in 4. The patient with the most severe VC is shown in Figure 3, who serves as a reminder that curvature greater than 30° can occur despite a distal meatus.

Other Sexual Dysfunctions

These men also told us other ways that hypospadias interfered with their sexual activities. For example, one man with a scrotal web extending up his penile shaft described how that thicker skin with hair, or the stubble from shaving, irritated his lover's vaginal introitus. The exposed urethral plate tissues, especially in men with MIP hypospadias, caused others discomfort during intercourse. Even a slight distal bend made it difficult for some to quickly reinsert their penis if it came out of the vagina.

Altogether, 1 of every 3 men reported sexual dysfunction from penile curvature or these other differences.

Abnormal Appearance

In addition to these functional concerns, nearly two-thirds of these men stated they were unhappy with the appearance of their penis, even though most were middle aged and some were in stable married relationships, many of whom had partners who said they were not bothered by how it looked. This was true whether they had been circumcised, as were half the patients, or not, since the abnormal appearance of the glans and meatus was their main concern.

Many recalled feeling inhibited to date as teenagers because of their different appearance, and a few who recently divorced wanted surgery to make the glans and meatus look normal before starting to date again. A few patients had unsupportive partners who didn't think they needed surgery, but stated they wanted to do it for themselves. Others had not previously been sexually active and would often present for surgery with one of their parents.

Emotional Disturbances

The study by Schlomer et al reported men with uncorrected hypospadias had worse SHIM scores and greater dissatisfaction with their meatus than other men. The curvature that a third of our patients had also causes more unhealthy mental days than others with a straight penis experience (Menon et al, 2016). Though not objectively studied, our patients described how their hypospadias impacted their general sense of well-being, and several summarized their motivation to have repair as a desire "to be whole."

With surveys finding that most male and female adolescents have viewed pornography on-line, certainly teens with uncorrected hypospadias know their penis is different—perhaps in contrast to earlier studies before internet pornography existed. But few are willing to disclose their difference to friends, much less want to discuss it with their mom and dad. Consequently, most face their concerns in isolation, much like their parents experienced when told their newborn son had a birth defect of his penis that they had never heard of before.

Then, when teens learn the hypospadias can be corrected the hope of becoming normal is counterbalanced by anxiety about surgery on their penis—and frustration, or even anger, when they realize this could all have been avoided by an operation in childhood that they would not remember.

For all the talk about allowing patients to make their own decisions regarding genital surgery, we have not yet met the teen who appreciated the postponement. Rather, many lash out at their parents, especially during the early postoperative period when discomfort is greatest.

This anger is less visible in adults. Nevertheless, some of the men we have repaired still refuse to discuss hypospadias with their parents, or even to inform them of their decision to have surgery. A few others came for surgery with their mothers, explaining that they wanted them to share in their pain. Some bring a parent to their surgery because they need help in the early postop days, and do not have a significant other to help them nor want to discuss their issue with a friend to ask for help, having to rely instead on an elderly parent to push them in a wheelchair for the few days they are recommended for bedrest post-operatively.

Surgery to correct hypospadias is more than a technical exercise in these patients. Emotional turmoil is so common, especially in teens, that we uniformly mention to both them and adults the availability of counseling to help them cope, and strongly advise they use it.

Distal Hypospadias Repair

Decision-Making

The goal for primary hypospadias repair in adults is the same as for surgery in boys: to make a normal penis, meaning straight, with a slit meatus at the tip of the glans, no visible scars outside normal skin and circumcision lines, and no lingering complications. We disagree with those who advocate making a subterminal meatus, since a meatus not normally enclosed by glans has continued likelihood for the urine spraying - which 80% of these men are already experiencing and is a prime motivation for them to want surgery.

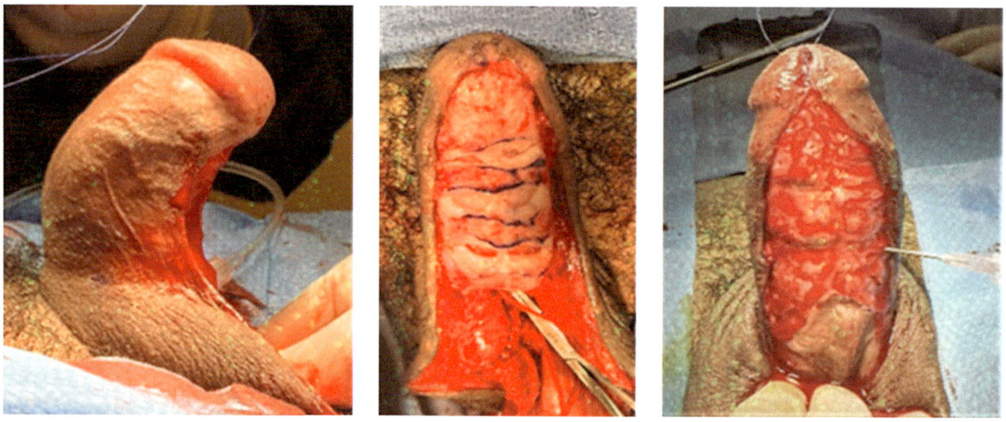

Figure 4. 3 Corporotomies in an adult.
A, VC greater than 30° after ventral degloving. B, appearance after 3 corporotomies. C, artificial erection after healing, 6 months later. No adult undergoing hypospadias repair has reported ED after healing these incisions

Surgeons who recommend subterminal correction justify it by the presumed increase risk for complications, especially meatal stenosis, when complete correction is done. However, as discussed below, we found results to be the same in adults undergoing hypospadias repair as it is in children despite conventional wisdom to the contrary. Meatal stenosis happens in less than 5% of patients after primary TIP repair (Pfistermuller et al, 2015), and in less than 0.5% in our practice, meaning higher occurrence likely indicates a technical error is being made by the surgeon.

The same algorithm for repair used in boys also applies to teens and adults. Most patients with uncorrected hypospadias have a distal meatus and a straight penis and so TIP repair is done. When VC measures 30° or more, 3 corporotomies are made for straightening, usually as part of a STAC-TIP 2-stage repair. We are comfortable that these ventral corporotomies straighten the curvature without causing erectile dysfunction in patients of all ages partly from our experience using them in teens and adults (Figure 4).

Preoperative Antibiotics

We do not administer IV antibiotics before TIP repair in boys. However, after several men developed purulent Enterococcus or gram negative urethritis during postoperative urinary diversion we started giving a single preoperative IV dose of Ampicillin and Gentamicin.

Surgical Procedure

The steps of distal TIP are done the same way in adults as in boys. The glans wings are developed along the visible margin to the urethral plate and then dissected laterally along the surface of the corpora. However, we have not found the extended glans wings dissection described for boys with a small glans < 14mm to be necessary in adults, although dissection should be done until there is no tension on them. Next, the urethral plate is incised throughout its length from within the meatus to its end junction with the glans, continuing down to the underlying corpora. Then the neourethra is stitched in 2 layers using a continuous, subepithelial 5-0 Vicryl beginning in approximately the midglans so as not to create iatrogenic meatal stenosis. The suture line is covered by a ventral dartos flap. Glansplasty is done using 4 or 5 interrupted subepithelial 4-0 Vicryl stitches, which creates glans fusion that is 8mm or more, averaging 10mm.

Management of the dorsal foreskin is often different in men, since it grows less in proportion to the penile shaft and glans during puberty and usually is not large enough for prepucioplasty. That situation gives the patient the choice between leaving the partial foreskin as it is, or removing it with a circumcision. Skin management without the option of foreskin reconstruction is another disadvantage to waiting until adulthood for repair.

Urinary Diversion

We insert a silver-coated antibacterial 12Fr foley, inflate the balloon and tie the catheter to the glans traction suture. Urinary diversion lasts 1 week.

Bandages

The penis is wrapped with adaptic and then Coban™, and then an outer bandage is added to immobilize it upwards on the abdomen as shown in Figure 5. A 1000mL leg bag is placed. This can all be pealed off after soaking in a shower or bath 5 days postoperatively. The catheter is removed 1 week post-operatively.

Postoperative Care

Medications after surgery include an oral narcotic (Norco), alternating with ibuprofen, Oxybutynin XL 10 or 15 mg once or twice daily as needed to control bladder spasm, daily Bactrim during urinary diversion, and Valium 10mg at night to make nocturnal erections less bothersome, since no medication prevents them.

Early in our experience with men we realized they were likely to develop scrotal hematomas if they ambulated the day of surgery. Strict bedrest for 24 hours, followed by limited ambulation the next few days alleviated that problem.

We recommend postoperative HBOT in smokers, diabetics, and other men with potential vascular disease even though they have not had prior penile surgery. Typically, 10-20 dives are recommended beginning the afternoon after repair. All men undergoing reoperation are recommended to have HBOT.

Results

We analyzed outcomes from both primary repairs and reoperations in adults and compared them to boys undergoing the same procedures during the study period. Eight adults had uncorrected hypospadias at a mean age of 23 years, ranging to 62, and urethroplasty complications (1 fistula) were no different than those in boys. The same was true in 61 adults undergoing reoperations. Therefore, we concluded that complications are not greater when surgery in done at an older age (Snodgrass and Bush et al, 2014).

However, the experience of surgery and recovery is very different in teens and adults versus infants and boys. As is generally true for any surgery in adults, postoperative pain is subjectively greater. Nocturnal erections are a particular source of worry to teens and adults, especially during their period of catheterization. There is no medication to prevent these erections, and the best remedy we have found is Valium at bedtime to make patients somewhat less aware and anxious about them.

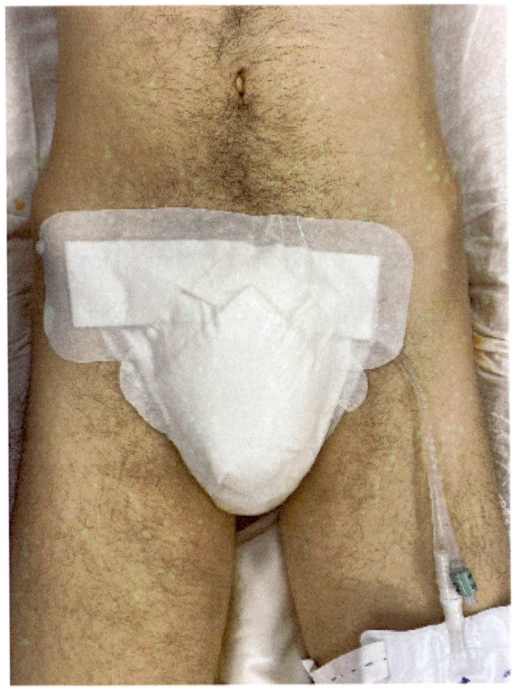

Figure 5. Adult postoperative bandage.

As already mentioned, some teens are likely to act out during recovery, especially towards their parents, speaking harshly, demanding frequent attention, seeming to want to make them share their pain. Parents often feel guilt for having delayed repair, setting up a cycle of in which they acquiesce to escalating demands. We suspect that those who recommend delaying surgery until puberty have not managed many teens undergoing hypospadias repair!

Despite these challenges during recovery, men report the repair makes their stream straight, compact and predictable, and their appearance normal. Their comments provide further insight into the impact hypospadias can have until it is corrected.

One year after distal TIP, the 22-year old shown in Figure 2 emailed,

> *You have remarkably changed my life for good, not only physically, but most importantly mentally.*
>
> *It has been a challenging journey my whole life as this has burdened me for over 16 years . . . while urologists advised it was only mild and I would be "fine", never comprehending the insecurity affect this condition has to someone's psychological health.*

Another man wrote,

> *I wish I could have afforded this during my adolescence years since I was so embarrassed with my condition.*
>
> *I was timid to be intimate with any girlfriend, because I was afraid I might hear the dreaded words, 'What's wrong with your penis?'*
>
> *That would have been devastating for this young man. Even as a grown man the embarrassment never goes away . . . such a relief not having to worry about it for the rest of my life.*

Hypospadias Reoperations

Does puberty create complications?

We reviewed teens and adults presenting with complications after childhood hypospadias repair to determine if pubertal growth caused new problems. Our series included 82 patients, of which 15 were Tanner 2-4 and the remainder Tanner 5 (Snodgrass and Bush, 2022).

Similar to adults with uncorrected hypospadias, the main complaints were urine spraying (60%), ventral curvature (40%), and dissatisfaction with penile appearance (25%). The main findings were glans/wound dehiscence (75%) and ventral curvature which averaged 50°.

Most of these patients presented with complications that developed during childhood after their repairs and were never successfully corrected. However, 15% developed new lower tract obstructive voiding symptoms, at an average age of 47 years, from strictures or meatal stenosis. Only 5% presented during puberty with new complaints, 2 with fistulas and another 2 having strictures.

Our results are nearly identical to those published by Lam et al (2005), in which 27 patients with proximal hypospadias were reviewed more than 10 years after surgery when each was Tanner 5. New complications diagnosed at that final follow up were found in 2 (7%), comprising 1 fistula and 1 stricture.

Another report which concluded follow up into puberty was necessary because of the risk for recurrent VC stated this occurred in 5% of their patients (Ekmark et al, 2013). However, their initial straightening was done by chordee excision, the authors stating this is so reliable that there was no need for artificial erection afterwards. Yet, as discussed in Chapter 1, Duckett proved VC most often persists despite thorough "chordee excision", and we published that 83% of patients presenting to us after chordee excision by other pediatric urologists had persistent or recurrent VC (Snodgrass and Bush, 2019). We also commented that this VC was usually not recognized in prepubertal boys by the original surgeon. Therefore, the *recurrent* VC Ekmark et al report was more likely *persistent* VC which simply became more obvious when the penis enlarged during puberty. Not one patient in our series stated they recalled having a straight penis which then bent during or after puberty. To the contrary, all recalled their penis being bent before puberty, as far back as they could remember.

Despite assertions that the "rapid growth" of the penis during puberty, which actually takes place over several years, can stress prior repairs and create new complications, we are not aware of any reported series documenting this occurrence.

Presentation

The most common complaints in our patients were urine spraying or stranguria, and penile curvature that included ventral, lateral and dorsal bends. Three patients had painful erections from short ventral skin after hypospadias repair, and 2 men had pain at the meatus during intercourse. Many were dissatisfied with the appearance of their penis, especially those with irregular skin from baseball stitching and/or pits and cuts in the glans from epithelial suturing. These were the chief complaint in a quarter of the men.

The most common findings were glans/wound dehiscence, ventral curvature, strictures and meatal stenosis, and fistulas. In addition, 12% had hair in the neourethra and lichen sclerosis was found in 1 patient.

Surgical Management

The goal in adult reoperations is the same as for all other hypospadias repairs – to make the penis normal. While that can be challenging after multiple failed operations leaving short skin and scars, penile skin can be lengthened and rehabilitated as discussed in Chapters 19 and 21, or replaced by skin grafts when it is too deficient or scarred for lesser maneuvers. Similarly, a meatus normally enclosed by glans can nearly always be accomplished despite prior injury, unless too much glans has been lost to technically create adequate wings.

Several factors help determine best management by reoperative TIP, inlay graft, or STAG/STAC repair (Snodgrass and Bush et al, 2009). Generally, those with dehiscence after a distal repair whose penis is straight undergo reoperative TIP when the urethral plate is not grossly scarred, and inlay graft or STAG if it is.

Those with complications after proximal repairs most often have more complex combinations of problems which often include dehiscence, ventral curvature, and meatal stenosis or neourethral stricture. VC $\geq 30°$ is straightened by 3 ventral corporotomies and STAC. Meatal stenosis and/or BXO usually requires STAG repair, while urethral strictures can be corrected by inlay grafting, or STAG when the lumen is nearly obliterated, as long as the penis is straight. However, most men with proximal hypospadias have persistent penile curvature $\geq 30°$. Many teens and adults with multiply recurrent fistulas also have persistent ventral curvature that needs to be straightened.

Most of these men also have deficient ventral penile skin, and surgeons should have a low threshold to perform STAC repair initially to reallocate and rehabilitate the skin before urethroplasty grafting, even when the penis is straight. Adults have far less collagen and elastin in skin than children, and penile skin subjectively does not tend to stretch to the same extent it will in children, even with hyperbaric oxygen therapy.

Postoperative Management

Care, including medications, bandages, and urinary diversion following reoperations is the same as described above for primary repairs in adults.

However, these men are more likely to have incisions continuing into the scrotum and a higher risk for postoperative scrotal hematomas. Initially, we kept these patients in hospital the first night on bedrest, but despite those orders nurses sometimes assisted them out of bed to the toilet, causing bleeding and a hematoma. Now we observe them in recovery a few hours and then discharge them with orders for 24 hours of bedrest. They are instructed to bring a wheelchair to the surgery center to use returning home or to their hotel, and to enter and leave the HBOT facility.

HBOT

The first patient we treated with HBOT was an adult with a recurrent fistula following numerous prior failed repairs. We now recommend all men undergoing reoperations have perioperative HBOT to supplement wound healing, following the same protocol as described for boys in Chapter 18. The first postoperative dive can be done later in the same day as surgery.

Results

As mentioned above, we found outcomes after reoperations in men were the same as in boys. At that time we reported complications in 25% of men (Snodgrass and Bush et al, 2014). Those were mostly fistulas and glans dehiscence, and our current rate for those combined is 12%.

Our graft take success is 92% for oral graft reoperations combined with HBOT, which is the same as for primary prepucial grafts without HBOT (Ahmed et al, 2024).

Is There Anyone Who Cannot Be Repaired?

Generally, no. Penile curvature can be straightened by removal of scarred tissues and release of tethering skin, plus 3 corporotomies when there is corporal disproportion. A neourethra can nearly always be made from oral mucosa grafts. Disasterous penile skin loss or scarring ultimately can be addressed with partial or total skin replacement using a skin graft. However, patients in whom external penile skin grafting is necessary will often have a more difficult course of hypospadias healing because of the impact tight skin has on urethroplasty complications, and external penile skin grafts do not have the same gliding/mobility as native penile skin.

The only tissue which cannot be regenerated or replaced with a similar substitute is the glans, and volume loss precluding creation of glans wings dictates the neomeatus must be left in a subterminal position.

Obviously, those boys or men presenting with horrific complications should be referred to the few surgeons with extensive experience managing such situations. Other surgeons should not suggest to the patient that his case his hopeless, because few are.

Key Points

Men with uncorrected hypospadias, and those with dehiscence after childhood repair, commonly present with urine spraying. Adults can also develop stranguria and urinary infections from strictures or meatal stenosis even into middle age. A third of these men with uncorrected distal hypospadias also have penile curvature, with an even higher percentage of curvature in men with complications following proximal hypospadias repair. Curvature can result in sexual dysfunction and body image concerns, but beyond that, can lead to higher rates of urethroplasty complications if not corrected. Accordingly, first straightening the penis is a mainstay of hypospadias reoperations in men, just like it is in children. Many who had childhood repair are bothered by skin irregularities, pits, and cuts in the glans that result from epithelial suturing and, therefore, surgeons should make every effort to prevent these avoidable issues.

These patients also present with emotional concerns from their hypospadias, showing that repair is best done in childhood. Experience managing these teens and adults emphasize that this birth defect can have life-long implications.

We reported that surgical results are similar in children and adults, and so repair can be done in men to make the penis normal. Many have come to us for correction when adult specialists said they would not risk making a terminal meatus.

References

Barbagli G, De Angelis M, Palminteri E, and Lazzeri M: Failed hypospadias repair presenting in adults. *Eur Urol* 49: 887, 2006

Bush N and Snodgrass W: Complaints of men with uncorrected distal hypospadias. Res Rep Urol 15: 425, 2023.

Dodds PR, Batter SJ, Shield DE, Serels SR, Garafola FA, Maloney PK: Adaptation of adults to uncorrected hypospadias. Urology 71: 682, 2008

Ekmark AN, Svensson H, Arnbjornsson E and Hansson E: Postpubertal examination after hypospadias repair is necessary to evaluate the success of the primary reconstruction. *Eur J Surg* 23: 304, 2013

Fichtner J, Filipas D, Mottrie AM, Voges GE, and Hohenfellner R: Analysis of meatal location in 500 men: wide variation questions need for meatal advancement in all pediatric anterior hypospadias cases. *J Urol* 154: 833, 1995

Hutton KAR and Babu R: Normal anatomy of the external urethral meatus in boys: implications for hypospadias repair. *BJU Int* 100: 161,2007

Lam PON, Greenfield SP, and Williot P: 2-stage repair in infancy for severe hypospadias with chordee: long-term results after puberty. *J Urol* 174: 1567, 2005

Schlomer B, Breyer B, Copp H, Baskin L, DiSandro M: Do adult men with untreated hypospadias have adverse outcomes? A pilot study using a social media advertised survey. *J Pediatr Urol* 10: 672, 2014

Snodgrass W and Bush NC: Persistent or recurrent ventral curvature after failed proximal hypospadias repair. *J Pediatr Urol* 15: 344, 2019

Snodgrass W and Bush NC: Do new complications develop during puberty after childhood hypospadias repair? *J Urol* 208: 696, 2022

Snodgrass WT, Bush N and Cost N: Algorithm for comprehensive approach to hypospadias reoperation using 3 techniques. *J Urol* 182: 2885, 2009

Snodgrass W, Villanueva C and Bush N: Primary and reoperative hypospadias repair in adults – are results different than in children? *J Urol* 192: 1730, 2014

Getting Better

Chapter 24

The Impact of Hypospadias Upon Families

Although surgeons focus their attention on the patient with hypospadias, the condition affects the entire family. Hearing their newborn has a birth defect is distressing to parents, especially when they have not previously heard of it - as is most often the case with hypospadias. There is fear of the unknown, and concern about treatment and the impact of both the condition and its management on their child's life (Fonseca et al, 2014). Parents may blame themselves worrying that they did something, or failed to do something, which resulted in the birth defect.

Making matters worse, parents of boys with hypospadias often face these concerns in isolation. Usually their parents have not heard of hypospadias either, and they are hesitant to discuss a genital problem with friends, wanting to protect the privacy of their new son.

These burdens arise from distal hypospadias, but are even greater when the hypospadias is more severe. Most distressing are the perineal cases when parents are told the newborn has ambiguous genitalia, or a micropenis. The worries those labels bring often persist even when the gender is confirmed male and the penis is measured to have a normal length.

Parents hope to find answers to their many questions during consultations with a pediatric urologist, but can leave frustrated when the entire visit is focused on surgery. Even when given time to mention other concerns, parents might ask what causes hypospadias and then be told about genetics and placental insufficiency and environmental toxins, when what they really want to know is if they somehow caused it to happen.

The decision for surgery is difficult for many parents, especially when the surgeon describes it as mostly "cosmetic". Their regret for agreeing to the repair when complications occur has been well-documented (Lorenzo et al, 2014). Less known is the worry that most still have even when surgery is successful (Snodgrass et al, 2021).

These stresses affect the relationship between parents. They also impact siblings, who worry about their brother after surgery and sometimes resent the attention given to him, especially when that disrupts planned events such as family vacations.

We were not very aware of these dynamics when we practiced at the university. Typical of pediatric urologists, our clinics were filled with children presenting with a variety of problems of which hypospadias seemed one of the most straightforward to diagnose and manage. We simply did not have much time to listen to the worries of parents, much less ask them about additional concerns they might have beyond the surgical correction.

This chapter reviews hypospadias from the parent's perspective to alert surgeons to their concerns - because to be experts in hypospadias care requires more of surgeons than just the technical performance of an operation. We are the primary care providers for all matters related to this condition.

Most of the information we present below was derived from the validated Impact of a Child with Congenital Anomalies on Parents questionnaire that was made available to caregivers through on-line social media (Snodgrass et al, 2021). There were 260 respondents, of which 80% were females. Their sons' hypospadias was reported as distal by 48%, proximal in 41% and unknown in 11%. Of these, 33% reported 1 operation, 22% 2 operations and 33% 3 or more operations. Another 13% of boys had not had surgery, either because it was not recommended by surgeons or not agreed to by the parents. According to the respondents, the repair successfully achieved a straight penis with the opening at the tip in 68% and not in 17%, with the remainder uncertain.

Key concerns identified from this survey, in other published reports, and in our discussions with parents include the following, divided into categories: no prior awareness about this birth defect, concerns about their son's health, the impact of hypospadias on their own relationship and the rest of the family, and decisional regret.

No prior awareness of hypospadias

86% of parents stated they had never heard of hypospadias before the diagnosis in their son. Though not asked by the questionnaire, most also report their parents are similarly unaware of this condition.

Isolation caused by hypospadias

Although not part of the questionnaire, many parents describe the sense of isolation they feel as a consequence of their son's hypospadias. Because it involves the genitals, many hesitate to discuss hypospadias with their friends, suspecting that they are not familiar with the condition anyway. Parents also worry about the response of day-care providers when they change the diaper and see that the penis looks different. Concerns for their son's privacy drives parents to conceive a different explanation for co-workers when they take off time for his surgery. The result is that many parents face the uncertainties and anxieties surrounding hypospadias without the support of their usual networks of friends and family.

Lack of knowledge about hypospadias

Inevitably, most parents turn to the internet for information about this birth defect. That can then lead to considerable confusion and even more anxiety regarding the best course of action for their son.

A small study interviewed 17 parents of boys with hypospadias who confirmed that the internet was their primary source used to gain information about the diagnosis, even though they admitted that what they read was often not clear and was possibly inaccurate (Chan et al, 2020). Parents also gain access to support groups through the internet and exchange information with other parents participating in those groups trying to fill gaps in their understanding. However, what they hear is not always correct, or might not apply to their son's circumstances.

The misunderstanding and misinformation in what they read increases the responsibility of urologists to allot time to provide accurate medical information during consultations.

Blame for the birth defect

In our survey, 57% of mothers and 38% of fathers wondered if they were to blame for their son's hypospadias. This increased to 78% in women who were given progesterone during pregnancy.

It is unusual for a parent to directly ask if he or she was responsible for their son's birth defect. Instead, they ask what causes hypospadias. If a mother received progesterone, especially in conjunction with IVF, she might ask about its relationship to hypospadias. Others may ask about soy products or other specific exposures, such as to pesticides or other potential toxins. Regardless, the underlying concern usually prompting these questions is what the parents might have done to cause the birth defect, and what can they do to avoid it happening again with another pregnancy.

Whatever other factual information surgeons may wish to provide during these discussions, we recommend they also mention that many parents asking these questions really wonder if they are to blame for the hypospadias. Acknowledging their worry frequently leads to tears revealing the depth of their guilt. Reassurances that they are not responsible lifts this burden – for example, the observation that most boys born to mothers who were prescribed progesterone are not born with hypospadias, and most boys born with hypospadias did not have in-utero exposure to progesterone, can greatly reduce the guilt felt by those who followed their OB's advice and took that medication. This is now a standard part of our new patient consultation.

Concerns for their son's health

58% of parents in our survey reported feeling sad about their son's hypospadias. Nearly two-thirds "worried a great deal" about his health and expectations for his future, *even when the hypospadias was successfully repaired.*

That number increased to 88% when there were complications after surgery.

Information regarding repair

As mentioned above, many parents have already studied hypospadias on the internet before their office consultation. In fact, we have been surprised how many have watched full-length unedited videos of hypospadias repairs and have read articles from the scientific literature. As a result, they may arrive already confused, and then be uncertain how to relate what they hear from the surgeon to what they have watched and read.

One of every five respondents in our survey wished the urologist would have spent more time explaining details of the surgery and the expected results. 78% of parents responding to Decisional Regret Score questionnaires in another study wished they had more information about hypospadias before surgery (Ghidini et al, 2016).

Parents of those with distal hypospadias often want to discuss the consequences of not having it repaired. Many are uncomfortable making a decision for surgery if they have read or been told the operation is mostly "cosmetic", as even a small risk for complications seems unreasonable if there are no medical reasons to recommend surgery, especially on a body part that few will see. This is the main reason the term "cosmetic" should never be used during hypospadias consultation. Instead, surgeons should use "appearance" or "aesthetic" when discussing what the penis should look like, and the correct terminology of "reconstructive surgery" for repair of a birth defect, which is never "cosmetic surgery" even if done primarily for aesthetic purposes.

Our survey additionally found that 33% of respondents had not planned on newborn circumcision, and wished there had been a discussion about prepucioplasty.

Furthermore, parents who seek more than 1 opinion often hear quite different explanations. For example, one urologist might examine a boy with distal hypospadias and declare the condition is minor with little risk for future bother if left alone, while another urologist explains their son is likely to have voiding problems if the defect is not corrected. Such opposite advice from experts is very distressing to care-givers trying to decide what is best.

Do childhood repairs last through puberty?

Another common concern is if a successful repair done in childhood is prone to come apart or develop new complications during puberty. This is often mentioned in social media groups, and sometimes by pediatric urologists, even though there is almost no published information supporting this belief, as discussed in Chapters 22 and 23.

Remarks that "rapid" pubertal growth could create new fistulas, recurrent penile curvature, or other complications prompted our review of teens and adults presenting with problems after their childhood repairs. We found that few new complications developed during puberty, and none of our patients with VC reported it developed during that time.

However, such comments raise doubts in parents about doing surgery in childhood if it is only going to come apart again during puberty.

Does hypospadias repair decrease penile sensation or inhibit penile growth?

Other reasons parents report being worried "a great deal" about their son despite successful hypospadias repair include warnings on social media that surgery decreases penile sensation and the resulting scars can restrict penile growth. Neither is true. We systematically query teens and adults who present with failed childhood repairs if they perceive abnormal sensation, and it is extremely uncommon to hear a patient has even a small area with decreased feelings. Similarly, it is very rare for patients to report a change in sensation after either primary repairs or reoperations.

We also inform parents that scars grow with the boy. Otherwise, the scar of the most common penile operation done, circumcision, would constrict the penis during puberty. Full-thickness skin grafts, unlike partial-thickness skin grafts, also have been shown to grow normally. Partial-thickness skin grafts should never be used on a prepubertal penis.

Impact on others in the family

Siblings

Brothers and sisters of a boy with hypospadias are also impacted by his condition. They worry when he returns home from surgery in pain, and are confused by the bandages and catheter they see when his diaper is changed.

Siblings can also resent the added attention their brother receives, and become angered if vacations and other family events are rescheduled to address a problem he is having.

Parents have also told us that even young siblings can develop their own embarrassment about hypospadias. For example, one mom related how an older brother answered a neighbor's question about upcoming surgery on his baby brother by saying he was going to have an operation on his back, even though he was well aware that his brother was having surgery on the penis.

Parents also wonder how they should explain hypospadias and surgery to brothers and sisters, and to the patient when he is old enough to understand. A patient's mother wrote How Down There Bear™ Got Repaired, an illustrated children's book about hypospadias repair that is available through Amazon and Barnes & Noble, to help with this.

Conflict between parents

Parents may not agree with each other regarding the best course of management for their son with hypospadias. Another study reporting the validated Decisional Conflict Scale questionnaire answered by each parent separately found disagreement in more than 1 of every 4 couples, even though strong conflict occurred in only 5% (Lorenzo et al, 2012).

Separation or divorce can complicate parent decision-making and settling on a course of action. None of the couples in the analysis by Lorenzo et al reported this situation, but the authors noted that parents already in conflict with each other likely face additional challenges coming to agreement regarding their son's birth defect.

Distress from surgery in older boys

Although most hypospadias surgery is completed before boys have much awareness of it, surgery delayed because of other medical conditions, waiting lists, and financial concerns, as well as failed repairs requiring additional surgery, can result in operations being done when patients are older. One set of parents have described how their son, realizing that another trip to the hospital means more pain, reacted by screaming, "I hate my penis!" Many have also commented how much more difficult it is to comfort their school-age son postoperatively than it was when he was younger.

Those advocating repair be delayed until boys are older likely do not realize the added stress that surgery in older boys brings to their parents and siblings. The difficulties that teens facing hypospadias surgery cause their parents was mentioned in Chapter 23. Additional study of these issues would be very helpful to guide the best care decisions for families.

Decisional regret

Preoperative consultations informing parents that distal hypospadias repairs are successful 95% of the time can add significant stress when their son develops a complication. As mentioned above, 88% of those parents answered our survey that they worried "a great deal" about their son's health as a consequence of a urethroplasty complication. In fact, 76% wondered if their son would ever be healthy. 40% complained that the surgeon did not explain things clearly, and many free-text comments complained that surgeons should disclose their personal results beforehand.

The guilt that most parents feel that their son was born with a birth defect is made even worse by the fear that they are somehow responsible for the complication. Did they not keep his wound clean? Did they allow the bandages to come off prematurely? Should they have applied more, or less, Aquaphor to the incision? That guilt increases if the surgeon suggests the complication occurred because the boy was constipated, or overactive, or pulled at his penis – anything that they might have been able to control.

Parents are also distressed to hear their surgeon say he or she almost never sees the complication their son has, as they believe something out of the ordinary must have happened and might not be able to be corrected.

It should not be surprising that parents sometimes regret their earlier decision for hypospadias repair, especially when a complication occurs. This was documented by one study of decisional regret (Lorenzo et al, 2012), but not another (Ghidini et al, 2016), which the latter authors attributed to better preoperative counseling.

Another factor leading to decisional regret is circumcision when the parents preferred an intact foreskin. A third of the parents answering our survey had not planned on circumcision for their newborn, and were later unhappy to learn that foreskin reconstruction was an option that was either not mentioned, or discouraged, by the surgeon. Lorenzo et al reported moderate to severe regret when circumcision was done even if the operation was otherwise successful. In contrast, Ghidini et al left the choice of foreskin management, circumcision or prepucioplasty, to the parents and reported no decisional regret resulting from this factor in their study. Consequently, those surgeons who do not wish to reconstruct the foreskin should refer those patients to someone who will.

Key Points

We had no idea of the extent that hypospadias can affect the entire family when our university-based practice allocated no more than 20 minutes for a new patient appointment, leaving only enough time to determine the extent of the condition, describe its management, and schedule surgery.

Even then we commonly heard parents say that they had never before heard of hypospadias until their son was born, but did not realize the fear and isolation that lack of awareness created. Nor did we know that when a parent asks what causes hypospadias, that their real concern is what they did, or failed to do, that led to this birth defect. Today we make certain to mention that they are not to blame for their son's hypospadias even when they do not raise this topic themselves.

In a practice devoted to hypospadias, we have learned that discussing "cosmetic" results causes some parents to question the appropriateness of surgery on a body part that they anticipate few will see. It is better, and more accurate, for surgeons to speak of "aesthetic" results or the "appearance" of the penis, and explain that hypospadias repair is "reconstructive surgery", which by definition, repair of a birth defect is. "Cosmetic surgery" is an incorrect term for hypospadias repair and should be avoided, even when a primary goal for surgery is a normal appearance.

It is also important that surgeons explain both the proposed surgery and the potential complications clearly, honestly disclosing their personal results. When complications occur, they should emphasize that the parents are not responsible and the problem can be corrected.

Similarly, realizing that many parents prefer the final outcome to be a natural-appearing penis, surgeons should ask how they want the foreskin managed. Certainly, surgeons able to repair hypospadias can also reconstruct the foreskin, or refer the family to someone who does.

Finally, surgeons can express greater empathy when they realize the emotional stress that hypospadias causes to the entire family. Simply acknowledging that fact helps parents realize their worries are widely shared and normal, and may give them greater confidence in their surgeon.

References

Chan KH, Panoch J, Cararoll A, WIehe S, Cain MC and Franket R: Knowledge gaps and information seeking by parents about hypospadias. *J Pediatr Urol* 16: 166, 2020

Fonseca A, Nazare B, Canavarro MC: Parenting an infant with a congenital anomaly: an exploratory study on patterns of adjustment from diagnosis to six months post birth. *J Child Health Care* 18: 111-2, 2014

Lorenzo AJ, Braga LHP, Zlateska B, Leslie B, Fathat WA, Bagli DJ and Pippi Salle JL: Analysis of decisional conflict among parents who consent to hypospadias repair: single institution prospective study of 100 couples. *J Urol* 188: 571, 2012

Lorenzo AJ, Pippi Salle JL, Zlateska B, Koyle MA, Bagli DJ and Braga LHP: Decisional regret after distal hypospadias repair: single institution prospective analysis of factors associated with subsequent parental remorse or distress. *J Urol* 191: 1558, 2014

Snodgrass P, Snodgrass W and Bush NC: Parental concerns of boys with hypospadias. *Research and Reports in Urology* 21: 73, 2021

Chapter 25

The Hypospadias Learning Curve

There are 5 publications describing the initial results of mostly distal hypospadias repairs done by recently graduated pediatric urology fellows in their independent practice. Of these, 3 reported a learning curve (Horowitz and Salzhauer, 2006; Rompe et al, 2013; Zubi et al, 2020), while the other 2 did not (Frimberger et al, 2008; Bush and Snodgrass et al, 2016).

A key question in those reporting a learning curve is whether improvement occurred though a repetition of steps done the same way, or by a technical change (or changes) in the way those steps were done which made the results better. If it was by repetition, then the next question is how many repairs need to be done to achieve benchmark success? If it was by changing how they performed steps in the procedure, would there have been a learning curve had those methods been taught and learned correctly during fellowship?

What is a learning curve?

The concept that the results of a process can change with experience was developed by industry. The typical outcomes measured are the time and the cost to perform the process. If a product is manufactured, the production efficiency also includes quality control, specifically how many correctly-made widgets are produced versus how many have defects and have to be discarded.

These principles have been applied to surgery. Most surgeons will perform a given procedure in less time and usually at less cost with increasing experience. However, both surgeons and patients are more interested in quality, and the most common measure of quality in hypospadias repair is the number of complications that occur postoperatively.

Benchmark results

A successful hypospadias repair makes the penis normal, meaning straight, with a vertical slit meatus properly located within the glans, the shaft symmetrically covered by penile skin, no visible scars outside the median raphe and circumcision lines, and no persisting complications. Even though this definition takes into account much more than the presence or absence of a complication, we can nevertheless establish benchmarks for success based on the initial rate of complications.

Benchmark Success for Distal Repairs

Complications should occur in less than 10% of distal repairs, as derived from the meta-analysis of distal TIP by Pfistermuller et al, 2015.

Benchmark Success for Proximal Repairs

There are fewer data from a larger variety of repairs, but it is reasonable to state that urethroplasty complications should occur in less than 25% of proximal repairs (Snodgrass and Bush, 2017).

All surgeons choosing to repair hypospadias should strive to achieve complications within these parameters, reviewing their own results and then making technical changes to improve them until they do.

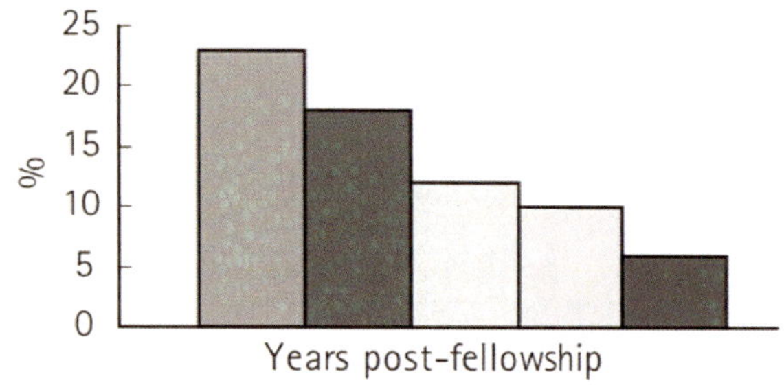

Figure 1. Near-linear decline in fistulas over time. Using a benchmark of 17% or fewer complications extrapolated for a series reported as mostly midshaft repairs, success was achieved after more than 70 cases during the 3rd year in practice.

Reported learning curves

Horowitz and Salzhauer used the rate of fistulas, rather than total complications, recorded in prospectively collected data during the first 5 years of independent practice to determine a learning curve. Their series is difficult to interpret since they said most of their 231 cases were midshaft and that a potpourri of repairs was used. They found a near linear decline in fistulas from 23% to 6% (Figure 1). If a benchmark between 10% and 25% is assumed for this series, success was reached in year 3 and the learning curve was more than 70 cases.

Rompre et al retrospectively reviewed 303 primary distal and midshaft/proximal TIP results for 1 surgeon during his first 9 years of independent practice. They reported the steepest part of the learning curve in the 250 distal cases was during the first 75 repairs, although the plot never reached the benchmark of 90% success. (Figure 2).

The authors also analyzed "non-distal" TIP repairs in 52 patients during the 9 years reviewed, finding a similar decline in complications. WS reported technical changes in proximal TIP which reduced complications from 55% to 13% (Snodgrass and Bush, 2011), but later realized that ventral curvature of 30° or more that most these patients have contraindicates TIP repair (Snodgrass and Bush, 2021).

Zu'bi et al (2020) retrospectively analyzed primary distal TIP repairs done by 1 surgeon over the first 14 years of his independent practice. They plotted a

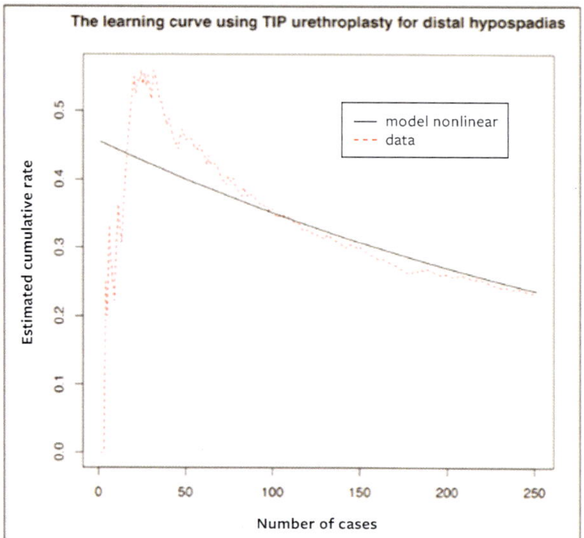

No. cases for distal hypospadias	50	100	200	300
Estimated cumulative rate (%)	40%	35%	27%	21%

Figure 2. Learning curve by cases for distal TIP repair. The curve shows complications peaking at approximately 55% and averaging 40% during the first 75 cases. Note that even at 250 cases complications still occurred at more than twice the suggested benchmark of 10% or fewer.

sharp rise in complications during the first approximately 120 cases (Phase 1), reaching 40%. Then the rate of complications plateaued at 20% for the next 100 cases, and finally decreased to 13% for the final approximately 200 cases (Figure 3). They considered Phase 2 as "competency" and Phase 3 as "proficiency" even though the final result remained above the suggested benchmark rate of complications as the standard which can be achieved.

In contrast, Frimberger et al summarized the results of 2 surgeons trained at different institutions during their first 3 years in independent practice. They found no significant difference in the volume of cases or outcomes between them. 80% were distal repairs, mostly TIP (75%) or MAGPI, with a complication rate, defined as fistulas, of 4%.

Bush et al reported the only series which directly compared the results of 5 former fellows in their early independent practice to those of their mentor during the same time period, all performing primary distal TIP repair. There was no significant difference

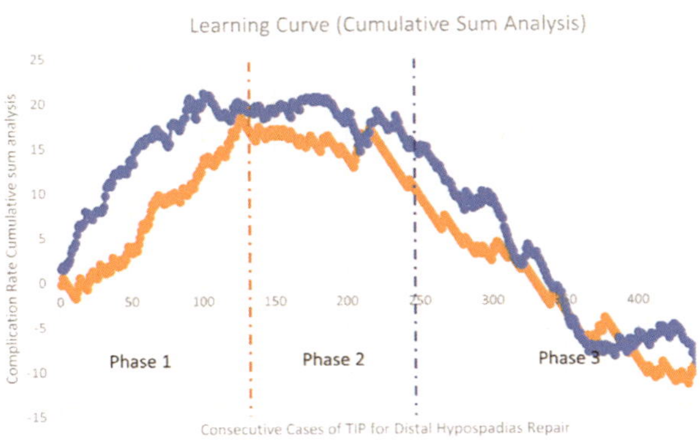

Figure 3. 3-phase learning curve for distal TIP repair. The orange line plots complications to case volume. Although not shown in the way the graph was generated, the initial rate of complications reached 40%, with a sustained decrease occurring after approximately 220 cases. Nevertheless, complications still developed in 13% of patients in phase 3, remaining above the benchmark.

---

in urethroplasty complications between the former fellows, or comparing them to WS, averaging 8% (5%-13%).

Factors explaining results

Repetition vs Technical Changes

The 3 series describing learning curves after fellowship training all attributed their initial complications to the difficulty of performing a complex operation optimally in independent practice, during a time interval that stretched from 5 to 14 years. 2 of the 3 surgeons never reached benchmark complication rates for mostly distal hypospadias surgery, which neither manuscript discussed. The concept of a standard that surgeons are expected to achieve is new to hypospadias repair.

Was the improvement they observed the result of more efficiently performing the operations over time? If so, one might expect the curves to more closely resemble each other, assuming that a given number of cases is needed for surgeons in general to reach their best performance. However, that varied for these 3 urologists from at least 70 to 250 repairs.

Although each attributed their improvement mostly to experience, they also admitted to making technical changes to their performance. Horowitz and Salzhauer did not use a dartos barrier flap during the first 2 years for distal repairs, and also tubularized the urethral plate too far distally in their earlier versus later cases. Since these technical changes influence the risk for fistula development, their improvement can be attributed to doing operations better rather than getting better through repetition of the same methods.

Similarly, Rompe et al wrote that "the operative technique remained the same over the years, *except for some minor adjustments*". Those included not incising the urethral plate too distally, presumedly into the glans, which decreased meatal stenosis. Zu'bi et al admitted their improvement could have resulted, at least in part, to technical modifications which included making the TIP incision deeper and adding spongioplasty to reduce tension on the glans wings approximation.

It is also noteworthy that the quickest improvement occurred for the surgeon who prospectively collected and reviewed his outcomes, presumedly because he recognized the need to do better sooner (Horowitz and Salzhauer). Would the 9 and 14-year learning curves found by the others have been shorter if they had reviewed their results sooner? Also, no learning curve was present from the trainees who learned distal TIP repair from a surgeon who prospectively maintained his outcomes and discussed benchmark success rates with them (Bush et al, 2016). Some, but not all, of the participants in that study maintained prospective distal hypospadias databases as well.

Successful Skills Transfer During Fellowship

Both surgeons reported by Frimberger et al presumably achieved benchmark complication rates in the first 3 years of independent practice, with the caveat that glans dehiscence was not reported. Although they trained in different institutions, they specifically attributed this success to a focus on learning to master a limited repertoire of techniques during fellowship and then meticulously applying what they learned in their practices.

Bush and Snodgrass et al described hypospadias training as a year spent mostly observing and assisting in a large number of cases, with discrete execution of key steps. The goal was to teach optimal performance of each of those steps, and the subsequent ability of these trainees to achieve the same results as their mentor early in their independent practices proved this complex surgery can be taught and learned without a steep learning curve.

Implications of learning curves

If the conclusions of the 3 learning curve reports are accurate, then surgeons graduating after fellowship will generate more complications needing more reoperations than usual during their first 70 to over 250 cases. In 2 of those studies, complications occurred in nearly half the initial repairs.

According to data collected from the US Board of Urology, the median number of distal hypospadias repairs done by certified pediatric urologists was 12 per year in 2008 (Kogan and Feustel, 2011). At that rate it would take newly graduated fellows between 6 and 25 years to approach benchmark success. Furthermore, the AUA reports that there are now 4 times more pediatric urologists, meaning the number of annual cases per surgeon has decreased and the time to gain benchmark success has likely increased.

A consistent theme throughout this textbook is that most hypospadias complications occur because of technical errors made by the surgeon. These mistakes are either learned during fellowship, and/or acquired in independent practice. The observation that 3 surgeons reported improved results after making technical changes known to reduce complications suggests they were not taught, or did not learn, to optimally perform the operations they used. The fact that the other 7 newly graduated surgeons achieved benchmark rates of complications without a learning curve shows they were taught and successfully learned how to do TIP in the best way.

Therefore, the most important factor predicting benchmark success repairing distal hypospadias early in independent practice is optimal fellowship training, rather than post-training experience.

Lessons for mentors and fellows

The most important lesson for mentors derived from these articles is that the mistakes they teach will harm more patients through the practices of the fellows they train. The most important lesson for fellows is that even the most reputable mentor might not do 1 or more key steps in a hypospadias repair in the best way, defined as the way creating the fewest complications.

To know if they are teaching optimally, mentors must periodically review their own results and not accept outcomes outside the benchmarks. Similarly, for newly graduated surgeons to know if they were taught and learned how to do hypospadias repairs correctly, they must periodically review their own results. Complications occurring in more than 10% of distal and 25% of proximal repairs should prompt a thorough review of how the surgeon, regardless of experience, performs the operation.

Too often faculty surgeons shrug off their complications as proof that their patients are unusually complex or reflect the pitfalls of teaching trainees. Similarly, practicing surgeons at all levels may blame complications on poor nursing by the parents, overactive patients, or even constipation. Complications should always be viewed as potential mistakes made by them.

Occasionally a mentor has commented that they know their outcomes could be better if they changed how they did a specific step, but they do not because "I'm satisfied with my results." We are not certain how best to respond to this statement, which does not follow the dictum of the Hippocratic oath for their patients. It also teaches a technical error to a new generation of young surgeons who will almost certainly repeat their mistake and harm others.

Teaching Fellows

We received no formal education in surgical mentorship from the university during our years on faculty. WS derived his teaching method for hypospadias surgery trying to balance the need to transfer knowledge and skills to fellows with his obligation to achieve the best result he could for each patient. Those potentially competing goals led to him perform most of every repair himself with the fellow assisting, observing him doing the same steps over and over in boys with differing anatomy. After several months, he allowed them to do a single step, and eventually a few steps, of an operation, but never a complete procedure beginning to end. Whether others agree with that approach is less the point than is the published fact that it worked

– his fellows graduated capable of duplicating his success with nowhere near his experience.

Some programs allow fellows to operate with minimal or no direct supervision. Regardless of the perceived merits of that approach, it potentially increases the likelihood for a trainee to carry mistakes into practice which were not observed and corrected by a mentor. Although it can be argued that limited performance of operations by fellows also limits the opportunities for mentors to recognize mistakes they might make, our results with 5 trainees showed that did not occur.

Hypospadias repair is difficult to learn. A year of intensive instruction in which the fellow both observes the mentor doing operations correctly and demonstrates ability to duplicate those steps under direct supervision is likely essential to transfer skills without a learning curve.

Life-long Learning

No other surgery done by pediatric urologists harms as many patients as does hypospadias repair. We encourage all surgeons to review their own outcomes to verify they are achieving benchmark success. We also advise newly graduated surgeons to not dismiss complication rates greater than the benchmarks as an inevitable learning curve, but rather to see them as warnings of technical mistakes they are making which can be corrected.

WS did not have a learning curve developing distal TIP. His first results published in 1994 are the same as his latest reported in 2010. This repeats the message that the operation reliably achieves benchmark results when its steps are done correctly.

Learning curve for proximal hypospadias

There is no published report regarding a learning curve for proximal hypospadias repair. This reflects several factors. First, the median number of these repairs done by certified pediatric urologists was reported by Kogan and Feustel (2011) to be only 3 per year. Such limited performance of a complex operation makes it difficult for surgeons to gain and then maintain optimal results. In addition, only in recent years has it been widely recognized that current outcomes from commonly used techniques, including 1 and 2-stage flaps and proximal TIP when VC is 30° or more are not satisfactory and certainly not meeting the benchmark stated above.

We are still learning how to best repair proximal hypospadias, having realized that proximal TIP should only be used when ventral curvature is less than 30°, and then having migrated from Byars flaps to Bracka grafts and then on to STAG and STAC. Throughout this process frequent review of our data has shown problems to be solved and operative steps to be revised. But this became most effective when we limited our practice to hypospadias repair and performed more than 25 times the reported median number of primary proximal repairs by US pediatric urologists annually.

Nevertheless, as we become increasingly proficient with STAC repair, we would anticipate that other surgeons taught these lessons who can apply them frequently should also achieve benchmark outcomes—possibly without a learning curve after training in the key steps.

Key Points

Newly graduated fellows who have been taught and have learned the optimal way to perform each step in distal TIP should quickly achieve the benchmark success of less than 10% complications without a learning curve.

There are no published data regarding a proximal repair learning curve. The rarity of severe hypospadias likely makes it difficult for even properly trained and experienced surgeons to achieve less than 25% complications - unless they have sufficient volume to perform the operation often enough to become proficient in all the steps applied to varying anatomy. In other words, there likely is a learning curve for these cases, and those with no more than the median of 3 cases a year probably cannot expect to see their results significantly improve.

Complications most often reflect technical errors made by surgeons. Every surgeon performing hypospadias repair should review his or her own results. Those with complications exceeding the benchmarks should review their performance step-by-step in comparison to how those with lower complications perform them and make adjustments to improve. Newly graduated trainees should not assume that they were taught steps in the optimal manner, unless their mentor knew his/her results and discussed this with them.

References

AUA Manpower Report, 2023

Bush NC, Barber TD, Dajusta D, Prieto JC, Ziada A and Snodgrass W: Results of hypospadias repair after pediatric urology fellowship: a comparison of junior surgeons to their mentor. *J Pediatri Urol* 12:162, 2016

Frimberger D, Campbell J and Kropp BP: Hypospadias outcome in the first 3 years after completing a pediatric urology fellowship. *J Pediatr Urol* 4: 270, 2008

Horowitz M and Salzhauer E: The "learning curve" in hypospadias surgery. *BJU Int* 97: 593, 2006

Pfistermuller KL, McArdle J and Cuckow PM: Meta-analysis of complication rates of the tubularized incised plate (TIP) repair. *J Pediatr Urol* 11: 54, 2015

Rompre M-PD, Nadeau G, Moore K, Ajjaoui Y, Braga LH and Bolduc S: Learning curve for TIP urethroplasty: a single-surgeon experience. *Can Urol Assoc J* 7: E789, 2013

Snodgrass W and Bush N: Staged tubularized autograft repair for primary proximal hypospadias with 30-degree or greater ventral curvature. *J Urol* 198: 680, 2017

Zu'bi F, Chua M, El-Ghazzaouli A, Kim JK, Shiff M, RIckardM, Blais A-S, and Farhat WA: Competence in tubularized incised plate repair for distal hypospadias: cumulative sum learning curve analysis of a single surgeon experience. *J Urol* 204: 1326, 2020

Chapter 26

Repairing Hypospadias Better

Countless articles begin with the statement that more than 200 repairs have been described for hypospadias. Of course, at any given time surgeons have chosen from fewer options, selecting a handful of favorites while advocates for each debated which was best.

WS has witnessed part of this evolution during the past 40 years. At the start of his career in the 1980s MAGPI and Mathieu were the preferred repairs for distal hypospadias, while transverse island and Byars flaps were the most commonly used for proximal hypospadias. But there were other options to these, such as the Barcat, Mustarde, and the Hodgson II that his mentor demonstrated just to show the fellow how they were done. After residency WS read about GAP, Koyanagi and staged graft distal repairs, though of these he only tried GAP and then abandoned it when every patient developed a fistula or dehiscence.

Innovators described these operations looking for better ways to create a neourethra that was more reliable, had fewer complications, and produced a more normal appearance than those which preceded them. Yet, in this list of techniques, only staged grafts routinely made a well-functioning urethra ending in a slit meatus at the tip of the glans.

Eventually, TIP emerged as the best operation functionally and aesthetically for distal hypospadias. Evolution of staged grafts into the STAC repair gives surgeons the best current means to repair proximal hypospadias of which we are aware. No other techniques so reliably achieve the goal of hypospadias repair to make a normal penis as do these. As a result, hypospadias repair is indisputably better today than in the past.

Nevertheless, problems persist, and many within the community of surgeons who undertake these repairs do not achieve the goals established at the beginning of this textbook: A straight penis with a vertical slit meatus normally enclosed within the glans, the shaft covered with symmetrical penis skin, no visible scars outside the ventral median raphe and circumcision line, and no lingering complications. In Chapter 25 we suggested surgeons should achieve these in more than 90% of distal and 75% of proximal repairs. However, we have also cited findings from the Dutch hypospadias study that 90% of surgeons have more than 10% complications after distal repairs. And all hypospadias surgeons know that complications following proximal repairs commonly exceed 50%.

The result is that more patients are harmed from hypospadias repairs done by certified specialists than any other surgery performed by pediatric urologists and surgeons. These failures can result in shame and embarrassment and frustration from a birth defect that lasts the lifetime of the patient.

How do we do better?

Acknowledge the Facts

Although every hypospadias surgeon has told families of boys born with this condition that it is a "common birth defect", the fact is that birth defects are not common. Only *one half of one percent* (0.5%) of newborn boys have hypospadias, and proximal hypospadias is a rare condition occurring in no more than *one tenth of one half percent* (0.05%).

Data collected from case logs submitted to the US Board of Urology in 2007 and 2008 by 230 certifying pediatric urologists showed that the median number of distal repairs was only 1 a month, with proximal repairs done 2-3 times a year (Kogan and Feustel, 2011). Today there are approximately 350 pediatric urologists while the birth rate in the US has decreased 15%, meaning the numbers of repairs by specialists have likely decreased.

Many studies report that the best results for challenging operations, like hypospadias, are achieved by high-volume surgeons. It is not known how many distal repairs a surgeon needs to perform each year to achieve success in more than 90%. WS published no complications in his initial series of TIPs during a time when he repaired distal hypospadias only 4 times a year. Frimberger et al reported less than 10% complications following distal TIPs in their first 3 years in practice doing an average of 15 cases a year. However, the Dutch Hypospadias Study (van der Toorn et al, 2015) found complications after distal repairs averaged 16%, with variation among participating surgeons from 4% to 63%. Whether those outcomes correlated with case volume was not stated.

Meanwhile it is difficult to argue that 2 or 3 repairs a year for the most severe hypospadias is sufficient to gain and then maintain expertise. Yet management of these patients has not been concentrated into the hands of fewer surgeons to give them the volume needed to improve results. Which means the current system of distributing these cases to any certified urologist who wishes to do them does not promote best outcomes for patients.

Another factor hindering progress is that few surgeons know their personal results, and those who assume they have few complications because they cannot remember the last time they encountered a fistula are not taking into account recall bias. We have consistently found that our results were not as good as we thought once we actually tallied them and realized we needed to do better. Surgeons who have not reviewed their outcomes are less likely to consider changes in management that would reduce complications, because they do not believe they need to.

It is also a fact that not all operations achieve the best possible results, yet surgeons continue using them. Some say a different operation has not yet passed the test of time, or that it does not make sense to them despite published data that prove their concerns unfounded. Initially surgeons worried the TIP incision would scar and create obstruction, and some still voice that objection 30 years later even though meta-analyses report less than 5% strictures in several thousand patients (Pfistermuller et al, 2015; Winberg et al, 2019). For at least some surgeons their low volume doing an operation that has a high potential for complications makes them reluctant to change from what they were taught.

That is especially true for proximal repairs where the stakes are higher and the difficulties achieving success are greatly magnified. We should not have been surprised when 3 papers from excellent pediatric institutions reported complications in over 50% of patients mostly repaired by Byars flaps, and rather than prompt a search for a better way, many surgeons around the US declared their results proved our expectations should be lower. Is that the best answer our profession has for the boys born with this condition?

A major part of our failure to successfully repair proximal hypospadias is a reluctance to change from chordee excision and dorsal plications, which do not correct the curvature that averages 70° and ranges to over 130° in these patients, and instead do ventral lengthening. Consequently, the most common complication after a proximal repair is persistent ventral curvature, and we found the tension that creates during erections caused urethroplasty complications in nearly 100% of those patients.

Even surgeons using the best repairs may not perform all the key steps optimally. They may have been taught wrong during training or misunderstood the author describing an operation that comes along after fellowship. For example, the most common technical error during TIP is failure to deeply incise the urethral plate, which then causes an increased likelihood for fistulas and meatal stenosis or urethral stricture. As we have said many times throughout this textbook, most complications happen because of errors made by the surgeon.

It is also important to acknowledge that there is no "minor" hypospadias. Even a distal repair is technically demanding with little margin for error. When complications occur, anything more than a fistula closure has at least double, or more, the risk for additional complications. In part this is because the same surgeon may make the same mistake the second time, and also because each operation impacts vascularity and wound healing. Which emphasizes the need to get the repair right the first time.

Finally, we cannot simply accept results that are below standard. Boys born with hypospadias want to become men with a normal penis, and when we fail to accomplish that it is the patient who has to live with the consequences, sometimes for a lifetime.

Simplify the Algorithm

Our data show that all hypospadias can be repaired using TIP when the penis is straight or has less than 30° ventral curvature, and STAC when there is bending of 30° or more. Which means the choice of technique is determined by objective measurement of curvature, and not a subjective assessment of the urethral plate and corpus spongiosum. Urethroplasty is done by tubularizing the incised urethral plate or a graft neoplate, slightly adjusted for the varying anatomy that hypospadias presents.

This algorithm removes the need for surgeons to select from a variety of operations and allows them to instead focus on doing these 2 repairs optimally. The fact that they share many key steps makes it easier for a surgeon to master them both.

Some object that such an approach forces an operation on the patient, rather than selecting one best suited for the anatomy. Yet the idea of surgeons relying on a limited repertoire is not a new concept. Duckett proposed the MAGPI, onlay flap and transverse island flap to repair all hypospadias, while Bracka advocated the 2-stage graft repair for all extents of hypospadias so that even the surgeon with limited volume could achieve good results.

Since TIP and STAC most reliably achieve the goal of making the abnormal anatomy of hypospadias into a normal penis, today they should be the repairs used.

Perform the Key Steps Optimally

The best way to perform each step in a hypospadias repair is the way that gives the best results. While that sounds obvious, the operative reports we read in patients who have complications most often describe technical errors. A colleague once told WS that if there are 30 pediatric urologists, there are 30 different TIP repairs. The tendency of surgeons to "modify" an operation to their own preferences can introduce errors. For example, not covering the neourethra with a dartos flap during a distal repair, which increases the risk of fistulas. Or, running the first layer of the neourethra in a proximal repair, when interrupted stitches give a lower fistula rate. Or, degloving and then declaring the flaccid penis is straight without doing an artificial erection. In the Dutch study, where most surgeons did not achieve the desired threshold success rate for distal repairs, the urethroplasty was performed in 1 layer in the majority of patients. Would the results have been different if 2-layer closure had been performed instead?

Throughout this textbook we describe these key steps done according to the best evidence. A surgeon who performs them differently must review his or her results to determine if they are within the highest standards, with less than 10% complications after primary distal repairs and less than 25% following proximal repairs. If not, changes should be made to do better.

Practice the 3 Ps

We recommend that all hypospadias surgeons start a simple database to record the patient's name, date of surgery, type of repair, primary or redo, date of follow up, and complications. That information can be entered into an Excel spreadsheet, or an electronic medical record, at the time of service. Then this prospectively collected data can easily be reviewed periodically and practice changes made as indicated to improve results. This **P**rospective data collection, **P**eriodic review, and **P**ractice changes for quality improvement has been the foundation of our hypospadias management for more than 20 years, and we continue to input data after each repair and follow up assessment.

For academic surgeons, this process continuously generates reliable data to ensure trainees are being taught best practices. It also suggests new hypotheses to test and gathers information to report and publish. But this works best only when the complications are defined in a similar, standardized manner by all participating surgeons. If glans dehiscence is completely ignored by some surgeons, and meticulously recorded by others, comparison of techniques and technical steps is virtually impossible.

Most importantly, the 3Ps inform surgeons if their results are as good as they think. WS has found many times that his were not, then tweaked his technique and reviewed results again to confirm they improved - all at the minimal cost of a few minutes to update the database between cases or after clinic.

Similarly, many urologists have told us at meetings and workshops that, having heard about the 3 Ps, they finally decided to test them and found, as we have, that their results were not as good as they assumed, either. So they made adjustments in their surgical technique, reviewed the new outcomes, and were pleased to see their results were better.

It astounds patients and parents to learn that most surgeons do not know their personal results for the operations they propose doing to them or their son. It also angers them to realize that the outcomes they were quoted were actually those of other surgeons who published them. Our profession cannot provide the best care for patients until surgeons know the current level of care they actually provide.

Specialize Proximal Hypospadias Repair

Proximal hypospadias is a rare condition that requires a complex repair to make the penis normal. Equal distribution of patients among certified pediatric urologists results in each performing only 2 or 3 each year, and so it is no wonder that published complication rates are so high.

WS performed all the proximal repairs at Children's Medical Center during his final years there, and left thinking that those 15 cases annually made him an expert. However, we quickly realized how much more there was to learn in our current practice which is mostly severe hypospadias surgery. That high volume showed us that grafts placed onto corporotomies are more likely to contract than those laid onto intact corpora, and that skin moved ventrally to cover the penile shaft cannot reliably help nourish the urethroplasty graft placed at the same time. Together these observations led to STAC repair, with healthier grafts and penile skin, and fewer urethroplasty complications, than any other method we have used or read about. Using STAC, we now expect to make a normal penis regardless of the severity of the hypospadias.

The minimum number of proximal repairs needed to properly perform STAC is not known, but we find it difficult to imagine that less than 2 a month would be sufficient. Furthermore, these operations require precision that we believe is better achieved by a team comprised of 2 experienced surgeons - rather than a surgeon assisted by a trainee or a nurse. Consequently, we recommend that centers designate a team to repair proximal hypospadias, providing those 2 surgeons with increased volume to gain more experience while monitoring their results to confirm they are achieving initial success in more than 75% of cases, and nearly 100% after closing a fistula or a glans dehiscence,

Even then, optimal care for boys with severe hypospadias may require regional centers specializing in these repairs. Our experience is proving that a center devoted to hypospadias surgery can attain high volume, improve results, and be financially viable.

Our profession owes patients a higher standard of care than it currently provides - and we can do better!

Future Directions

Only when surgeons reliably do the best techniques in the best ways and assess them using standardized, uniform outcomes measures, can we look to an even more complex topic in hypospadias repair: wound healing. The fact that publications consistently show 5-10% of boys heal with complications despite using a technique that successfully repairs over 90% of patients suggests an underlying difference in wound healing. Using a different example, urologists have all observed that inguinal incisions usually heal leaving a fine, often difficult to see scar, yet a few closed the exact same way produce a thickened, raised scar.

While that is mostly an aesthetic concern, the few boys who consistently contract a urethroplasty graft or develop hypertrophic skin scars present challenges to ever achieving a good functional outcome.

Unfortunately, wound healing currently is difficult to objectively assess. We have found that measuring the area of skin grafts is one reproducible means that can identify the few who heal differently. However, measurements of shaft skin flaps have so far proved too subjective.

Furthermore, even if a problem can be objectively identified there may be no current remedy. For example, at least one report indicates a specific androgen receptor mutation increases wound healing complications, but at this time there is no intervention to counteract that effect. Meanwhile, genetic testing remains haphazard and so the prevalence of such factors that can cause complications despite optimal surgical technique cannot be known.

The best intervention we have found that improves wound healing is HBOT. Perhaps there will be a role for other adjuvant therapies such as stem cell or platelet rich plasma infusions, or drug therapies. We are currently recording outcomes in patients with eczema to determine if that impacts their hypospadias wound healing. If so, then perhaps systemic dupilumab to decrease associated inflammation might decrease complications.

We close the second edition of *Hypospadiology* with this discussion to emphasize again that surgeons must first examine their own surgical technique to reduce complications, so that they can then identify outliers who might have altered wound healing. Only then can progress be made to improve results in those patients.

References

Kogan BA and Feustel PJ: What can we learn from pediatric urology certification logs? *Urology* 78: 147, 2011

Van der Toorn F, de Mooij K, Nijman R et al. The Dutch hypospadias study: complications and prognostic factors after distal and mid-type hypospadias repair. Abstract presented to ESPU, Prague, 2015.

About the authors

Dr. Warren Snodgrass and Dr. Nicol Bush are co-founders and directors of the Hypospadias Specialty Center, devoted to the surgical care of patients of all ages with hypospadias. They are the most published authors in the history of hypospadias repair, with over 50 peer-reviewed scientific articles, numerous book chapters, and their own textbook *Hypospadiology*, now in its 2nd edition. Their YouTube channel provides additional teaching through both lectures and surgical videos.

Dr. Snodgrass is best known as the originator of TIP repair, the most commonly performed distal hypospadias repair worldwide. He also developed the 3 corporotomies for straightening severe penile curvature. He and Dr. Bush modified the 2-stage graft repair for proximal hypospadias into the STAG procedure, and then evolved that further to the STAC repair – a game-changing operation for both primary and reoperative hypospadias. Dr. Snodgrass relates this history in his memoir, *No Margin for Error: A Surgeon's Struggle Repairing Hypospadias.*

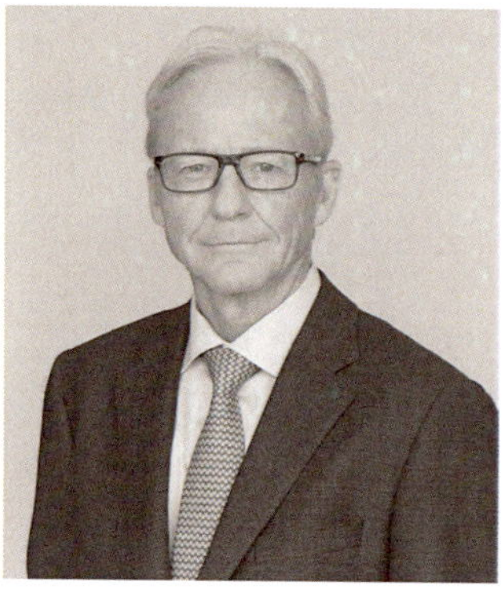

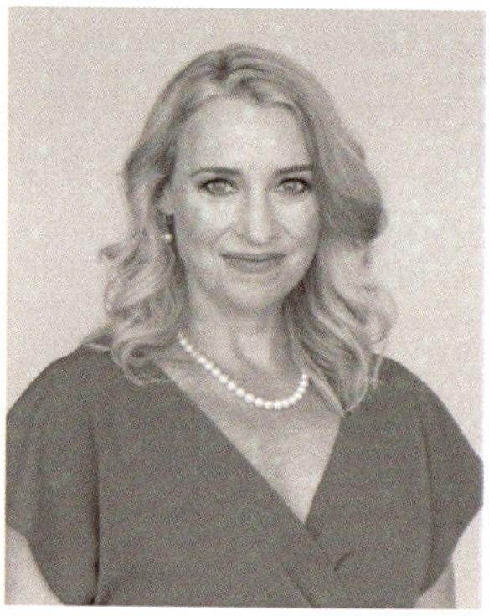

The authors are also well-known for their commitment to evidence-based practice and their use and advocacy of self-assessment to improve surgical outcomes. Dr. Snodgrass started a quality improvement database in 1999 to document every hypospadias operation, and Dr. Bush has a masters degree in Clinical Science which guides their analyses.

Their innovation, vast experience, and self-assessment to get better are evident throughout *Hypospadiology*, Second Edition.

www.ingramcontent.com/pod-product-compliance
Lightning Source LLC
LaVergne TN
LVRC101546220926
848486LV00041B/385

* 9 7 9 8 9 8 9 4 2 3 5 7 6 *